Fertility Counseling: Case Studies

Fertility Counseling: Case Studies

Second Edition

Edited by

Sharon N. Covington
Shady Grove Fertility, Rockville, MD

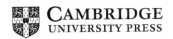

CAMBRIDGE
UNIVERSITY PRESS

University Printing House, Cambridge CB2 8BS, United Kingdom

One Liberty Plaza, 20th Floor, New York, NY 10006, USA

477 Williamstown Road, Port Melbourne, VIC 3207, Australia

314–321, 3rd Floor, Plot 3, Splendor Forum, Jasola District Centre, New Delhi – 110025, India

103 Penang Road, #05–06/07, Visioncrest Commercial, Singapore 238467

Cambridge University Press is part of the University of Cambridge.

It furthers the University's mission by disseminating knowledge in the pursuit of education, learning, and research at the highest international levels of excellence.

www.cambridge.org
Information on this title: www.cambridge.org/9781009014304
DOI: 10.1017/9781009030175

First published 2015
This second edition published 2023

A catalogue record for this publication is available from the British Library.

Library of Congress Cataloging-in-Publication Data
Names: Covington, Sharon N., editor.
Title: Fertility counseling. Case studies / edited by Sharon N. Covington. Other titles: Case studies | Fertility counseling.
Description: Second edition. | Cambridge ; New York, NY : Cambridge University Press, 2022. | Replacement in part of Fertility counseling / edited by Sharon N. Covington. 2015. | Includes bibliographical references and index.
Identifiers: LCCN 2022024069 (print) | LCCN 2022024070 (ebook) | ISBN 9781009014304 (paperback) | ISBN 9781009030175 (ebook)
Subjects: MESH: Infertility – psychology | Reproductive Techniques, Assisted – psychology | Counseling | Case Reports | BISAC: MEDICAL / Mental Health
Classification: LCC RC889 (print) | LCC RC889 (ebook) | NLM WP 570 | DDC 616.6/92–dc23/eng/20220615
LC record available at https://lccn.loc.gov/2022024069
LC ebook record available at https://lccn.loc.gov/2022024070

ISBN 978-1-009-01430-4 Paperback

....

Case studies are based upon relationships and teamwork that exists with both our clients and our colleagues. I am eternally grateful for the many patients I have worked with over the years who have entrusted me with their care, some for a single meeting and others for 30+ years. I am also profoundly indebted to the trusted colleagues who have supported, educated and guided me along the way. Too numerous to mention by name, these mental health professionals as well as the physicians and staff at Shady Grove Fertility have provided me the "wind beneath my wings". With deep appreciation, I dedicate this book to all of you: It has been an honor and a privilege to be on this journey with you.

The secret of change is to focus all of your energy, not on fighting the old, but on building the new. **Socrates**

Contents

VI Practice Issues

Online resources are available for download at www.cambridge.org/covington-case-studies
Password: CaseStudies2023

Preface

A case study approach to learning is one of the most effective tools in many fields, including medicine and mental health counseling. It provides a link between theory and practice, allowing for an in-depth, multifaceted exploration of complex issues in real-life settings. I have heard consistently over my many years of teaching that clinicians relate best and often learn more from the stories we tell about our work with patients than from all the didactic material they read. Bridging clinical concepts and real practice is essential in internalizing knowledge.

The *Case Studies* volume of *Fertility Counseling* integrates the foundational material of the *Clinical Guide* with common situations that arise in clinical practice. While the cases presented in these chapters are made up from a compilation of clients rather than individual stories, they nonetheless represent key components and issues that occur in fertility counseling. The authors are all highly skilled clinicians with years of knowledge and have generously shared not only their experiences in working with fertility patients, but also how they felt about these experiences. Transference and countertransference are key counseling concepts discussed in both volumes and are critically important to address in these cases, because many fertility counselors come to the field as a result of their own personal experience with reproductive loss. Every patient we see has a reproductive history and story that influences the course of therapy, as does the therapist.

I am grateful for and deeply appreciative of these vibrant case studies and the authors' willingness to share their feelings about the impact of this work. Their personal experiences enrich the case material, making it highly relatable for the reader. An essential element in every case is the importance of the therapeutic relationship, and as psychologist Carl Rogers noted, the empathic, genuine and unconditional positive regard the therapist brings to it. As I went through each of these cases, there were so many that resonated with patients I had seen over the years as well as the thoughts, reactions, feelings I had about them and their struggles. I felt I learned a great deal from the concepts and case analysis presented in both volumes, which is one of the things I value most in my almost 50 years as a clinician: to have the honor and privilege to continue to learn and grow from all those I work with.

Sharon Covington
December 2021

Contributors

Linda Applegarth, EdD
Clinical Associate Professor of Psychology
The Ronald O. Perelman/Claudia Cohen Center for
Reproductive Medicine
Weill Medical College of Cornell University
New York, NY, USA

Lauren Megalnick Berman, PhD
Licensed Psychologist,
Fertility Psychology Center of Atlanta, LLC,
Atlanta, GA, USA

Kate Bourne, BSW
Private Practice, Melbourne, AU

Laura Covington, MSW, PhD
Clinical Social Worker,
Shady Grove Fertility and Covington & Hafkin and
Associates,
Washington, DC, USA

Marilyn Crawshaw, PhD, CQSW
Department of Social Policy & Social Work,
University of York, York, UK

Eileen Dombo, MSW, PhD
Associate Professor and Assistant Dean & PhD
Program Chairperson, The National Catholic School
of Social Service, The Catholic University of America,
Washington, DC, USA

Carrie Eichberg, PsyD
Licensed Psychologist, Boise, ID, USA

Jane Ellis, BA, CQSW
Donor Conception Network, London, UK

Megan Flood, MA, MSW
Licensed Independent Clinical Social Worker,
Washington, DC, USA

Elaine Gordon, PhD
Clinical Psychologist, Independent Private Practice,
Santa Monica, CA, USA

Maya Grobel, MSW
Licensed Clinical Social Worker, Private Practice,
CEO of EM•POWER donation LLC,
Los Angeles, CA, USA

Kimberly Grocher, PhD
Clinical Social Worker, Independent Practice, NY, NJ,
MD, and FL
Lecturer, School of Social Work, Columbia University;
Lecturer of Social Work in Psychiatry, Weill
Cornell Medical College; Adjunct Professor, Graduate
School of Social Services, Fordham University,
NY, USA

Sarah Holley, PhD
Professor, Clinical Psychology, San Francisco State
University, and HS Assistant Clinical Professor,
Department of Psychiatry and Behavioral Sciences,
University of California, San Francisco, San Francisco,
CA, USA

Astrid Indekeu, PhD
Licensed psychologist, sexologist, private practice,
Hasselt, Belgium, Fellow at Centre for Sociological
Research, KU Leuven, Leuven, Belgium

Janet Jaffe, PhD
Co-founder and Co-director of the Center for
Reproductive Psychology, San Diego, CA

Mia R. Joelsson, MSW
Clinical Social Worker
Shady Grove Fertility and Independent Private Practice
Gaithersburg, MD, USA

Loree Johnson, PhD
Licensed Marriage and Family Therapist,
Independent Practice, Los Angeles, CA, USA.

Laura Josephs, PhD
Clinical Assistant Professor of Psychology at the
Center for Reproductive Medicine, New
York-Presbyterian Weill Cornell Medical Center,
New York, NY, USA

Nancy Kaufman, LCSW, LP
Licensed Clinical Social Worker and
Licensed Psychoanalyst, Independent Practice,
New York, NY, USA

Erika Kelley, PhD
Clinical Psychologist, Department of Obstetrics
and Gynecology, University Hospitals Cleveland
Medical Center; Assistant Professor, Departments of
Reproductive Biology and Urology, Case Western
Reserve University School of Medicine,
Cleveland, OH, USA

Sheryl Kingsberg, PhD
Clinical Psychologist and Chief, Division
of Behavioral Medicine, Department of Obstetrics
and Gynecology, University Hospitals Cleveland
Medical Center; Professor, Departments of
Reproductive Biology, Psychiatry and Urology, Case
Western Reserve University School of Medicine,
Cleveland, OH, USA

Susan Klock, PhD
Professor, Departments of Obstetrics and
Gynecology
and Psychiatry, Northwestern University Feinberg
School of Medicine, Chicago, IL, USA

Kristy Koser, PhD
Licensed Professional Clinical Counselor,
Aporia Counseling & Psychotherapy, PLLC Berlin, OH,
USA

Irving Leon, PhD
Adjunct Associate Professor of Obstetrics and
Gynecology, Michigan Medicine,
Ann Arbor, MI, USA

Jeanne O'Brien, MD
Reproductive Endocrinologist and
Chairperson, Ethics Committee
Shady Grove Fertility, Rockville, MD, USA

Lauri Pasch, PhD
Professor, Department of Psychiatry and Behavioral
Sciences
University of California, San Francisco
San Francisco, CA USA

Brennan Peterson, PhD
Professor, Chapman University

Departments of Marriage and Family Therapy &
Psychology
Crean College of Health and Behavioral Sciences
Orange, CA USA

William Petok, PhD
Licensed Psychologist, Independent Practice,
Baltimore, MD, USA

Rachel Rabinor, MSW
Licensed Clinical Social Worker, Certified in Perinatal
Mental Health
Independent Practice, San Diego, CA, USA

Arabelle Rowe, MSW
Diplomate Member, Association for Behavioral and
Cognitive Therapies.
Greenwich Psychotherapy & Associates, Greenwich, CT,
USA

Mary Riddle, PhD
Associate Teaching Professor of Psychology, Department
of Psychology,
The Pennsylvania State University,
University Park, PA, USA

Patricia Sachs, MSW
Licensed Clinical Social Worker,
Shady Grove Fertility and Covington & Hafkin and
Associates
Rockville, MD, USA

Tara Simpson, PsyD
Licensed Psychologist,
Shady Grove Fertility and Covington & Hafkin and
Associates
Rockville, MD, USA

Margaret Swain, RN, JD
Attorney in Private Practice,
Baltimore, MD, USA

Carol Toll, MSW
Licensed Clinical Social Worker,
Shady Grove Fertility and Covington & Hafkin and
Associates
Rockville, MD, USA

Uschi Van den Broeck, PhD
Clinical Psychologist and Family Therapist,
University Hospitals Leuven, Gasthuisberg,
Leuven University Fertility Center (LUFC), Leuven, BE

Karen Wasserstein, PsyD
Licensed Psychologist,
Shady Grove Fertility and Covington and Hafkin &
Associates
Bethesda, MD, USA

Laura Winters, MSW
Licensed Clinical Social Worker
Private Practice, Chatham, NJ, USA

Katherine Williams, MD
Clinical Professor of Psychiatry, Stanford University
School of Medicine

and Director of the Women's Wellness Clinic, Stanford,
CA, USA

Landon Zaki, PsyD, PMH-C
Licensed Psychologist
Bloom Therapy
San Francisco, CA USA

Julianne E. Zweifel, PhD
Department of Obstetrics & Gynecology
University of Wisconsin School of Medicine & Public
Health,
Madison, WI, USA

Collaborative Reproductive Healthcare Model: A Patient-Centered Approach to Medical and Psychosocial Care

Nancy Kaufman and Loree Johnson

Introduction

Nancy Kaufman: I was trained as a psychoanalyst and have been practicing in New York City for more than 30 years. When my own fertility struggles went from years of hopelessness to renewed possibility, this not only changed the course of my life, but of my work as well. To help those struggling through the loss toward a new future became the focus of my practice. I see individuals, couples and lead groups for those pursuing family building using donor assistance, which is my particular area of research interest.

Loree Johnson: I was trained as a systems therapist and have worked in community mental health and private practice during my 25-year career. As with many clinicians, my practice evolved as I experienced recurrent pregnancy loss and complicated grief. Initially unaware that infertility and loss disproportionately affected women of color, I noticed the shortage of medical and mental health professionals of color within the field of fertility counseling and how that added a layer of struggle to my journey. As a result, I am passionate about supporting individuals and couples struggling with infertility and loss, especially in communities that feel invisible and are underrepresented within the field.

The two cases presented in this chapter are a composite of various clients we have seen in our practices that illustrate many aspects common to the experience of the infertility journey. They represent diversity in clinical thought, style and training. We think that together they are an excellent companion piece to portray the many different lenses within the field of fertility counseling and reproductive medical treatment.

The Case of Leah

Leah came to see me 10 years ago in my private psychoanalytic practice. A 37-year-old, married female, originally from Israel, she was about to begin her first IVF cycle at a major metropolitan fertility program.

Leah was extremely anxious about the procedure and reported a long history of anxieties surrounding health and medical issues, which she recognized added to her present feeling state, as did her work as a scientist in an extremely stressful job. We agreed to work together weekly in supportive psychotherapy to help her manage the stress of her impending infertility treatment (see Chapter 3 in the companion *Clinical Guide*).

I immediately felt drawn to her. Highly educated, articulate and insightful, she presented as an ideal client. Leah understood that her personal history and her particular character were responsible for adding to her understandable current anxiety. She wanted to know herself better in order to manage through this period. I was eager to work with her. Little did either one of us realize the long journey we would be embarking on together.

Leah and I formed a working alliance very quickly. The sessions became a refuge for her – a quiet, safe place where she could let her guard down and her feelings out. Each week, after having contained them in order to function in her life, they came pouring out in my office.

Initially, I was concerned that I wasn't offering her enough. But I began to see how the safe space to unleash this torrent of feelings with a nonjudgmental listener enabled her to manage a stressful job and navigate an increasingly complex medical situation while remaining integrated.

Her first IVF was unsuccessful as were several more, followed by a very early miscarriage. Her options were beginning to narrow; her defenses to unravel.

Treatment during this phase was first to help her deal with and recover from each loss and disappointment so as not to have them build on each other, as well as to help her determine what her next steps should be and how to navigate them. As is often the case with infertility patients, each new loss can reawaken prior losses, both fertility-related and life losses in general (see Chapter 21 in the companion *Clinical Guide*).

Leah experienced her infertility as a narcissistic injury [1]. Coming from a family that prided itself on having many children, she faced the additional burden of feeling she was letting them down, as well as her

husband and herself. In her mind, Leah was not succeeding in her role as a woman, a wife or a daughter.

Because of my own history of infertility losses, I felt
especially connected to Leah and her pain. I often felt the
desire to offer hope but was aware that helping her stay
with her feelings of despair is what could actually better
help her heal and move toward her own feelings of hope.
I was able to "hold" these feelings for her [2], because they
mirrored my own past feelings of hopelessness. This
familiarity enabled me to understand her rather than
judge her, and she felt accepted for all of her feelings
even when she felt "crazy."

The rollercoaster of hope and despair continued as
another pregnancy was achieved but was short-lived and
resulted in another miscarriage. After another period of
mourning Leah, along with her husband Ari and their
team of doctors, determined that the next step would be
considering the use of donor eggs (see Chapter 22 in the
companion *Clinical Guide*).

The next years of treatment dealt with this realization,
which initially felt like an insurmountable hurdle. Leah
spoke openly about her distress and her inability to move
forward. At the same time, she recognized that while she
moves very slowly when it comes to dealing with painful
changes, in the end, she is always able to proceed. This
awareness allowed Leah to keep working toward her
overarching goal of motherhood.

She anguished over this decision, grappling with
her fear that she was giving up too soon in achieving
a pregnancy on her own. She worked through this by
separating the loss of her genetics from her desire to
become a mother and ultimately was able to move
ahead with donor assistance.

I recognized that her defense system easily became
overwhelmed and her slow approach to moving forward
was actually a necessity to remain integrated. Defenses
are, of course, constructed to protect fragile parts of the
ego [3]. For Leah, I understood that her avoidance of
moving too quickly served as protection against a deeper
fear of being psychically weakened and of regressing.
Therefore, I supported her defenses rather than try to
break through them and moved at her pace.

Like many other infertility patients, Leah felt betrayed
by her body and anguished over the repeated failures in
achieving a pregnancy. She would often ask, "What happened to my child? I can't find my child," illustrating,
clearly, that a longed-for child can be emotionally present
even when physically missing [4].

In order to come to terms with her feelings regarding
the use of donor gametes, Leah joined a support group for
those struggling on similar journeys (see Chapter 5 in the
companion *Clinical Guide*). Additionally, she began seeing
an acupuncturist as another means to control her anxiety.

It was also during this time that we had several sessions that included her husband (see Chapter 4 in the
companion *Clinical Guide*). Slightly older, from the same
country and also in the same high-stress profession,
Ari had been a kind and supportive partner during their
15-year marriage. He was, however, more traditional in
his thinking and needed more time to get used to the idea
of using donor gametes.

Once they each moved through the various stages
toward acceptance of using donor gametes, Leah and
Ari came to the realization that they wanted to use a
directed/known donor. They wanted to meet the donor
and have the experience of knowing her as a person and
to understand her motivation for donating. They actually
hoped to maintain ongoing casual contact throughout the
years to normalize the method of their children's conception story, provide answers to any questions as their
children grew up and to always have updated medical
information. They saw an ongoing relationship as a way
to express their gratitude to the young woman who would
make their family possible (see Chapter 9 in the companion *Clinical Guide*). As scientists, they also understood
that recent developments in consumer genetic testing
had rendered the notion of anonymity obsolete (see
Chapter 13 in the companion *Clinical Guide*).

Leah and Ari found an agency willing to facilitate this
kind of ongoing relationship, after which the painstaking
search for the "right" donor began. When they could not
proceed with their first chosen donor, they once again felt
heartbroken and unable to imagine finding anyone else. But,
in time, as they moved from seeing the donor as
a replacement for Leah, they were able to accept another
suitable donor.

I found that in treating Leah I would sometimes take
a more active role than I normally would in treating
nonfertility-related clients. Sometimes I provided support and encouragement, took part in role playing to
help her get used to difficult conversations and corrected
misinformation. While I continued to work with her on
a deeper level to understand how her current losses had
re-traumatized her and awakened internalized fears from
her early history, sometimes more active participation on
my part proved to be essential.

Leah spoke English fluently, but it was not her first
language and so was not the "language of her emotions" [5]. After years of working together I became
accustomed to the lyrical rhythm of her speech and

the deeply conveyed emotions she expressed. When she occasionally misused a word, I understood her intent and felt immersed in her world. If she could not think of the appropriate English word to explain something I would ask her to say it in her native language. Rather than a barrier, the flow of language in our sessions, which were conducted in English, felt like another point of connection between us.

Leah was a deeply religious woman and often saw her infertility through this lens: "It is up to God to give me a child, when He is ready." This thinking served to give Leah hope and was a way to explain the injustice she deeply felt.

A recurrent theme, however, was that Leah felt she was committing a sin by pursuing fertility treatments and feared she might be severely punished. Despite feeling plagued by this thought, she continued to seek out religious leaders until she finally found one who understood her faith as well as her deep desire to become a mother. When this rabbi gave her his blessing, Leah decided to accept his words, but it was years before she felt able to practice her religion again.

This religious aspect aroused strong feelings in me. I did not share Leah's views but was I helping her commit a sin? Would I be responsible if she experienced some kind of "punishment?" Sometimes she wondered whether the repeated failures to become pregnant *were* that punishment. Was I responsible for that? Some of these feelings were what I believed to be common self-examination, but mainly I believed they were "induced feelings" [6], namely that they were Leah's feelings rather than mine and were induced in me through the powerful transference connection between us (see Chapter 8 in the companion *Clinical Guide*).

After struggling to find a donor with whom they felt compatible, Leah and Ari forged a very positive connection with Frannie, the donor they ultimately chose. Leah worked very hard to keep her fears under control and was able to maintain a close and collaborative relationship with Frannie [7]. Talking through each fear with me allowed Leah to voice her concerns without taking them back to the donor and potentially damaging that relationship.

Following a first failed donor egg cycle and additional heartbreak, they were successful on the second attempt and began the new journey of finally being pregnant. After an anxiety-filled but otherwise normal gestation, Leah's mother-in-law came to assist them in taking care of their newborn son. It was not an easy time. Leah was filled with panic, anxiety and feelings of inadequacy, finding herself in an unfamiliar role while totally sleep deprived (see Chapter 23 in the companion *Clinical Guide*).

During this time, Leah and I continued our work on the telephone (see Chapter 25 in the companion *Clinical Guide*). With her permission, I contacted a psychiatrist who specialized in postpartum issues so that she would have someone to consult if necessary (see Chapter 7 in the companion *Clinical Guide*).

I was also concerned about myself. Would I be responsible if something happened to her? What if something happened to the baby? I found that I was thinking not only of them but also of my own potential culpability in this situation and how best to protect myself (see Chapter 27 in the companion *Clinical Guide*). Leah elected not to see that referral, but she did begin to find other ways that helped her begin to feel more and more in control.

It was my understanding that during this period her mother-in-law, who had come to "help," was actually undermining Leah's confidence at every turn. Her mother-in-law criticized Leah's attempts to care for her baby and virtually took over, leaving Leah feeling even more inadequate. She was so tired and demoralized that she could not put up much of a fight. But the stronger she became the more she saw how this dynamic had affected her and had always been operating in her relationship with her own mother as well. This terrible period actually began a new awareness for Leah, helping her to establish a new sense of self as the mother of her child, separate from both her own mother and her mother-in-law.

When her second child was born two years later using the same donor, Leah felt much more confident as a mother and was able to maintain firmer boundaries with her mother-in-law, who once again came to help. She was able to carve out space for herself as the mother and caretaker of her new baby, while her mother-in-law was given the role of helping her older child as a grandmother.

For many years, Leah had attended a support group focusing on disclosure issues in donor-assisted reproduction. Initially, she worried whether she would be able to tell her children their story without feeling overcome with grief at the losses she had suffered. Hearing how others in the group had worked through similar feelings helped her feel prepared and empowered. Her primary identity had shifted away from being an infertility patient to that of a mother.

Leah's son knew of the donor, Frannie. Although they lived in different states, they remained in contact, just as Leah and Ari had hoped. Their experience together was so positive, in fact, that Frannie was also the donor for their second child 2 years later (see Chapter 14 in the companion *Clinical Guide*).

Leah now wanted her son to begin to understand the role that Frannie had actually played in his life, so one day, when he was 3 years old, Leah decided to tell him the story of the day he was born:

I waited and waited and finally we found Frannie and she gave us a part of herself that we needed to help make you. Then I carried you in my tummy and out you came. The doctor said, "Here is your son!" and he put you in my arms and I finally met you and I was so happy. Her son was delighted with this story and begged, Tell me again! [8]

What is apparent is that Leah communicated to her son the joy and love she felt at his birth and about Frannie's involvement. As a result, this young boy's first awareness of having been conceived using donor assistance was joyful and positive. His mother transferred those feelings to him in telling the story in this way. A happy and positive foundation had been laid to incrementally build upon this story.

In a recent session, Leah recalled the overwhelming feelings she had when difficult issues once arose with the donor:

*What really changed things for me was when I was angry with Frannie and instead of telling **her**, I told you. Then I saw that my feelings actually had changed. I wasn't angry anymore and was able to speak with Frannie in a calmer way. That's when I really understood that I could change.*

This was one of those rare moments in treatment when a clinician truly believes in the therapeutic process. I felt relieved and proud of Leah and of the hard work we had done together (see Chapter 21 in the companion *Clinical Guide*).

Our session occurred the week after I began writing this chapter when she spoke in this very unusual way, which outlined exactly how therapy had helped her. What might I have been unknowingly communicating to her, or was I listening differently . . . for different things?

The following week Leah again unconsciously cooperated by providing me with the final paragraph for this case study. In speaking about a nonfertility-related traumatic situation she had to contend with, she said:

For most of my life I felt I could never move forward. Never move fast enough to get the things I wanted. And I always feared that would mean I would lose everything.
But I did move forward.
I did get what I wanted.
And now I know that it is possible.
That I can do it.

And I will keep moving.
No matter what happens.

I always believed that Leah (and my other patients) **could** do what felt impossible, perhaps because I knew that 24 years ago I had done the very same thing (see Chapter 19 in the companion *Clinical Guide*).

In writing up this case I became acutely aware that the patient's culture played little (conscious) role in our treatment relationship or in her reporting of her infertility experience. Was this a blind spot on my part? Did my ignoring this affect her willingness to bring up the issue in our treatment? Interestingly, Leah recently described how she sometimes feels mistreated by medical personnel when they hear her accent. I wonder if my growing awareness of the role that race, ethnicity and difference can play in medical treatment allowed this important dimension to finally enter the treatment room (see Chapter 18 in the companion *Clinical Guide*).

Nancy L. Kaufman

The Case of Mia and Julian

Mia, age 37, and Julian, age 39, have been married for nine years and together for 15 years. Mia is a college professor, and Julian is a marketing executive. They met through mutual friends at a distant family member's family function. During their courtship, they connected around their love of travel and spent hours sharing stories of their various adventures. Julian appreciated Mia's passion for teaching and research and her dedication to her students. Mia found Julian's sense of creativity endearing and inspiring. They enjoyed traveling together while growing their respective careers.

Even though they came from different backgrounds – with Mia identifying as White and Julian identifying as Puerto Rican – they connected in their shared ambition to advance their careers. Mia was on track to finish her Ph.D. with hopes of becoming a tenured professor, and Julian worked at a marketing agency with hopes of starting his own one day. Outside of work, they enjoyed spending time with family and friends and celebrated loved ones as they grew their families.

After getting married, Mia and Julian agreed to wait a couple of years before starting to try for a baby. As part of their conception journey, Mia stopped taking all birth control that she had started in college. They proceeded to monitor Mia's cycle, identifying her "fertile window," and figured that pregnancy would happen *"naturally"* soon after. However, after two years of trying, Mia and Julian started to feel frustrated.

Mia wanted to seek medical help, but Julian was reluctant. They fought about when and how to seek help, which usually ended with Julian's attempts to reassure Mia that pregnancy would happen "*as it was supposed to.*" Finally, Julian relented, and Mia scheduled an appointment with a reproductive endocrinologist (RE). Julian's hesitance for seeing a doctor manifested around scheduling conflicts for the initial consultation, which resulted in him missing the appointment and Mia attending alone.

Mia reviewed with Julian what transpired in the consultation, covering her medical history and the diagnostic tests required of both of them. Mia completed her blood work quickly while Julian lagged in making his appointment. This pattern triggered Mia's frustration as she perceived Julian's lack of motivation and action as disinterest in starting a family.

After stalling for a few months, Mia requested counseling with me to address her concerns about starting treatments and the frustration she was experiencing in her marriage. During our initial telephone call, I sensed a hesitation to include Julian in the process. Mia mentioned Julian's hesitance in seeing a therapist, because seeking mental health services was frowned upon in his community. Mia stressed the importance of finding a therapist of color with whom Julian could connect to make the process as smooth as possible (see Chapter 18 in the companion *Clinical Guide*). I validated Mia's desire and concern and discussed how Julian's hesitance could exist for many reasons and how having a perceived cultural connection may help reduce barriers in the counseling process [9].

Even though Mia initially expressed a desire to seek help individually, I encouraged her to bring Julian to our first counseling session, as infertility is a shared experience in a couple's relationship. This meeting would serve as an opportunity to provide collaborative care for their shared concerns (see Chapter 4 in the companion *Clinical Guide*). To Mia's relief, Julian attended, and I immediately established a rapport with each of them, centering around how they felt being in therapy. Mia expressed her comfort with counseling as she had done a few sessions before. Julian sighed heavily and shifted in his seat.

Sensing Julian's potential discomfort, I preemptively acknowledged how talking to a stranger about deeply personal issues can be challenging, which prompted Julian to share:

It's hard talking to an outsider about deeply personal issues between my wife and me. She's a lot more open than I am.

It's easier for her to talk about this stuff, whereas it's not for me. No one in my family or community – that I know of – has had any issues trying to conceive. I've only heard of **other** *people having fertility issues. You know what I mean?*

As I inquired about Julian's use of the word "other," he referred to members of the White community. Julian's experience felt similar to mine as a Black woman, wherein infertility has also historically been viewed as an issue that affected white individuals, not people of color [10,11]. Between the continued existence of this fertility stereotype and Julian's discomfort with therapy, I normalized his attitudes as part of our rapport building [12].

Subsequent meetings with Mia and Julian were used to explore the history of their relationship, including their individual and shared perspective about their fertility journey. I held space for them to discuss being in counseling as a biracial couple discussing their fertility journey. The discomfort they displayed at the beginning softened when sharing how they met and fell in love. Seeing Mia and Julian's tenderness in their reflection was a moment I wanted to highlight, as they both reported feeling exhausted and frustrated by their consistent fights. When couples become mired in conflict and distress, as can be the case with infertility, those tender moments can be fleeting. Reflecting on these memories can serve as a powerful intervention in reducing feelings of disconnection and distress.

As I began to see the pattern with their frustration and their fights, it became clear that Mia and Julian were feeling overwhelmed, scared and sad. Mia was rattled by her initial medical diagnosis of premature ovarian insufficiency (POI) [13]. Julian's posture shifted as he finally discussed being diagnosed with a low sperm count. Underneath the anger toward each other was a sense of shock and disbelief. They expressed concern about the weight of simultaneously managing two fertility diagnoses, which posed a greater perceived obstacle to their fertility journey than they had previously imagined.

Upon exploring their sense of shock even further, Julian shared:

Not only did I think that fertility issues did not affect people like me, I thought the complete opposite. All my life, I've heard male family members make references to their masculinity, taking pride in it and talking about their children almost like a product of their masculinity. Now it makes me question if I'm less of a man because of [my diagnosis]. I thought I would be like the other men in my family. This is embarrassing!

I wondered if Julian's "hesitance" at various points of their journey was connected to his embarrassment and shame. He shared:

I struggled with going to the doctor and getting tested. If the tests came back conclusive – which they did – I didn't know how I would face reality. I felt ashamed.

Julian's feelings felt palpable and familiar. When viewed through a cultural lens, the expectation and pride of procreating with ease highlighted the long-held hyper fertile stereotype that exists in both our respective communities. The historical narrative that has consistently defined Black women as "sexually promiscuous" and "fertile" [14] has also shaped the perception of Latin men as hypersexual [15].

Discussing how race and culture impact the clinical picture – particularly the intersection of fertility and mental health – is a delicate process [16]. Even though Julian may have perceived me as an ally, a fellow person of color, I wanted to ensure that I did not assume we had more commonalities than discussed, regardless of common backgrounds. Therefore, I phrased my questions generally, checking in to see what felt true for Julian. I was keenly aware of how vocal Julian was about his struggle. Knowing how challenging it is for Latinx men to discuss their feelings about their fertility, especially through a cultural lens, I wanted to capture as much of Julian's voice as possible while I could (see Chapter 15 in the companion *Clinical Guide*).

I also noted how Mia listened intently to Julian's distress and shared her own. She described how she felt similarly to Julian as she questioned her femininity because of her diagnosis. She went on to mention:

While I've tried to be sensitive to Julian's perspective, it hasn't always been easy. I thought his missing our consultation with the RE and lagging on getting tested meant that he didn't want a baby as much as I did. I tried to be open to hearing his side, but it didn't seem to make as much sense as it does now. I love his family and culture, but I know how different my experience is from not having grown up in it. As a result, I never fully appreciated how he might feel.

I held space for Mia and Julian to reflect on what it was like hearing and sitting with the other's pain around their respective diagnoses and what that reality meant for them as an interracial couple. Since Mia's frustration with Julian stemmed from her perception of his hesitance in following through with tests as part of their treatment, I found expanding our understanding of what lay underneath that hesitation imperative while in the therapy room.

Mia's ethnic background of English, Dutch and French heritage appeared to have little bearing on her perception of her fertility, as it did for Julian. She described her family as open-minded and noted that she was unaware of any close or distant relatives with fertility issues, except for a cousin who suffered a pregnancy loss in her first trimester. Mia seemed aware of Julian's struggles with shame but acknowledged that listening to him share in session felt different. She appeared much more attuned and sensitive to his struggle, which was reflected in her body language and attempts to comfort Julian when she sensed his distress.

Mia described a point in their conception journey that had previously served as a point of contention in their relationship. Julian wanted her to see a healer in his community known to help couples conceive through herbal, body, and spiritual work. This suggestion by Julian and his family felt odd at first, but Mia obliged, not fully understanding their insistence on seeking "alternative" help. She mentioned that:

I had heard Julian and his family members mention healing practices that were completely unfamiliar to me. These practices were deeply spiritual and characteristic of their family, even if not recognized by the larger medical system. I had also heard passing references to skepticism of doctors in general, but their insistence on meeting with a [community practitioner] makes more sense now.

We processed how these suggestions were rooted in a sense of mistrust of the medical community. Julian shared how he had witnessed and heard stories of loved ones being overlooked or mistreated when they sought care, sentiments that I heard as well [17]. Due to the overall mistrust, seeking help for physical or mental health issues was considered taboo. Therefore, Julian's initial hesitancy at the start of treatment was far more complex, as the act of seeking help evoked feelings of shame and conflicted with cultural and familial messages (see Chapter 18 in the companion *Clinical Guide*).

As Mia and Julian navigated their reactions to their diagnoses, shock, disbelief, and shame waned and yielded glimpses of relief. They had an explanation for why Mia had not become pregnant for the past few years. Now they had an answer and a plan. They could work with their doctor to determine the best course of action, which at this point looked like IVF with her eggs, with the potential to move to donor eggs (see Chapter 9 in the companion *Clinical Guide*). Mia mentioned some concerns about moving forward with donor eggs, which triggered some anxiety. However, I validated her concern and encouraged her (and Julian) to pursue a second medical opinion for reassurance about their diagnoses and treatment plan.

In the meantime, we discussed their doctor's initial recommendations for lifestyle changes to help them optimize their chances for pregnancy while contemplating their decision. Admittedly, Mia and Julian were overwhelmed thinking about the addition of vitamins and supplements recommended for both of them. In addition, Mia commented that they would need to reduce their alcohol intake for the time being. However, they both agreed to be as aggressive with their changes to give them the best chance at IVF working. Their plan also entailed a repeat semen analysis for Julian after a few months of vitamins and lifestyle changes, giving them immediate feedback about how well his changes worked.

Meanwhile, their couple's sessions were wrought with conflict about what changes to make. Mia expressed frustration with Julian's lack of consistency with adhering to their nutritional and lifestyle changes. Upon further exploration, Julian expressed a sense of frustration for making the changes that felt "forced." I acknowledged that frustration, since making dramatic lifestyle changes during medical treatments could be challenging.

Mia and Julian sought a second opinion from a clinic that confirmed the first clinic's diagnosis of POI. However, they were willing to try one cycle with Mia's eggs before moving on to donor gametes, which felt important to the couple. We also processed the protocol recommendations and their reactions.

The doctor discussed the protocol, which involved minimal stimulation due to her high follicle stimulating hormone (FSH), after explaining the rationale behind the minimal stimulation protocol and how it would potentially take longer to gather enough eggs to use for embryos to test further. Mia and Julian were a bit deterred by the prolonged timeframe and cost, but felt comforted by using fewer medications and potential stress on Mia's body.

We met periodically during Mia's stimulation protocol, which occurred over several months. Following their doctor's opinion, I helped them manage expectations about how many eggs to expect with each cycle, from one to three per month instead of 7–14 that they had heard was expected with full IVF protocols.

Over the next eight months, Mia and Julian were able to create and "bank" nine embryos, three of which tested normal after preimplantation genetic screening (PGS). Before transfer, Mia underwent an endometrial receptivity analysis (ERA) test to identify receptivity. After determining the proper window of progesterone for transfer, they started looking forward to their first transfer date.

Using the relaxation skills discussed in session, we identified skills for Mia and skills for Julian to support Mia (see Table 1.1). In addition, we identified a list of strategies for different scenarios during which either of their anxieties surfaced, with prompts of what would be helpful at specific times.

With cautious optimism, Mia and Julian approached their first transfer. They felt good about the process but were disappointed that their pregnancy test results came back negative. Even though we are trained as clinicians to maintain emotional distance from our clients, fertility counseling is unique because many of us have personal stories that brought us to the field. I walked right along the path with Mia and Julian and felt excited and hopeful for them. However, the disappointment and helplessness I felt upon learning of their negative beta were palpable. As a supportive person in their lives, I had to honor my disappointment, but not at the expense of holding space for them to process and grieve as needed.

Julian appeared to take the negative result harder than Mia, at least according to Mia's report. Usually stoic and reserved, Mia shared the look on Julian's face when they heard the news together. They knew their clinic would call with the results, and they waited to listen to the voicemail together. They could tell by the tone in the nurse's voice that the news was not good.

I helped Julian and Mia grieve the loss of their failed cycle and the unexpected waves of grief that accompanied receiving that negative result. They unknowingly shared elements of disenfranchised grief where they expressed feeling less entitled to their sadness because they never actually received a positive pregnancy result [18]. Julian even asked, *"How do I grieve the loss of something I never had the chance to see grow?"* Mia gently nodded and followed up by saying, *"I was so attached to this little embryo from the very beginning. Knowing that I'll never meet this little being is devastating."*

Mia went on to share that finding a place to share their loss, outside of counseling, was difficult because they were met with confusion and insensitive comments from friends and family who questioned how they could mourn the loss of something that wasn't a "living being." As a fellow loss mother, I could relate to the immense sadness from never knowing one's child or who they would grow up to be. Additionally, I could empathize with the isolation associated with not having grief acknowledged by one's community. The counseling

Table 1.1 Promoting resilience and managing anxiety during fertility treatments

- Emphasize skills and attitudes that promote resilience
  - Relaxation techniques
  - Adaptive coping strategies
  - Finding strength and power in acceptance
- Encourage social connections/support through friends, family and religious community, and therapy/support groups
- Encourage self-advocacy with their medical team
- Process sense of disenfranchised grief

room was used to process the presence and power of disenfranchisement as part of their grieving process, which appeared to allow them more space to grieve (see Chapter 19 in the companion *Clinical Guide* and Table 1.1).

Julian and Mia decided to wait a few months before proceeding with another transfer. After almost 4 years into their conception journey, they expressed feeling emotionally exhausted and needing to rest. Subsequent sessions focused on validating their decision to embrace their need and allow them time to process the stress of the journey and the sting of the initial loss to pass.

In addition to grief, we used that time to discuss how their sexual relationship had shifted over the years. Julian noted that sex used to be a fun way for Mia and him to connect, but now it felt like a burden. Julian also stated that he struggled with the expectation of "performing on-demand" and experienced difficulty with sexual performance [19] (see also Chapter 6 in the companion *Clinical Guide*). Mia also acknowledged distress in their sexual relationship and loss in sexual desire. I normalized the impact of stress in trying to conceive, psychologically and emotionally, and its impact on their relationship [20]. We discussed strategies to make their intimate relationship fun again, now that they had a break from treatments.

I am also aware that in this write-up Julian's story and voice appear more present than Mia's. This imbalance was not purposeful, yet born out of a desire to capture as much of the male perspective as possible, which is often missing in the fertility literature. I wonder if the absence of Mia's voice may reflect how she felt during the counseling process with me. I also noticed that I did not fully explore how it felt for Mia to have a therapist of color and subsequently be "outnumbered" in the room.

Furthermore, I am keenly aware that there are still nuances to explore when clients seek counseling from someone of a similar background. Having a shared cultural experience as part of an underrepresented group, racially or ethnically, does not presume a lack of differences. Even though there may be a general level of common cultural experiences and understanding, clinicians of color should remain curious as we would hope our White counterparts would.

Loree Johnson

References

1. Bernstein J. Current trends in the treatment of narcissism: Spotnitz, Kohut, Kernberg. *Modern Psychoanal* 2013;**38**(1):25–49.

2. Burns LH. Infertility as boundary ambiguity: one theoretical perspective. *Family Process* 1987;**26**:359–372.

3. Covington SN. Personal communication, 2021.

4. Kernberg OF. *Severe Personality Disorders: Psychotherapeutic Strategies*. New Haven, CT: Yale University Press, 1984.

5. Roland A. Induced emotional reactions and attitudes in the psychoanalyst as transference in actuality. *Psychoanal Rev* 1981;**68**(1):45–74.

6. UKEssays. Holding and Containing – Winnicott (1960) [Internet]. November 2018. Available at: www.ukessays.com/essays/psychology/holding-and-containing-winnicott.php?vref=1 [last accessed June 19, 2022].

7. Mindes EJ, Covington LS. Counseling known participants in third party reproduction. In: Covington SN, Ed. *Fertility Counseling: Clinical Guide and Case Studies*, 1st Ed. Cambridge: Cambridge University Press, 2015, 136–149.

8. Benward JM. Disclosure: helping families talk about assisted reproduction. In: Covington SN, Ed. *Fertility Counseling: Clinical Guide and Case Studies*, 1st Ed. Cambridge: Cambridge University Press, 2015, 252–264.

9. Zayas LH, Torres LR. Culture and masculinity: when therapist and patient are Latino men. *Clin Social Work J* 2009;**37**:294–302. https://doi.org/10.1007/s10615-009-0232-2

10. Alvero R. *Pilot Study: Why Latinos Don't Seek Fertility Treatment*. Denver, CO: University of Colorado Advanced Reproductive Medicine, 2014.

11. Ward EC, Wiltshire JC, Detry MA, et al. African American men and women's attitude toward mental illness, perceptions of stigma, and preferred coping behaviors. *Nurs Res* 2013;**62**(3):185–194. https://doi.org/10.1097/NNR.0b013e31827bf533

12. National Alliance on Mental Illness. Identity and Cultural Dimensions: Hispanic/Latinx. Available at: www.nami.org/Your-Journey/Identity-and-Cultural-Dimensions/Hispanic-Latinx [last accessed June 19, 2022].

13. Driscoll M, Davis M, Aiken L, et. al. Psychosocial vulnerability, resilience resources, and coping with infertility: a longitudinal model of adjustment to primary

ovarian insufficiency. *Ann Behav Med* 2016;**50**(2):272–284. https://doi.org/10.1007/s12160-015-9750-z

14. Roberts D. *Killing the Black Body: Race, Reproduction and the Meaning of Liberty*. New York, NY: Vintage Books, 2017.

15. Mastro D, Behm-Morawitz E, Ortiz M. The cultivation of social perceptions of Latinos: a mental models approach. *Media Psychol* 2007;**9**(2): 347–365. https://doi.org/10.1080/15213260701286106

16. Nuñez A, González P, Talavera GA, et. al. Machismo, marianismo, and negative cognitive-emotional factors: findings from the Hispanic Community health study/Study of Latinos Sociocultural Ancillary Study. *J Latina/o Psychol* 2016;**4**(4):202–217. https://doi.org/10.1037/lat00000

17. Washington H. *Medical Apartheid: The Dark History of Medical Experimentation on Black Americans from Colonial Times to Present*. New York, NY: Doubleday, 2006.

18. Lang A, Fleiszer AR, Duhamel F, et al. Perinatal loss and parental grief: the challenge of ambiguity and disenfranchised grief. *Omega* (Westport) 2011;**63**(2):183–196. https://doi.org/10.2190/OM.63.2.e

19. Read J. ABC of sexual health: sexual problems associated with infertility, pregnancy, and ageing. *BMJ* (clinical research ed.) 1999;**318**(7183):587–589. https://doi.org/10.1136/bmj.318.7183.587

20. Bokaie M, Simbar M, Yassini Ardekani, SM. Sexual behavior of infertile women: a qualitative study. *Iranian J Reprod Med* 2015;**13**(10):645–656.

Reproductive Psychology and Fertility Counseling

Susan Klock

Introduction

I am a clinical psychologist who has focused specifically on women's reproductive health my entire career. My training has been as a clinician-scientist so my practice includes evidence-based clinical work, and I also continue to conduct clinical research in the area of assisted reproductive technologies. I work in a multidisciplinary, academic medicine infertility practice with individuals and couples going through IVF, gamete donation and gestational surrogacy. My theoretical orientation is cognitive-behavioral although I find that in working with couples, I frequently rely on my family systems training as well.

I was drawn to the specialty of reproductive psychology during my internship when I was fortunate enough to have a rotation in the Department of Obstetrics and Gynecology at the institution where I completed my training. As part of my rotation, I worked in the infertility clinic and I found that the diversity of clinical cases, the complex psychological, social and ethical challenges were so engaging and interesting that it guided my career path from that time on.

The following case presentations represent common clinical issues in my work. The patients discussed are a fictitious composite and the cases reflect salient approaches discussed in the *Clinical Guide* volume chapter.

Hannah and Mark

Hannah is a 37-year-old, married attorney who has a 4-year-old son. Hannah and Mark met while she was in law school and he was in graduate school. The couple married when the patient was 28 and both partners agreed to postpone trying to have a child until they were established in their careers. The patient began working for a prestigious law firm immediately after law school, but after 3 years she left and joined another firm that purported to have better work–life balance. Shortly thereafter she conceived and had an uneventful pregnancy, delivering her son at term.

When their son was 3, Hannah and Mark began trying for a second child. Both partners agreed that their ideal family size was two children and that they would like them relatively close together in age. The patient had noted that the transition to first-time parenting was "good – but hard sometimes" as she struggled with being pulled away from time with her son by the constant demands of her legal career. She also described a "superficial" work–life balance culture at her firm. She elaborated that while the company policies were in place to provide adequate time off, most attorneys did not take advantage of the time off because the productivity goals for advancement were difficult to meet. Hannah also noted that she felt pressure to manage the impression that she was "strong enough" to raise her son and work the requisite hours in the mostly male dominated workplace.

The couple tried on their own to conceive but after a year they consulted with Hannah's obstetrician who, after some initial lab tests, recommended that the couple see a reproductive endocrinologist (RE). The initial work-up indicated the only finding of concern was a low-normal AMH and mild hypothyroidism. The patient started on levothyroxine and, once her thyroid levels were within normal limits, she began three cycles of clomiphene citrate and intrauterine insemination (IUI). After the IUI cycles were unsuccessful, their RE recommended that Hannah and Mark undergo in vitro fertilization (IVF). The couple completed a series of appointments in preparation for IVF. Hannah and Mark met with their RE to review the medical process and sign the consents; the nurse to review the time frame and procedures; the pharmacist to review the medication regimen and practice injections; and the clinical health psychologist to review their treatment history and to provide psychoeducational consultation regarding stress and coping with the IVF treatment process.

During the first interview Hannah was quiet, displaying slight psychomotor agitation and frequently repeating that she did not want to participate in the interview. She maintained intermittent eye contact and answered questions with one- or two-word answers. Mark provided information about their reproductive history. Hannah's affect appeared depressed but she denied any current symptoms of depression. When asked about her psychiatric history, Hannah reported that she had had an episode of depression during law school. She described the depression developing as the pressures to succeed during law school mounted and as competition with her fellow students heightened. She reported that she experienced low mood, loss of interest in activities, poor concentration, insomnia and fragmented sleep and passive suicidal ideation. When asked about the suicidal ideation at that time, Hannah described feeling like she "didn't want to be here anymore" but she also noted that she did not have any intent or plan. She had shared her struggle with a friend who referred her to a therapist but Hannah reported that she didn't have time for therapy, so she met with her internist who prescribed fluoxetine. The patient reported that the medication provided her with relief, she was able to finish law school and discontinued the medication after approximately 1.5 years. We discussed the impact of a previous episode of depression and the likelihood of an episode of depression developing during infertility treatment [1]. We reviewed the signs and symptoms of depression [2] and it was recommended that Hannah contact me if she noticed any of her symptoms returning.

The couple completed their first cycle of IVF. They had a fresh embryo transfer and were able to freeze two additional embryos. The first cycle was unsuccessful, as were the two subsequent frozen embryo transfers (FETs). After the last FET, Hannah called to set up an appointment because she noticed symptoms of her depression recurring.

At the first therapy appointment, we reviewed her current symptoms of depression, which were low mood, initial insomnia with fragmented sleep and irritability. Her affect was depressed and angry, her eye contact intermittent and her speech was halting, with bursts of content followed by silence. Her thoughts were logical and sequential. I suggested we meet weekly, but she resisted and said she would only have enough time to meet twice a month. I did not think this was optimal but I wanted her to feel as if she had control in the therapeutic relationship because she seemed hesitant to engage. I had to remember that the overall goal was to facilitate her engagement in the therapy, not about my expectation for what would be "best" for her. We began with twice-monthly appointments, with the option to meet weekly depending on where she was in the treatment process. We continued to meet twice a month for a year as she completed three more cycles of IVF.

We began the therapy by focusing on her experience of the infertility treatment process, which allowed me to understand her appraisal of the infertility experience and her ways of coping. She described her anger and dismay at her inability to get pregnant again. She expressed her hostility toward "needing" psychotherapy to help her cope. She had previously been able to "handle everything" and was upset that she could not "handle" the unsuccessful attempts to get pregnant. The anger was typically expressed at the beginning of the session and then she would begin describing how sad she was that she was not able to get pregnant.

The central theme for the first several months of treatment was focusing on the cognitive and behavioral ways of coping with IVF. From a cognitive perspective, we focused on differentiating the things she could control and the things she could not. We explored in a very detailed way that she could not control how her ovaries responded to the medication, how her estrogen level would rise nor how many eggs would be retrieved. In order to help her engage in problem-focused coping, we explored how she could control how she managed her time at work, when she exercised, and how she modified her sleep habits. It became apparent that she was chronically sleep deprived due to working late after her son was in bed. We then focused on stricter boundaries around work and leisure time, with a re-framing of "success" at work, e.g., she could still be successful at work by meeting, not exceeding, work productivity goals. Additionally, her low mood corresponded to the treatment process with worsening moods during the stimulation phase of the IVF cycle and after an unsuccessful pregnancy test.

In the middle phase of therapy, we discussed that infertility was the first time in her life that she could not meet a goal by working hard. This became the central theme in the therapeutic work as she grieved the loss of control and the loss of a potential second child. During this time, she also began discussing her feelings of loss of self-esteem and not perceiving herself as strong and capable. The loss of self-esteem began to extend to her perception of herself at work and questioning whether she was a good lawyer. She frequently discussed work conflicts and issues in which she second-guessed herself and her decision-making. Previously, she had been confident and assured at her work, but the experience of IVF failure seemed to have infiltrated her self-esteem at work. As she went through the IVF treatment, I also awaited the results of her cycle but I did not check the results before I met with her. I felt it was important to have a spontaneous response to her reporting of the outcome during our sessions. We processed her feelings and I provided cognitive reframing and challenged her beliefs with examples of her competencies at work.

Hannah also identified the loss of her sense of being physically healthy. She often felt bloated, uncomfortable and moody during the first half of the IVF cycles, she gained weight and experienced continual discomfort with the medication injections. The feeling of loss of being physically healthy was compounded by her frequent clinic visits required by the IVF treatment process. Additionally, she talked about herself as an "invalid" who could not exercise or engage in physically rigorous activity due to the treatment restrictions.

Another loss that she identified was the change in her relationship with her son. She described feeling that her involvement in IVF had taken her concentration away from her son and that she wasn't being the "best" mother to him as she could be. I challenged that assumption by reminding her of the examples of her effective parenting that she had shared with me during the course of the therapy. During this time, I felt as if our therapeutic alliance was becoming more established. I learned to identify the pattern of an angry outburst or silence at the beginning of a session but after several minutes of silence, Hannah was able to begin discussing the topic on her mind that day. It was important for me to remain quiet as she had time to prioritize what she wanted to discuss. I was often uncomfortable sitting in silence but I felt it was important for her to be able to have the time and space she needed to have a safe holding space for her thoughts and feelings.

Hannah and Mark decided to end treatment after 2.5 years without an ongoing pregnancy. They had remaining frozen embryos but both partners agreed that they had tried enough and were ready to move on from this part of their lives. Hannah began exploring other areas of focus for her life, primarily spending time with and doing activities with her husband and son. She began describing them as "a complete family of three." Additionally, after about 6 months, she began identifying the positive aspects of having one child, such as ease of travel, less stress trying to manage work–life balance and more time for her to spend on her pro-bono advocacy work. Our sessions tapered down to once a month and largely focused on other areas of life, except for one time when a close co-worker announced her fourth pregnancy, Hannah felt the old sting of loss, but quickly moved through it.

As Hannah's therapist, I viewed her experience through the series of losses she experienced and focused our therapeutic work on processing the feelings related to the losses and identifying ways of coping with the losses and rebuilding those areas of herself that she felt had been damaged. The loss of the dreamed for second child, the loss of self-esteem, loss of health and loss of some facets of her relationships were identified. The sadness and grief of those losses seemed to be expressed as anger initially, which took patience and stillness to manage. I felt it was important to give her space to experience the anger and

grief before moving into the more active coping part of the session. As the end phase of the therapy began, Hannah increased the time interval between appointments, which felt appropriate as she separated from the clinic and our therapy. At the end of treatment, when patients have reached a level of closure, I feel content to see them move on because I view my role as a guide or helper through the treatment experience. I view my work as time-limited because I believe that the patient's growth and development makes my role (happily) obsolete.

Kristin and Mike

Kristin, 34, and Mike, 36, had been married for 2 years before they started trying to conceive. Kristin was a nurse and Mike was an accountant. Kristin had chronic asthma and anxiety; Mike was healthy without any pre-existing conditions. They presented to the fertility clinic with unexplained infertility. Kristin had attributed their fertility problems to herself, due to her asthma and the stressfulness of her job as an ICU nurse. Kristin completed her fertility work-up and Mike had a semen analysis, which came back indicating azoospermia. He was then referred to the consulting urologist who confirmed the diagnosis. Mike was told there were no medical or surgical options for him. The couple was devastated by the diagnosis. They were referred for a routine psychological consultation to explore their options, including child-free living, adoption, and parenting via gamete donation.

Kristin and Mike were seen for their first appointment. Mike was visibly uncomfortable; his affect was irritable and depressed. He made intermittent eye contact and spoke very little. Kristin appeared anxious and became tearful at the start of the appointment. Kristin began describing their situation as Mike retreated further from the conversation, at one point checking his messages on his phone. I asked Kristin to pause, as I asked Mike how he was doing. He retorted, "How do you think I'm doing? I can't believe this is happening. This is the worst thing that has ever happened to me." He further explained, "I don't like shrinks and I don't need a therapist, I'm just not going to do this." When asked what the "this" was, I assumed it was the psychological consultation, but he was referring to conceiving using donor sperm. He said he could not bring himself to have "another man's baby" and that if he couldn't be the biological father, then he wouldn't be a father. Kristin continued to cry and try to convince him it would be his baby and they needed to get started in treatment because she "wasn't getting any younger." As a psychologist and fertility counselor, I felt strong empathy with their pain. I felt like Mike's anger was a reflection of his deep pain associated with his diagnosis. Even as he expressed his dislike of "shrinks," i.e., me, I did not take this personally, I just experienced it as an aspect of his pain. Further, I felt impatient with Kristin's urgency to begin treatment before Mike was ready. I have seen this dynamic frequently in couples using third-party gametes. The fertile partner often doesn't appreciate the amount of time and psychological processing the infertile person needs to make the transition to accepting gamete donation.

The purpose of the psychological consultation for couples considering gamete donation is to help them process their feelings regarding their diagnosis and to explore the rewards and challenges of family building via donor gametes. The first goal with Kristin and Mike was to help them communicate their thoughts and feelings about Mike's diagnosis with one another. Kristin's intense emotional reaction to Mike's diagnosis had been the focus of their conversations, with very little time or space for Mike to express how he felt and to process his grief. From a posttraumatic growth perspective, Mike needed the opportunity and a safe place to manage and work through his emotions. The psychological consultation and subsequent supportive psychotherapy provided this space for Mike and Kristin to grieve the extraordinary loss of a shared biological child. My secondary goal was to help them make a decision about their family building plan.

We set up a series of four appointments to begin discussing the above goals. During these meetings we discussed their families of origin and their individual and couple plans for family building. Kristin had stated she always knew being a mother was a very important goal for her. She was very close to her sister and brother and "couldn't imagine" not having children of her own. Mike was one of four children in a strict, religious family. He described not being close to his parents or his siblings. He had hoped to have children with Kristin but it was never a top priority. He was focused on his career and advancing within his firm. During these initial visits Kristin did most of the talking and emotional expression. She tried to use the majority of the time in the session to discuss her feelings – how this diagnosis affected her, her plans and her feeling of having to get pregnant around the same time as her friends to "keep up." She needed frequent redirection to allow Mike the space and time to talk in order to facilitate the posttraumatic experience and processing of his emotions. Mike benefited from prompts and questions to elicit his thoughts and feelings about the situation. By the end of the fourth session, we agreed to

pause while the couple completed this assignment – each partner was to identify the pros and cons of the three options we had discussed (adoption, donor sperm use, and child-free living), and we would reconvene in 3 weeks.

At the next session we reviewed each partner's assignments. Kristin indicated that she was not sure she could ever be happy if she wasn't a parent but that she was open to donor sperm use or adoption as a path to parenthood. She reassured Mike that he was her priority and that she would express her preferences but would defer to him on the final decision-making because his diagnosis affected him profoundly. In this way Kristin exhibited her substantial social support of Mike, which was also a needed component of his posttraumatic adjustment and growth. By putting Mike's needs ahead of her own in relation to this decision, Mike indicated that he felt supported and loved by Kristin. In terms of the fertility treatment, Mike indicated that his primary concern was that a donor-conceived child wouldn't really be "his" but he also would do anything to make Kristin happy. We explored Mike's ideas about what made a man a father. Using his own relationship with his father as an example, he reflected on the fact that he was not close to his mother or father and they were his genetic progenitors. Alternatively, he had a close relationship with a mentor at work who he felt really knew him and with whom he had discussed his infertility. His mentor had provided another facet of social support that was crucial to Mike's adjustment. These conversations led to an in-depth discussion of the "nature versus nurture" discussion that is common with couples considering gamete donation. It was during this session that Mike agreed to look at a sperm bank website for the first time. We set strict boundaries around the experience, because Mike stated, "Just because I'll look, I don't want Kristin to think I'm ready or this is a go." We agreed that the couple would look at two different banks for 30 minutes each, then stop. They were also assigned the task for individually writing down the characteristics they would prioritize in a donor.

At the follow-up appointment 2 weeks later, Mike was tearful when discussing how emotional it was for him to look at the donor websites. Kristin was patient and empathetic as his grief came to the forefront and the rest of the session was spent processing his grief. The following week we continued to process his grief and he also began describing what characteristics would be necessary if they were to use a donor. For him, ethnicity, physical resemblance and education were the top priorities. Kristin agreed and they again went back to the donor websites and began to look for a donor that might be acceptable to both of them. They were seen every other week to continue to process their feelings about donor conception and for Mike to adjust to the decision. After several months, Mike came to the decision that he would rather be a parent via donor than to not be a parent and therefore agreed to begin the donor selection process. This represented posttraumatic growth and adjustment after the devastating diagnosis of Mike's infertility.

The couple planned to maintain privacy about donor conception with their friends and family, except the confidant that Mike had shared it with and Kristin's sister. It took them several months to select a donor and begin IUI treatment. Kristin conceived after their fourth cycle with a twin pregnancy. They were seen for two sessions for support in the first trimester, then ended therapy with the understanding that they could return as needed. Kristin delivered healthy twin girls.

The couple returned to therapy when the twins were 5 years old to begin discussing the disclosure process. Kristin had read children's books to the twins that explained donor conception [3,4] but Mike was afraid that the girls would reject him or their relationship would change if they disclosed their donor conception. Kristin felt the girls needed to know because she had learned through her online research that children should be told at an early age. We explored Mike's resistance and began trying out different scenarios around disclosing and not disclosing. Mike suggested telling the girls when they were 21. We explored the possible consequences of that option and he soon realized that that scenario might be more emotionally difficult for the girls. In this discussion, the concept of what was best for the girls, not Mike, emerged and was framed as one of many thousands of parenting decisions that were difficult but in the best interest of the children. It also became clear that neither Mike nor Kristin had the words to use to describe to the children how they were conceived, a very common experience. We spent time in the session practicing the specific words to use to tell them. We also discussed the "matter of fact" neutral tone that would be helpful to maintain in discussing donor sperm use, because if Mike and Kristin expressed shame or discomfort about it, the girls would pick up on that and in turn may feel shame or discomfort about their donor origin. This discussion was aided by information on the Donor Conception network [5] and the children's books. We also discussed that they should be aware of times when it would be natural to bring up the topic of conception, such as when the children inquire about family or resemblance or stories of how they were born. After agreeing in principle that they would disclose, it was just a matter of time before one evening, during story time, they together told the girls. Mike later described feeling overwhelming anxiety and then a rush of relief when the girls took the information in their stride and returned to their bed-time routine. We discussed that disclosure is a process over time, but now the foundation had been set for further, more detailed discussion as the girls grew and their intellectual understanding of reproduction deepened.

Working with Kristen and Mike illustrated an example of posttraumatic growth after a diagnosis of azoospermia. Mike moved through the stages of grief and loss with the strength of his own resilience, expression and processing of his emotions and social support from Kristin and other trusted friends. He was able to come to a new place of understanding the priority of parenting. He applied that new understanding to the situation and used it to decide to pursue parenting via donor sperm. His understanding of the role of a parent grew to prioritize the ongoing parent–child relationship over the genetic contribution. In order to facilitate Mike's adjustment, I often re-directed Kristin's emotional expression to allow Mike the time and space he needed to discuss and process his feelings. And, while I work in an infertility clinic, I do not believe it is my role or job to convince people to use donor gametes to conceive. Instead, my role as I see it, is to help patients explore the facets of the decision and help them come to a consensual decision regarding their family building plan.

References

1. Holley SR, Pasch LA, Bliel ME, Gregorich S, Katz PK, Adler NE. Prevalence and predictors of major depressive disorder for fertility treatment patients and their partners. *Fertil Steril* 2015;**103**:1332–1339.

2. American Psychiatric Association. *Diagnostic and Statistical Manual of Mental Disorders*, 5th ed. https://doi.org/10.1176/appi.books.9780890425596

3. Nadel C. *Daddy, Was Mommy's Tummy Big?* London: Moonkind Press, 2007.

4. Celcer I. *Hope and Will Have a Baby: The Gift of Sperm Donation*. Croydon: Graphite Press, 2007. Available at: www.hopeandwill.net [last accessed August 4, 2021]

5. Donor Conception Network. *Our Story*. Donor Conception Network, London, 2002. Available at: www.dcnetwork.org [last accessed August 4, 2021]

CASE 3   Fertility Counseling for Individuals

Linda Applegarth and Arabelle Rowe

Introduction

Linda Applegarth [LA]: As a psychologist who also has a personal history of infertility, I have been treating fertility patients for nearly 40 years. I never fail to be moved by their emotional pain, shame, frustration and profound sense of loss. At the same time, I am equally impressed and moved by these patients' resiliency, psychological strength and ability to utilize a wide array of resources and social support as they strive to build their families. After working with Resolve, Inc., and establishing a private practice in Northern California, I was privileged, 35 years ago, to join the clinical faculty and medical team as Director of Psychological Services at the Perelman Center for Reproductive Medicine at the Weill Medical College of Cornell University in New York City. My primary professional goal has been to serve the psychosocial needs of fertility patients and work to mitigate their emotional anguish while also helping to build a sense of hope, strength and resolution.

Arabelle Rowe [AR]: I am a clinical social worker with extensive experience on both sides of the Atlantic, having trained and worked in London as a *guardian ad litem* prior to my move to the United States (US). For the past 15 years, I have worked at New York Presbyterian Hospital (NYPH) in Westchester County, New York, on psychiatric inpatient units with a wide range of diagnoses, including working as a clinician on the Women's Unit that encompassed both peri- and post-natal depression, anxiety and psychosis in the context of women's behavioral health across the life span. I was overcome by the prevailing sense of loss experienced by patients who were away from their families as they faced the crisis of hospitalization. Yet, I never failed to be impressed by the strengthening and solidity of family ties which were a key factor in recovery. At NYPH, I co-founded and co-led a year-long CBT training program for clinical staff. I am a Diplomate member of the Academy of Cognitive and Behavioral Therapies, and a member of the British Association for Behavioural and Cognitive Psychotherapies. My experience in working with patients with fertility struggles is limited, but my background and training has provided me with a keen interest and insight into the pain and often silent suffering of those pursuing fertility treatments. I am humbled by these patients' strength, competence, and coping as they navigate the uncertainty and fear of their journeys to parenthood.

We have chosen to present a case together from the perspective of two different, but effective, theoretical treatment approaches [1]: Psychodynamic Therapy [LA] and Cognitive-Behavioral Therapy [AR]. The case of Sarah is fictitious and a composite of common clinical issues clients struggle with in individual fertility counseling.

Sarah: A Case Study from Two Treatment Perspectives

Sarah, age 33, is a well-respected Canadian artist who has received a special grant to teach art at a competitive university in New York City. Her husband, James, a successful graphic designer, has been able to join her. They have been married for 4 years, together for 7 years. She described a stable, supportive marital relationship. Sarah is the middle of three children; she has a younger sister and older brother. She is from a family of highly educated professionals. Her father and siblings have each obtained Ph.Ds. She describes her parents as happily married.

Sarah and her husband have been attempting to conceive for the past 3 years. The diagnosis, "unexplained infertility," has confounded the couple as well as their physicians. They have completed several IVF cycles in Canada and New York and have done both fresh and frozen embryo transfers. As a result, Sarah has had two "biochemical" pregnancies. More recently, she suffered a 12-week pregnancy loss following an embryo transfer. It is this loss that brought Sarah into psychotherapy. For several weeks, the pregnancy continued despite the knowledge that it was no longer viable. Coincidentally, Sarah learned that her sister, Ann, in western Canada, was pregnant and due to deliver near the same time that Sarah's lost baby *would have been* born. As a result, she is unable to talk with her sister, or other family members, about Ann's pregnancy because of the intense emotions she experiences. An additional compounding factor has been the recent announcement that Sarah's brother's fiancé is also pregnant.

Sarah's physician, a reproductive endocrinologist, has suggested that she and her husband try another IVF cycle. Sarah has refused, saying that the process has been too difficult emotionally. At Sarah's initiation, the couple has subsequently consulted with an egg donation program; yet, Sarah also expresses uncertainty and sadness about this option.

Sarah described herself as being very close to her family, especially her sister. Yet, when they now speak to one another, Sarah feels distant and alone. Her family members know of Sarah and James's loss, but have also refrained from talking about it with Sarah – they have also apparently felt uncomfortable talking about Ann's pregnancy. Conversations have been superficial and often empty.

Upon presentation, Sarah's emotional pain was palpable. She wept on and off during the treatment hour. She described feelings of shame and loneliness. She spoke of the "cruelty" of her infertility experience – and envisions a future of never again feeling emotionally connected to the family she loves. Sarah openly fears that her sister, her brother, and her parents "will not believe" the depth of her emotional anguish – and will essentially tell her that she is "overreacting" and to "get over it" – and to move on. Thus, her sadness and sense of loss appeared to come not only from losses she has experienced through infertility, but also from the breakdown of close family relationships.

DSM-5 Diagnosis: *Major Depressive Disorder, Moderate*

A Psychodynamic Treatment Approach [LA]

My work with Sarah began with a thorough family and psychosocial history. Because of the difficulty Sarah had historically talking with others about her condition, she was surprisingly able to speak openly about her thoughts and feelings. We were able to establish a good working alliance early in the treatment. My personal goal with her was to create a safe, trusting place, free of judgment. After several evaluative sessions, Sarah and I were also able to collaborate and to articulate treatment goals [2]:

1. To resolve the infertility by making family-building decisions about which she was psychologically and emotionally comfortable;
2. To share her feelings with family members, especially with her sister;
3. To re-establish more comfortable relationships, in general, with family and friends; and
4. To ameliorate her depression.

Clearly, these goals are intrinsically intertwined. Within this context, it was important that I, as the therapist, also foster positive expectations of the treatment outcome [3] and help to develop a strong therapeutic alliance.

Sarah was fully committed to treatment; however, she was, as expected, both consciously and unconsciously resistant to change. For example, it was important to explore her refusal to be a part of an infertility support group. This meant bringing unconscious material into consciousness, and ultimately to point out her need for emotional connection to others while at the same time fighting against it. What did this type of avoidance mean on a more deep-seated level?

It was my contention that Sarah's unconscious mental activity was affecting her thoughts, feelings and behavior with respect to her notions about her infertility. Thus, it was important to explore her family relationships within the context of her earlier life experiences.

Although there was an emphasis in treatment on the issues that Sarah was dealing with in the "here and now," it was also critical to learn more about her views about her parents and their impact upon her as a child. It was my belief that some of her unconscious thoughts and feelings were causing her to suffer emotionally as she and her husband struggled to become parents themselves.

My goal as a clinician was certainly to gain a better understanding of what was going on in Sarah's unconscious that might be contributing to her distress, while at the same time establishing a safe, supportive relationship to explore these issues. I learned over the course of several sessions that her parents openly expressed their high expectations of each of their children with respect to succeeding academically and professionally. It was also important to follow family and social traditions that included marriage, children, owning a home and being an active family member – regardless of geographic location. Sarah was ultimately able to articulate that she felt she was a disappointment to her parents, and that she had let them down.

Several months into treatment, Sarah was able to articulate that seeing and talking with her mother was especially painful. She commented that she had slowly become aware that her mother's sole purpose in life, despite her other accomplishments, was *motherhood.* Her mother's pride in her children was pivotal to her identity and sense of self-worth. Sarah was tearful as she spoke of this, and her anguish about the idea of not being a part of her mother and sister's exclusive "club" was most distressing. Infertility was not only about being deprived personally of parenthood; it was also about being emotionally disconnected from those with whom she was most attached. On so many dimensions, infertility was about failure – and shame.

As a result, the therapy began to focus on the things that gave Sarah good feelings about herself and her abilities. We spent time in session talking about her creativity and "productivity" as an artist. This had not faltered during her infertility treatments and was ultimately a source of stress and anxiety reduction. Additionally, we spent several sessions talking about Sarah's relationship with her husband. He had been her sole source of emotional support, but it became clear that he had often found it difficult to meet her emotional needs and mitigate her distress. It was hypothesized that if she could better articulate with him how he could be most helpful to her in times of distress, he would be able to attend to her in a more meaningful and helpful way. They both also began to make a more concerted effort to enjoy New York City life, including attending art exhibits and theater – and occasionally reaching out to friends.

Eventually, my time with Sarah allowed me to address the transference issues in our relationship. I also considered how my own countertransference might inform me in better understanding Sarah's psychodynamics. Her feelings for me were warm and positive, as evidenced by her ongoing commitment to treatment and affect. I believe that I became the mother figure that she craved: a caring, listening, and nurturing parent, free of judgment or expectations. On occasion, I found myself confronted with feelings of frustration and helplessness as I heard Sarah's inability to manage her anguish. My own feelings allowed me to make interpretations and "suggest" that her own family also felt helpless to assist Sarah on an emotional level. Sarah's inability to talk about her struggle to have a child kept her isolated and distant – and angry.

These dynamics were clearly illustrated at the birth of Sarah's sister's child. Essentially, her sister sent her a text message about the birth – and few details were provided by any family members. As she spoke of this, Sarah began to weep. She yearned to be a part of the family's celebration, but also recoiled at learning more about the joy they were experiencing. We spent several sessions focused on these conflicted feelings. Several weeks later, Sarah contacted the Donor Egg Program she had reached out to a year earlier. She commented that she was feeling sad but less invested in having a child who was genetically hers. Her open wish to leave her pain behind (and move on to the donor egg option) was especially compelling – for her and for me.

Although the Donor Egg Program indicated initially that they did not have a suitable match for her, Sarah was contacted a month later and told that a match had been found. Embryos were created and frozen, and Sarah and her husband planned to undergo a single embryo transfer within the next few weeks. She verbalized a sense of hope and optimism, albeit with caution. Our work will continue as she moves forward with family-building options and struggles to rebuild important family relationships in psychotherapy. Our strong working alliance and powerful positive transference in the relationship have led to Sarah's greater self-understanding and proactive decision-making.

A Cognitive-Behavioral Treatment (CBT) Approach [AR]

At the time Sarah contacted me, she was devastated by recent news of her younger sister's pregnancy and this was compounded by the fact that her brother's girlfriend was also pregnant. Establishing a strong therapeutic alliance with Sarah was essential for effective, structured, collaborative, time-limited CBT. Likewise, psychoeducation on how depressed mood may fluctuate as we addressed the emotional, cognitive, and behavioral components of her depression was important. In the intake session Sarah scored 28 on the Beck Depression Inventory-II (BDI-II) [4] and eventually she was diagnosed with major depressive disorder, moderate.

The overall goal for Sarah was to help her identify maladaptive thought patterns, develop alternative cognitions, and act in a more adaptive manner to mitigate her depression. We collaborated on a *descriptive case conceptualization* to highlight these links [5]. The central problem of her own infertility was very painful to Sarah, so we did not start with this. Instead, we focused on targeting her depression with *behavioral activation*, using activity monitoring and scheduling, to amplify that action precedes motivation. Consistent with a *strengths-based approach* [6], we incorporated some of Sarah's favorite activities (baking, hiking) and countered Sarah's report "I never enjoy anything anymore." Experiencing and acknowledging pleasure helped balance her negative belief and served to highlight ways to look at alternative explanations for her thoughts. We also explored how her responses were maintaining the triggers in both the long- and short-term. For example, Sarah's withdrawal from family only served to increase the isolation she felt and was a barrier to her goal of feeling more connected with them.

We collaborated on a *thought record* where the event was her younger sister being pregnant. Her automatic thought "She is only 30 years – I SHOULD have become pregnant then" led to emotions of shock, sadness and guilt, with behaviors of crying and inability to speak with her sister directly. Another thought was "All my friends from university are getting married and having kids now," which was accompanied by further thoughts of being peripheral/different and the emotion of sadness. Sarah herself was able to identify her *cognitive distortions* of all-or-nothing thinking ("If I am not pregnant now I never will be"), mind reading ("My family are avoiding me"), overgeneralizations ("Everyone I know is pregnant"), and catastrophizing ("My life will have little meaning without a child").

Sarah was able to recognize her propensity to selectively focus on the negative, thereby eclipsing other positive aspects which proffered a different conclusion. She was able to understand the rigidity of her thoughts and shift to more flexible views that pregnancy was a possibility as she was still in the fertility program, that she herself was limiting contact with her family, and that many of her friends were not pregnant. Although difficult, Sarah was able to give some fleeting credence to the possibility that she could still have a meaningful life utilizing third-party reproduction (egg donation) or living a full life without children.

Witnessing others becoming pregnant, her own pregnancy loss, and the image of never becoming a mother herself led to depressed mood. This was reinforced by her behaviors of reduced communication with others, withdrawal, withholding information, and avoiding images of babies and pregnancy on social media. *Imaginal exposure* was introduced to counter Sarah's low distress tolerance of learning about or seeing other pregnancies. After this we moved to *in vivo exposures*, starting with planned, deliberate readings on this subject and eventually to the social media platforms where content and pace were less predictable. Eventually, Sarah expanded her tolerance yet again by meeting with friends who are now parents themselves. She has more cognitive flexibility to recognize the value of reconnecting and strengthening bonds of friendship without the tinge of her own perception of judgment or fear of intrusive questions from friends.

To deepen our understanding, we developed a longitudinal case conceptualization of her *conditional assumptions, core beliefs and coping strategies*. A key facet of this was understanding how Sarah structured her experiences by identifying the rules determined by these assumptions. Sarah's conditional rules included the need to: be perfect at all times; elicit approval from others; be in control at all times; and show no vulnerability. Her core belief was "I am worthless and incompetent" in the context of loving but critical parents. Following from these, Sarah engaged in safety coping behaviors of appeasing others, diligently applying herself to all tasks to maintain an image of perfectionism, avoiding harsh judgment from others, and preserving approval, particularly from parents. We challenged the imperative stance of having to be perfect, the faulty logic that her love from her parents was conditional on perfectionism, and her own perception of her violating this rule should she let her standards falter. With *guided discovery*, Sarah reported that she would feel worthless and incompetent and thus her coping strategy of being in control at all times avoided possible exposure of herself as incompetent.

Sarah was unable to identify how her "should" statement originated but she did recognize that her behaviors were maintaining this negative cycle. She was collaborative with exploring costs and benefits of this assumption and able to see that her high standards, effective as they may have been in her formative years in staving off perceived rejection from parents and others, no longer had utility. She was able to accept that doing "the best I can" in all areas of her life was a more logical and realistic tenet. We also noted that Sarah was blaming herself for not getting pregnant. Addressing this cognitive distortion was done by *reattribution*, examining all external factors as well as biological factors involved to attenuate the thought. This was a successful intervention to balance Sarah's thoughts.

We explored her feelings of not being understood by anyone. She could see how these thoughts and feelings had driven her behavior of withholding from her family the extensive IVF treatment she had endured due to her painful feelings of shame and not wanting to impose any burden on her parents or siblings. Helping Sarah to consider sharing some of her current distress over her infertility issues with her family was important, as this potentially opened her to receive longed-for validation and conversation and curiosity about her struggles with getting pregnant. Sarah is currently considering attending an overdue family reunion where she will see all family members and we are focusing on strategies, such as developing a "coping card" in anticipation of negative feelings and cognitions that may occur.

We looked at several *thought records* to confirm that these were patterns in Sarah's cognitions and behavior, and explored costs and benefits of maintaining her core beliefs. The use of *inference chaining* – challenging the evidence for and against a belief – here was productive. If the belief was not true, Sarah would have more hope. She was able to acknowledge that her current belief fueled her depression and hopelessness, reinforcing her belief that "it will always be this way." *Mindful detachment* (learning to observe the thought, not engage with it), breathing, and muscle relaxation were all helpful behavioral exercises to target these thoughts to even out tensions. We also looked at other areas of Sarah's life where she had successfully tolerated uncertainty (e.g., the anticipated reaction from others on her art installations) to clarify her ability to accept risk and build a more balanced view of her self-competence.

With more *cognitive flexibility*, Sarah was able to adopt a new core belief that she was worthy, capable and did not need to seek reassurance/approval from others. This led to a revision in her maladaptive conditional assumptions with new rules enhancing acceptance of herself as always doing her best, even if not perfect or pregnant. By harboring less fear of judgment from others (and herself), Sarah recognized that she did not need to be in control at all times, that she is able to manage risk, and that there were definite benefits to these adaptive assumptions. This shift in cognitions was also evidenced by Sarah's own report of "worrying less" and a score of 22 on the BDI-II. Sarah's ability to modify her thoughts led to an improvement in her symptoms and addressing her dysfunctional beliefs in the middle stage of our treatment together led to a more enduring change. With *covert rehearsals and role-plays* in session, Sarah was able to consolidate her confidence in her new core beliefs that led to more functional assumptions about her life, with or without children.

As a cognitive-behavioral therapist, I found myself impressed by Sarah's motivation for change as well as by her interest in this evidenced-based approach. However, there were some countertherapeutic issues, as Sarah initially expressed trepidation as to how this behavioral treatment approach could help with her deep-seated depression. It was therefore incumbent upon me to collaborate with Sarah in flexible and creative ways to counter her ambivalence. Finally, as we progressed though the goals and objectives of treatment, I found our collaborative work to be not only helpful to Sarah, but also a meaningful and positive experience for me as her therapist.

Summary

As colleagues with different theoretical approaches to individual adult psychotherapy, we nonetheless have endeavored to demonstrate the efficacy of both types of treatment modalities for Sarah, a fertility patient suffering from depression. We believe that this was best done by describing the specific techniques and processes inherent in each approach as they applied to Sarah's feelings, thoughts and behaviors. The main focus of psychodynamic therapy was the attention to Sarah's unconscious processes, including a focus on her transference and on Linda's countertransference. The goal was to bring forth past memories, relationships, and experiences that could provide a better understanding of current behavior and feelings. Increased insight and awareness led to Sarah's confidence to make important changes.

The cognitive-behavioral therapy was based on the notion that changing Sarah's maladaptive thinking could lead to important changes in feelings and behavior. This structured approach could also help her understand how her cognitions influenced her actions and helped her to modify problematic behaviors, and to make appropriate and productive decisions – and to feel better.

Ultimately, however, it is our belief that one of the primary ingredients for change in therapy is the *working alliance* between patient and therapist. The positive and caring relationship that we were able to build with Sarah during the treatment was paramount to her emotional and psychological growth – and to resolution in her fertility journey.

References

1. Leichenring F. Comparative effects of short-term psychodynamic psychotherapy and cognitive behavioral therapy in depression: a meta-analytic approach. *Clin Psychol Rev* 2001;**21**:401–419.

2. Leichsenring F. Psychodynamic psychotherapy: a review of efficacy and effectiveness studies. In Levy RA, Abion JS, Eds. *Handbook of Evidence-Based Psychodynamic Psychotherapy: Bridging the Gap between Science and Practice*. New Jersey: Humana Press, 2009, 3–27.

3. Cabaniss DL, Cherry S, Douglas CJ, Schwartz A. *Psychodynamic Psychotherapy: A Clinical Manual*, 2nd ed. Oxford: John Wiley & Sons, 2017.

4. Beck AT, Steer RA, Brown GK. Manual for the Beck Depression Inventory-II. San Antonio, TX: Psychological Corporation, 1996.

5. Padesky CA. Collaborative case conceptualization: client knows best. *Cogn Behav Pract* 2020;**27**(4):392–404.

6. Padesky CA, Mooney KA. Strengths-based cognitive–behavioural therapy: a four-step model to build resilience. *Clin Psychol Psychother* 2012;**19**(4):283–290.

CASE 4 | Fertility Counseling for Couples

Kristy Koser

Introduction

I entered the field of reproductive psychology shortly after completing my own journey to conceive through multiple IVF attempts and ultimately success via surrogacy. I was acutely aware of the disarray infertility creates, as I was beginning to see others actively trying to conceive in my practice. I knew their desire, pain, loneliness and hope in a very intimate way. I found water in my eyes more often with my fertility-related clients, along with a deeper determination to encounter their human experience outside of just the run-down of fertility-related treatment. Along with my own experience of infertility and its enduring battles, I also knew the impact it could have on the couple relationship. I had been training, teaching, and specializing in couples therapy for almost 10 years in private practice before I had to really start practicing what I "preached" when my own relationship had to stretch in new ways to accommodate the fear and grief that was emerging. My personal experience, combined with my professional training, greatly impacted my rationale for treating the couple relationship during fertility distress. It was hard to know where one partner's experience started and the other's ended. So much of a couple's experience during infertility begins to linger in everyday decisions, conversations, and subtle bids for connection, and it often goes unnoticed.

My general couples therapy treatment approach relies heavily on attachment theory and emotionally focused therapy (EFT). I have found this orientation also lends nicely to fertility counseling [1]. Couples are usually under some amount of distress, at times significant, which creates a barrier to effective communication and the inability to secure little emotional safety in the relationship. John Bowlby [2] introduced attachment theory and its value in conceptualizing a couple or individual's response to proximity, consistency, safety and security in relation to a caregiver or romantic partner. This conceptual lens, along with evidence-based interventions from EFT, has been shown to help couples learn to stay emotionally engaged even when they get stuck in their communication cycle, activating each other's attachment styles and impacting their perception of stress throughout the fertility journey [1,3].

When working in the field of reproductive psychology, there is a guarantee of encountering many painful feelings and complicated processing. Rarely can anyone make a guarantee in the realm of reproduction. However, the feelings associated with it are bound to create a lasting impact on the individuals and the potential future child. In your office, couples can show up stuck in their negative and misattuned communication cycle, grid-locked in making necessary treatment decisions for the future. They can also emerge in deep grief over the loss of a pregnancy or the news that there is little prospect for a genetically related offspring. Whatever the case, it is likely the couple is feeling an immense amount of pain and suffering. However, the difficulty is often helping the couple process this pain together without the usual coping skills of turning inward and dealing with it each on their own. In the following fictitious case study, Brock and Molly present as a typical couple in fertility treatment: exhausted, desperate, and feeling disconnected. While this example is a heterosexual couple, many of the issues and dynamics parallel in same-sex couple relationships.

It is paramount in these situations to work *within* the relationship, not just with each individual. In reality, it is important to consider and to communicate that the couple's relationship is also your client, so that you are in fact holding three entities in the room. This mindset helps to bring the clinical focus and interventions back to the couple's bond and exercise the challenge of turning toward each other during this time, instead of away. My interventions in the case study while subtle, help to remind the couple they are in this together, while also addressing some of the individualized feelings that fuel their tendency to want to isolate or withdraw. This case study example presents a one-time consultation with this couple, although it is likely they will need to be seen again throughout their fertility journey. In this one-time session example, several theoretical conceptualizations and interventions are discussed, along with illustrating a starting place for fertility counselors to begin addressing therapeutic issues as opposed to only providing supportive counseling with couples. I utilize attachment theory in the case study as a theoretical lens to better understand the feelings that are likely fueling their disconnection, rooted far before the experience of infertility and now activated during such a crucial time.

The Case of Molly and Brock

When Brock and Molly walked into my office, they had just concluded their second in vitro fertilization (IVF) cycle, resulting in another disappointment. Molly, 34, a successful real-estate agent and Brock, 36, a fire fighter, had been married 8 years. They were patients of a local reproductive endocrinologist for the past 2 years, starting first with noninvasive treatment and progressing quickly toward IVF. I had a brief conversation with Molly on the phone about their reproductive history and learned they had experienced a variety of fertility treatments and had a miscarriage during an IUI cycle. The latter was devastating for the couple to process. Molly and Brock decided to pursue counseling, with the support of their physician, before determining how to proceed building their family.

When the couple entered my office, they appeared nervous and quickly took their seats. I looked at both of them and said, "*I know from the paperwork, and from the brief conversation with Molly on the phone, you've been through a lot these past 2 years. I'm curious how your relationship has weathered all those unpredictable ups and downs?*" I start first by asking about their relationship, making it clear I consider what they went through – and are still going through – to be something a couple experiences together. Although it can be common for one partner to feel the brunt of the infertility experience, the impact of the process is significant for both parties. Typically, men are not as involved in the day-to-day tasks of fertility treatment and may feel excluded from the reproductive medical process [4]. Therefore, including the male partner in counseling helps to reconnect the couple as a pair, a team, facing infertility together. Working within the couple relationship during fertility treatment is essential in helping to create a cohesive narrative about the experience in order to integrate this painful time into their relationship history, since "... infertility is a dyadic, rather than an individual problem ..." ([5], p. 394).

Molly and Brock quickly agreed it had been difficult to find the right words to comfort and understand each other's experiences. They reported feeling discouraged not only with their recent fertility failure, but with the emotional distance that had emerged in their relationship. Brock spoke first, looking hesitant and uncomfortable, "*I think we are doing better now; we tend not to think about the past and try to stay really positive for the next cycle.*" Molly looked straight ahead numbly, clearly experiencing something different. Our eyes met and I asked, "*Would you agree with that statement, Molly?*" Her eyes filled with tears and she said, "*Sometimes, although it's really hard to just keep staying positive. I really try to not let my emotions flood out all over the place. I know that makes Brock overwhelmed. But somedays I just can't do it, I'm consumed with anger and sadness.*"

I follow up with, "*It sounds like you both have been doing your best to keep afloat, and in doing so, it's looked different for each of you, maybe missing each other's needs or feeling alone in the process. Am I getting that right?*" Molly quickly added, "*I feel incredibly alone.*" Brock didn't look over at her. He stared straight ahead, suddenly appearing like he wished to disappear into the couch he was sitting on.

I broke the silence by saying, "*So much emotion is brought to the surface with infertility that we sometimes think it's best to keep it to ourselves or figure it out on our own. It can be hard to reach for our partner in those moments. Feeling alone can also look different for each person. Brock, have you felt lonely in this process too?*"

Brock glanced quickly at Molly and said, "*Yes, it feels strange to say, because nothing is happening to my body. But, it's really hard to watch Molly go through everything physically and then be so disappointed. I feel like I can't relate, so I don't try. I just go quiet and assume my role is to stay positive.*"

What I was noticing is supported by other research suggesting that emotional avoidance can be met with emotional pursuit, leading to more distress for the partner originally attempting to avoid [3]. I follow up with, "*So when you feel alone Brock, you go quiet, retreat inside and, Molly, when you feel alone, what do you do?*"

Molly looked at Brock and said, "*Well, I'm pretty vocal about it. I often wait for Brock to say something reassuring to me, or comforting, so I keep showing my emotions. I know he hears me crying at night or knows about how hard it is to hold my new niece. But he never says a thing, just looks right through me, like I don't exist.*"

"*And in those moments, you feel alone. Like you don't exist to Brock, is that right? What else comes to mind in those moments?*", I ask.

Molly's eyes start to water again and she looks away. "*I just get scared, so fearful and my head starts to spin,*" she said.

I respond with, "*Fearful and alone. Those are big feelings. And part of you longs for Brock to help you hold those big feelings?*" She nods. "*Can you help me understand what comes to mind when the fear shows up?*"

Brock is listening carefully to Molly's response. She says, "*I fear I will not be a mom, that I waited too long, and now this is the consequence. I fear we will have to use an egg* donor, and I worry about what Brock thinks of this. Is this all my fault? All this pain and suffering feels like my issue and I should just deal with this myself. It feels like I'm doing this to us and to him."

As I listened to Molly talk about the fear that is often present for couples undergoing fertility treatment, it became clear that how she is expressing that fear gets lost when it comes in contact with Brock's feelings of helplessness and inadequacy, thus fueling their misattuned communication cycle and the narrative that it's better to just keep these feelings inside. This pursue/withdraw scenario can keep couples spinning, lacking the ability to make the important and necessary decisions while in treatment.

Even with all this heightened emotion, what is imperative in this moment of therapy is for each party to realize that continuing to view the other as being incapable of understanding their emotional experience will slowly erode whatever level of emotional connection was there before fertility treatment began. It is in this moment that couples have the choice to use this painful experience as an opportunity to repair and strengthen their emotional bond, or allow the fear and isolation to take over and suffer the consequences.

I responded to Molly, "*It sounds like this fear gets really big for you and you start to spin, asking yourself all kinds of questions about your worth and wonder how Brock sees you. Those are big questions to hold on our own.*"

"*Brock, did you know all of this is surfacing for Molly in those moments? That she is actually looking for you to come closer when those fears get too bi*g," I asked. Again, I want to remind Brock how important he is in this fertility process, not just helping to create their future child, but in building a stronger connection with his wife during the treatment. In my clinical experience, the supporting partner can often feel lost or unsure of how to best support the partner being treated. They may get complicated messages about how to help and how to give space, ultimately leading to giving up or just remaining silent.

Brock shared, "*I don't know how much to intervene. I know it's painful for her, so I don't intrude. Of course, I see the tears and subtle depression, but I stand back, trying to stay positive. It's so hard to watch her hurt and feel so helpless. I don't want to burden her with my pain.*" In this moment, I am helping Brock become aware that his usual way of coping with hard feelings may not be the most conducive to protecting the feelings of his wife, and in fact, she may need a response from him that is entirely different.

"*Right, it's so hard to watch the person you love most hurt so badly,*" I responded. "*Even your profession as a fire fighter shows how much you want to rescue and keep others safe, so I bet it's excruciating to not know how to help. She is hurting because of something you can't fix, there is no way to talk or buy your way out of this pain, so what is there for you to do? And yet, she keeps reaching. What would it be like to share some of the helplessness you feel when she hurts, and how you want to comfort her and yet don't want to intrude?*"

Brock went on to share how hard it has been to know where he belongs in this family-building process. He felt silly, at times, that his major contribution is providing a sample of sperm, while his wife is taking time off from work, sick on the couch, bruised from injections and feeling an array of hormonal shifts. Brock decided his best course of action was to get out of the way – cheer from the sidelines – but in doing so, he couldn't reach Molly when she needed it most. He was emotionally too far away. He couldn't help prop her up and gently usher her to the unidentifiable finish line. Instead, he watched helplessly and she suffered quietly. Molly felt this was her burden to carry, that she must just "push through" each day and cycle, feeling guilty for needing anything more.

We have learned that a diagnosis of infertility can sometimes activate attachment-seeking behavior and that more securely attached individuals can experience less distress during fertility treatment [6]. This research implies that "couples recover more successfully from the grief, loss, and disconnection heightened by the diagnosis and treatment of infertility, if the couple relationship is safe, secure, and partners are emotionally accessible" ([1], p. 28).

Molly shared, "*I feel selfish needing him this much, I know he is busy and I feel so needy and weak. Sometimes all I need is a hug or a text or something small and I don't know why I can't just get over it and keep 'powering' through.*"

I replied, looking at both of them, "*All that work to keep each other at a distance, far away from seeing and feeling the pain each of you feel, comes at a cost. How much suffering do you need to endure before you do not consider comfort as selfish? I think you have paid the price repeatedly through this process. It's okay to ask for comfort, especially from each other. This pain is not your punishment.*"

This last statement seemed to resonate with them. While they may not have consciously considered suffering or pain as punishment, it can be a common feeling going through fertility treatment [7]. That somehow the pain of it all is penance for some past transgression or that more suffering now equals more substantial joy in the future. What's at risk with this perspective is the complacent feeling that "I don't need others ... they won't understand ... or I need to deal with this on my own." There is a cost to this mindset. While most couples think it protects them and their relationship to keep these more difficult emotions at bay, it only allows for disconnection to emerge.

Brock looked at his wife and shared, "*I guess we've been missing out on our relationship the last 2 years. We've been so focused on building our family, we've totally neglected these other parts of our life. We've been so focused on missing out on being parents, that we've missed out on our marriage, the thing we already have and also work hard for.*" This tunnel vision is common for couples in fertility treatment. The cycles, medication, lab results, even down to the hours counted between injections, can make it feel regimented and obsessive. It is consuming for most individuals, and the tunnel vision can lead individuals to miss the incredibly successful scenarios that are present on a daily basis. Helping couples reframe and readjust that perspective can be helpful. Tunnel vision has a cost, and the expense is usually the couple's relationship.

I look back at both of them and say, "*Maybe sharing those feelings with each other would help you both feel less alone or like an outsider in this? Maybe sharing those feelings would allow an opportunity for you to break this negative cycle you get into?*"

I want to encourage them to start turning to each other in times that typically elicit the desire to turn away. I also want to help them find creative solutions for how to notice and start remediating the direction of their communication cycle when they sense they are headed to opposite emotional corners. If I can help create some "emotional muscle memory" in my office, it could help them later when the emotional stakes feel high at home.

I turn to Molly and ask, "*Can you turn to Brock and share that even when you are hurting and in pain you need Brock there with you? That you feel comforted by his presence, even if he doesn't know what to say, just to know he is there?*" This prompt to share deeper feelings allows for new options to emerge, which may help break out of the negative, isolating, misattuned manner of communication couples get stuck in. This strategy is something a fertility counselor can help untangle and can provide concrete, positive coping strategies when couples feel overwhelmed and disconnected.

Molly turned and shared, with tears in her eyes, the longing to have Brock be close through this process even though she often displays the opposite. She carefully explained how she can't always be strong, and that when she feels shame about their infertility, she needs to be reminded she is lovable and wanted.

This emotional sharing and attuned communication from Molly allowed Brock to feel needed, which was the very antidote to his helpless and inadequate feelings. Reminding Brock there are ways to help hold the pain of this process, without "fixing" it, could provide relief to both of them. In doing so, it highlights Molly's exhaustion from carrying the "mental load" of infertility and the longing for permission to not have it all figured out. This gives opportunity for Brock to step in to this emotional space in a new way, knowing that his touch, words, or presence have an impact and he can be an active part of this complicated process. Suddenly both parties have "room" in the other's existence, there is no longer the need to be operating in their separate corners, but instead an invitation to come share the same emotional space together.

Reflection and Summary

It has been suggested that how each partner relates to their own attachment style, and to each other's attachment style, can impact how they respond to the stress of infertility [3]. Therefore, fertility counselors will be encountering attachment dynamics and relational patterns that have been established far before the experience of infertility. It is likely those attachment histories will impact how they respond to each other in times of distress, which include infertility. A fertility counselor can assess a person's attachment history by listening to how they speak and reflect of other close relationships in the past; their experience of others attempting to care for them; or the lack of attunement, predictability and consistency they experienced as a child and/or as an adult. All of these opportunities open the door for further exploration of those experiences and their impact on the perception of emotional accessibility in their current relationship.

Over the years as I sit with couples, I am reminded often that infertility is something that effects both individuals, regardless of who is enduring the treatment or who is more emotive in session. The emotions of a couple, spoken or unspoken, are so palpable in the therapy room, and illuminating the human experience of a sometimes cold, procedural process cannot be ignored. When I have two faces staring back at me with tears, fear, and desperation, I am reminded how much is at stake, that their world is upside down. It is in this human connection with each other and at times with me, that couples begin to redefine what is success. And, what we end up discovering is that perhaps success is not just about bringing home a baby. It becomes more about the ability to make decisions, to tune in to themselves and their partner, to face fear and shame, guilt and anger in order to make sense of the trials to become parents together.

References

1. Koser K. Fertility counseling with couples. A theoretical approach. *Family J: Counseling Therapy Couples Families* 2019;**28**(1):25–32.

2. Bowlby J. *Attachment and Loss: Volume 2. Separation: Anxiety and Anger.* New York, NY: Basic Books, 1973.

3. Donarelli Z, Kivlighan DM, Allergra A, LoCoco G. How do individual attachment patterns of both members of couples affect their perceived infertility distress? An actor-partner interdependence analysis. *Personality Individual Differ* 2016;**92**:63–68.

4. Grace B, Shawe J, Johnson S, Stephenson J. You did not turn up … I did not realize I was invited …: understanding male attitudes towards engagement in fertility and reproductive health discussions. *Hum Reprod Open* 2019; 2019:1–7.

5. Read SC, Carrier ME, Boucher ME, Whitley R, Bond S, Zelkowitz P. Psychosocial services for couples in infertility treatment: what do couples really want? *Patient Educ Counseling* 2014;**94**:390–395.

6. Lowyck B, Luyten P, Corveleyn J, D'Hooghe TM, Buyse E, Demyttenaere K. Well-being and relationships satisfaction of couples dealing with an in vitro fertilization/intracytoplasmic sperm injection procedure: a multilevel approach on the role of self-criticism, dependency, and romantic attachment. *Fertil Steril* 2009;**91**:387–395.

7. Daniluk JC. Strategies for counseling infertile couples. *Counseling Dev* 1991;**69**:317–320.

Fertility Counseling with Groups

Rachel Rabinor and Landon Zaki

Introduction

Rachel Rabinor: After my own personal challenging experience with secondary infertility, I committed to starting a support group when I got to the "other side." Despite all the wonderful resources I discovered and relied on throughout my journey, what I yearned for most was a hand to squeeze, a shoulder to cry on, and other knowing nods that could offer support through some of the hardest times. I started my first support group in 2016 and have been running groups ever since.

My initial social worker training in the person-in-the-environment framework continues to provide a useful multifaceted perspective in assessment and treatment. I'm trauma-informed and integrate my training in EMDR, The Daring Way™, cognitive, interpersonal and mindfulness-based therapies. I operate a private practice in San Diego, California, specializing in reproductive and perinatal mental health.

Landon Zaki: My journey to the field of fertility counseling also grew out of personal experience – in my case, as a birth trauma survivor, NICU mom, and perinatal patient. I felt compelled to transform my trauma into something more and realized that I connected deeply with the grief, loss, and trauma that many fertility patients endure. When I decided to start a reproductive psychology practice in 2018, I knew it was more than just a job for me; fertility counseling felt like a calling and has since become a passion. I am a cognitive-behavioral psychologist by training and integrate cognitive-behavioral therapies with mindfulness and compassion-focused practices in my work with perinatal and reproductive mental health clients. Running fertility support groups continues to be one of the greatest joys and rewards of my work.

This chapter uses case studies to discuss clinical issues that present challenges to running support groups, and guidelines for when someone may be best served by a different type of support. The approach utilized throughout this chapter is the mind-body group, based on the extensive research of Alice Domar, which we have independently been facilitating for the past 5 years.

Groups referenced in this chapter were time-limited, six to seven sessions. Psycho-education and

cognitive-behavioral, relaxation and expressive arts techniques are integrated into an emotive-interactive framework. This format was researched independently by both authors and chosen due to the efficacy in decreasing rates of depression and overall distress [1]. The cases described are entirely fictitious; any resemblance to someone, living or deceased, is purely coincidental. It has been compiled from several sources to illustrate issues that typify reproductive trauma and loss. The "I" in the therapist's narrative reflects both authors' collective experiences.

Challenges to Starting a Fertility Support Group

Join me in this exercise. Take out your journal, or open the notes on your phone. Make sure you pause to reflect and write down your thoughts.

Imagine you are starting a group.
What feelings come up as you sit with this experience?
Where do you feel them in your body?

There are many reasons you may want to run a support group. Perhaps you benefited from one at some point in your life. Maybe the institution where you work has asked you to lead this group. Maybe like me, you yearned for a group when you needed it most and now you're in a position to offer support to others.

The common concerns are about logistics – how do I market the group? Should it be open-ended or time-limited? Open or closed? Can I mix a group of participants using third-party reproduction with someone who's yet to start IVF?

What came up for you when you answered the questions above? Underneath many of those concerns there is often a deeper reason. Was it fear that has prevented you? Did you have a negative experience facilitating a group in graduate school or earlier in your career? Do you fear not knowing "enough," or feeling ill-prepared to serve such a diverse population when you have had only your own experience? Or maybe you've had no personal experience with infertility and you're wondering if you're qualified to run a group on the topic.

Perhaps you're reading this chapter, hopeful that one more article, consultation or CEU course will provide the missing information you need and then you'll be ready. You're not alone. We've been there. In fact, according to

The addenda referred to in this chapter are available for download at www.cambridge.org/covington-case-studies

Valerie Young, as many as 70% of people experience this feeling – imposter syndrome [2].

Imposter Syndrome

Questioning our worth, fear of being found a fraud and making excuses for one's success are the three hallmarks of imposter phenomenon (IP), as it was originally coined by Paulina Clance in the late 1970s [3]. The shame of perceived inadequacy and fear of failure can keep us stuck and cause us to procrastinate. It can also result in high levels of anxiety as we overthink and over-work in order to avoid being found out.

I, Rachel, first encountered the imposter syndrome during my years struggling with secondary infertility. I felt ashamed of "complaining" about being unable to conceive a second child because I had successfully conceived my first! My shame prevented me from joining online forums and getting the available support I so desperately craved. These feelings surfaced again as I started planning my first support group. What would participants think if they knew I "only" experienced secondary infertility? Was I unworthy of the role of leader because of my first successful pregnancy and birth? Did my own success minimize my pain of secondary infertility or negate my ability to empathize with those unable to conceive at all? How would my personal experience impact my therapeutic style and what about the question of disclosure: How much do I need to share? How much do I want to share? We've reviewed these issues in the *Clinical Guide* companion chapter and a deeper discussion is available in Janet Jaffe's chapter on counter transference and self-disclosure in the first edition of *Fertility Counseling* [4].

And while I, Landon, was motivated and enthusiastic about starting a group, I too struggled with this piece. Not having experienced infertility myself, I felt somehow "inauthentic" and "unqualified" to lead an infertility support group. Part of me also felt guilty having children. What would I say if clients asked how I got into this work? Would I talk about my reproductive trauma or engage some "information management strategy" to keep my story from becoming known? I grappled with if and how to share my own personal experience, and worried if not having infertility would devalue my role as a group leader.

The feelings associated with imposter syndrome can show up again and again as we grow. Transitions are natural triggers for self-doubt [5]. Take writing this chapter for example: a first for me, Rachel. With it came those familiar feelings of self-doubt and criticism as I wondered repeatedly, *Do I even know enough to write this chapter?*

The shame of being found out can stop us from striving toward our goals, it keeps us small. Brené Brown says that vulnerability is the key to getting past these limiting feelings: wholeheartedly embracing shame and vulnerability is the pathway to joy and authenticity [6]. It is certainly a risk to try something new. To start a group, write a chapter, begin a new job. These are all risks of varying degrees that require courage as we vulnerably step into the discomfort that arises and embrace what we're inspired to do in the world.

Cathartic Healing and Groups: The Courage to Show Up

Sara's Shame, Stigma and Isolation

We know that group sharing is an antidote to shame, and shame is what keeps individuals experiencing infertility so isolated and also what makes a group such a valuable part of healing. As Brené Brown says, "If you put shame in a Petri dish, it needs three things to grow exponentially: secrecy, silence and judgment. If you put the same amount of shame in a Petri dish and douse it with empathy, it can't survive" [7]. My work with Sara* speaks to the power of groups in healing the shame and stigma of infertility.

Sara*, a Mexican human rights attorney, was a self-proclaimed feminist. At 35, she met Sam, an American living in Mexico. She had no interest in having children. They fell in love, married and agreed to remain childless. Two years after their marriage, they moved to the United States (US), at which point she changed her mind. Now she yearned to be a mother.

After being unable to conceive for 2 years, she and Sam began to explore assisted reproductive technology (ART). They started with three rounds of intrauterine insemination (IUI) and then moved on to in vitro fertilization (IVF). It was after her second failed transfer that she called me for individual counseling.

In our first session I quickly learned how Sara's conservative Mexican culture and her Catholic upbringing had colluded in creating a climate of shame that had kept her silenced. Raised Catholic, Sara had turned away from the church in her late twenties. Upon learning about her struggle to conceive, Sara's mother, a devout Catholic, urged her to return to the church, rather than seek help from a reproductive endocrinologist. Believing that infertility resulted from her split with the church, her mother prayed for her, repeatedly evoking religious liturgy, such as "God has a plan" and "You need to have faith". Sara felt stigmatized, minimized, blamed, unsupported, and conflicted about how to maintain a relationship with her mother.

In the midst of Sara's struggle, her younger sister suddenly announced her own pregnancy. Her sister was unwed and the pregnancy was unplanned. Sara was devastated. Her mother, while trying to be empathic, offered platitudes and shared clairvoyant visions of the bond between the two pregnant sisters. Being unable to conceive was an undeniable stigma in her mother's world. Sarah felt alone, isolated and unwelcomed.

During the intake process I had mentioned my next 6-week support group would be starting, but Sara had initially declined. Sharing with strangers was not part of her culture and besides, she was caught in a web of shame and guilt: her infertility was her fault because she had waited too long.

After a spontaneous pregnancy quickly ended in miscarriage, Sara became depressed and I was worried: She was unmotivated at work, once a source of inspiration. She was spending weekends in bed while her husband worked long hours. I began thinking once again about encouraging her to join a group. I wasn't entirely sure if she was well enough to participate, but I knew she needed community and was in no position to create that in her current state. My years of running groups had validated what Yalom describes as the curative power of empathy afforded by the group setting, and I was hopeful Sara would consider.

Although I was concerned that Sara's depression might limit her ability to participate and would demand too much from others, I took a risk and once again raised the possibility of joining. I validated her feelings of hesitancy, articulated the power of sharing, being heard and supported by group members. I normalized her fear and longing for connection. To my surprise, Sara agreed to join the group. Later I would learn that what had changed her mind was the strength of our connection.

The Power of Empathy and Human Connection

Just hours before the first group, I received a text message from Sara that she wasn't sure she could make it. She was having a hard day and couldn't imagine how she would make it through the group without crying. I called and left a voicemail, encouraging her to show up; normalizing the fact that many group members fear becoming too emotional, and that her fear was a common reaction. "There's no such thing as too emotional," I told her. She came.

I spent the first group trying to establish a climate of safety and building group cohesion. Using an exercise from my training in Brené Brown's The Daring Way™ allowed me to promote connections and to normalize negative emotions and group fears (see Addendum 5.3 for more details on this process). "How could you not feel jealous?", I asked one woman who expressed fear that she was a bad person because she didn't want to attend her sister-in-law's baby shower. I validated other "shameful thoughts" I knew to be the norm. I was excited to see group members opening up and sharing.

This first group generally brings to light what I've come to see is an omnipresent fear: "What happens if someone in the group gets pregnant?" It is my role as the leader to speak about what's unspeakable, so I present my "rule:" if someone gets pregnant, they will sit out the following group. This gives the group time for accessing and expressing the necessary processing. Grief is inevitable and I know it's important for it to be expressed. My goal is to offer hope and assurance that this group will not be one more place where they would feel unable to speak what needs to be said and left out and left behind.

Sara came into my office the following week for our individual session, glowing and gushing. She was amazed at how comfortable she had felt with the others. Since the group session she had been texting with one member and had made a walking date with another. As she repeatedly remarked at how positive and reassuring it felt to be among other women who understood what she was going through, I could sense her excitement. It was a great joy to share what felt like a big win for us both.

Over the coming weeks, as she navigated the next steps in her fertility journey alongside the unfolding plans for her sister's baby shower and upcoming wedding, Sara found the group to be a pillar of support, a respite where she felt held and nurtured. She willingly shared her reaction to the feelings of judgment from her best friend who thought she should be happy and needed to get over the envy and sadness. Within the group, she felt both seen and heard for what she was going through, and self-compassion for the many losses she endured and continued to process.

Sara's relationship with other group members continued to support her long after the group formally ended. A common offshoot of these groups is that often strong relationships are formed. Not only did participation in the group expand her support network, but it offered her a forum to role play tough conversations she wanted to have with her family about how they could support her during this difficult time. As described in the *Clinical*

Guide companion chapter, the social context of disclosure matters. Disclosure to empathetic and supportive others can reduce stigma and shame and increase a sense of normalcy and belonging.

Sara's experience in the group highlighted just how isolated she had become due to infertility. While medical appointments continued to consume her free time, she began to prioritize her wellness. She made an effort to spend more time outside, to exercise, nourish her mind and body with healthy foods that were not only prized for their reputation as fertility-friendly foods, and perhaps most important for Sara – connecting with her new friends.

Take-Away Thoughts

In each group I always emphasize the courage it takes to show up. Sara knew me and trusted me before joining the group, but so many others who join a group do not reach out until they feel desperate, lonely, isolated and unseen by their community. My job is to help them realize there is nothing to lose in taking this leap and offer them hope that a support group can be a turning point in their infertility story. As trained mental health professionals, we are at times their lifeline, and a group offers a connection where one is desperately needed.

Addressing the Elephant in the Fertility Group

When Kate Became Pregnant

Two years later, just days before a new group series was to begin, I received a call from Kate. I learned quickly that Kate had been through six cycles of IUI and three rounds of IVF in the past 5 years. The results had all been disappointing – two miscarriages and many failed cycles. One embryo remained, which would be her fifth and final transfer, and was scheduled after the second group session. This meant if she became pregnant, we would know before our fourth group. Would she be a good fit, I wondered?

I anticipated difficulties. A pregnancy was always tricky to navigate, and if she didn't become pregnant, she'd be devastated. And if she did become pregnant – that was always difficult for other members. Dealing with this situation is a predictable part of running infertility groups. We scheduled our intake appointment for the following day, and that Friday afternoon I found her in my waiting room with the other five group members.

The night before the group I had revisited our first session notes. I wondered how she would fit in and how to best raise the worries, concerns, fears and hopes that are always evoked when we discuss the topic of how I will keep the group a safe space in the likelihood someone gets pregnant.

As it typically went, we spent that first group session discussing goals, establishing trust and addressing the elephant in the room – what if someone gets pregnant. This conversation is always complex. On one hand, it brings a sense of hope into the room as each member imagines for a moment that this will be them. On the other hand, it evokes dread, as members disclose how hard it would be to witness yet another person leaving them behind. This group was no different. A few individuals mentioned that they were actively trying, including Kate, and a couple of people noted that they would be happy for the pregnant person. A few members stayed quiet: I wondered if they were unsure of their feelings or felt reluctant to express what they may have felt were "negative" thoughts.

The second session arrived and Kate was vulnerable, sharing her anxiety about the upcoming transfer early the following week. Two other members had been through transfers and empathized with Kate. They shared coping strategies for the 2-week wait and laughed at the rituals they've engaged in, like eating pineapple and McDonalds fries, while wearing cute socks during the transfer. Unsurprisingly, this seemed to be a bonding moment and my heart swelled a bit.

Beth, a 37-year-old group member, sought support around the guilt she was feeling about not wanting to spend time with her brother and sister-in-law, who was 8 months pregnant. Beth had conceived at the same time, but then had miscarried. Now she grappled with how to cope that her sibling was having a baby and she wasn't. She felt guilty for not wanting to see them and disappointed that her mother didn't understand why she didn't want to participate in family meals. She shared how this brought up painful memories from childhood where her brother was catered to and she felt shunted aside. She wasn't sure how she'd manage once her new niece or nephew arrived. She wasn't alone, she learned. Meredith, a woman in her early thirties, had had a very similar situation with her younger sister who had been pregnant 2 years earlier. Veronica's best friend was also currently pregnant.

As the group ended, members shared their well-wishes with Kate and said they'd reach out to check in on one another before our next group. I felt a warmth at how they were connecting and offering support already. This was just what the group was designed for: to support individuals through their struggle. Some women could hold babies but couldn't stand being around pregnant people, while others could tolerate the opposite. They don't always feel the same but they can often empathize with one another in a way that's unique to those who've experienced reproductive trauma and loss.

And then it happened. On a Monday afternoon, Kate sent me the email confirming her first beta was positive. As expected, she experienced a mix of emotions – ecstatic and yet terrified given her history of miscarriage. I empathized with what it would mean to be pregnant and not have the support of the group and others who understood the magnitude of this moment. It's well established that pregnancy anxiety after infertility rivals that of infertility itself (see Chapter 23 in the *Clinical Guide*). I know this both first hand and also due to the abundance of research that corroborates this reality [8]. But I was getting ahead of myself. It wasn't yet firmly established that she would leave the group.

Emailing me in advance of the group was my request, which I communicated during our first session. It seemed important to process the news with Kate before sharing with the group in person. We spoke by phone the following day, both about the variety of emotions she was experiencing and also the next steps.

Once she received her second beta confirming a viable pregnancy she would email the group, and sit out the next session. Being cognizant of the many ways clients have been surprised and triggered by family, friends and social media posts, I find this strategy helpful, allowing them time to process independently before coming together as a group to discuss.

Pregnancy and Group Processing

The topic of Kate's pregnancy brought both a sensitivity and emotion to our fourth session. I provided a framework for the session, inviting and encouraging feedback from all participants and communicating how we would move forward. After the session, I said I'd email the group and request individual email responses about comfort and safety with Kate's return to the group. I affirmed that if anyone felt uneasy, I would help Kate connect with other supportive resources in the community. The group would continue without her.

The conversation was slow. Nina was the first person to speak and shared her joy for Kate and comfort with her return to the group. She talked about what a caring and supportive person Kate was and that she needed support now too. I flinched internally, worried how this would sit with the others. Someone else talked about the hope that it brought, that if Kate can become pregnant perhaps they too would be so lucky. Then Beth bravely and candidly shared how triggered she was, and how difficult it was for her to be happy for others when she was in so much pain. Group members empathized with Beth and I hoped this could be a corrective experience for her, showing that her feelings were expectable, normal and important and not discredited as they were in her family of origin.

I emailed the group later that day, requesting their input on welcoming Kate back. I waited nervously for their replies to trickle into my inbox. I wondered how the group would navigate this hurdle. My goal was to help balance the group's needs, and Kate was certainly part of the group. But the group needed to be a safe place for all members to share openly about their experience. How would hearing Kate's worries about her pregnancy impact the rest of the group who longed to have those concerns? And yet, would asking Kate to leave the group be yet another loss? She sought this group for support and though becoming pregnant was the first obstacle, it wasn't the end of her story.

Beth was the first to reply – the group wouldn't feel safe for her if Kate returned. She shared additional thoughts about leaving the group herself, feeling ashamed by her reaction, wishing she could be more like Nina who was compassionate and warm and didn't seem triggered like she was. We spoke by phone later that day and I validated her concerns about not wanting Kate in the group. She recognized Nina's words had triggered her, bringing up childhood wounds; the same feelings she recently shared about dinner at her mother's. I reminded Beth of the group's empathic responses, hoping to provide more balance to her inner dialogue.

After I received the remaining email responses, I sent a message to the group that I had spoken with Kate and connected her with another group and resources in the community. When the group reunited later that week, Beth courageously shared that she had almost left the group. She acknowledged the feelings that had been unearthed in our last session, her anger toward her mother who had and continued to prioritize her brother. But this outcome felt different, she told us. Beth shared that unlike her experience with her family, she felt recognized and validated by the group process.

Take-Away Thoughts

Encountering a pregnancy in a short-term group can be unsettling, derailing the group from its overarching purpose of providing support for the infertility journey. The primary goal of a support group is to create a space that fosters connection and decreases feelings of isolation and loneliness. This group always has three pillars as I describe it: support, skills and facilitated conversations about some of the many issues known to cause distress during infertility. While a pregnancy may feel like a derailment, it's actually an opportunity. Members are given the opportunity to advocate for themselves and share their feelings about a difficult situation that happens all the time in their private lives. But these conversations occur in the safety of our group environment, guided by a leader who is attentive to these issues.

The Power of Groups

The responsibility of the group leader can feel daunting at times. The work to recruit participants and form a short-term group can be overwhelming, requiring a great deal of time and energy. However, the group experience itself holds a power that is both energizing and transformative, outweighing the inherent challenges of managing such a dynamic experience. The battle of infertility is lonely and isolating, especially when it is lengthy, as it is for so many. Offering a holding space that fosters safety, community and an opportunity to connect with one's own resiliency are invaluable to those in the midst of their struggle and will not be forgotten. As the old adage goes, "Sorrow shared, half the pain; joy shared, twice the gain."

References

1. Domar AD, Kelly AL. *Conquering Infertility: Dr. Alice Domar's Mind/Body Guide to Enhancing Fertility and Coping with Infertility.* London: Penguin Books, 2004.

2. Young V. Thinking your way out of imposter syndrome [Internet]. 2017. Available at: www.youtube.com/watch?v=h7v-GG3SEWQ [last accessed June 19, 2022].

3. Clance PR, Imes SA. The imposter phenomenon in high achieving women: dynamics and therapeutic intervention. *Psychotherapy (Chic)* 1978;**15**(3):241–247.

4. Jaffe J. The view from the fertility counselor's chair. In: Covington SN, Ed. *Fertility Counseling: Clinical Guide and Case Studies.* Cambridge: Cambridge University Press, 2015, 239–251.

5. LaDonna KA, Ginsburg S, Watling C. "Rising to the level of your incompetence": what physicians' self-assessment of their performance reveals about the imposter syndrome in medicine. *Acad Med* 2018;**93**(5):763–768.

6. Brown B. Daring greatly: how the courage to be vulnerable transforms the way we live, love, parent, and lead. Unabridged. New York, NY: Penguin Random House Audio, 2019.

7. Brown B. Listening to Shame [Internet]. 2012. Available at: www.ted.com/talks/brene_brown_listening_to_shame [last accessed June 19, 2022].

8. Stevenson EL, Trotter KJ, Bergh C, Sloane R. Pregnancy-related anxiety in women who conceive via in vitro fertilization: a mixed methods approach. *J Perinat Educ* 2016;**25**(3):193–200.

Sexual Therapy Primer for Fertility Counselors

Erika Kelley and Sheryl Kingsberg

Introduction

Erika Kelley: My initial training as a clinical psychologist focused on understanding the impact of interpersonal violence on women's health, including sexual functioning. This highlighted to me the complex interplay of biopsychosocial factors affecting women's health, and drew me to an interest in understanding women's health across reproductive stages, including in pregnancy, postpartum, and menopause. My role as a behavioral health psychologist in the Department of Obstetrics and Gynecology at University Hospitals has provided me opportunities to work in an interdisciplinary setting to promote women's health across these reproductive stages. Understanding the impact of infertility diagnoses and treatment on women's mental (and sexual) health has been a natural extension of my interest in this field.

Sheryl Kingsberg: My work with fertility patients began when I joined the Division of Behavioral Medicine within the department of OBGYN at University Hospitals Cleveland Medical Center/Case Western Reserve University School of Medicine in 1991. Our department had one of the pioneering fertility programs and the department chair and reproductive endocrinologists recognized the value of having reproductive mental health professionals on the team instead of as outside referrals. I am trained as a behavioral medicine psychologist, which reflects a clinical focus on treating, usually with a cognitive-behavioral framework, the psychological consequences of medical conditions. While my clinical and academic position within OBGYN included treating a wide range of women's health conditions (e.g., sexual dysfunction, postpartum mood disorders, gynecologic cancers, pregnancy loss, menopause), infertility was a perfect fit for my training and clinical and research interests.

This clinical case example represents a compilation of cases we have seen in practice, demonstrating how sexual function is driven by a multitude of factors, but by a collaborative and interdisciplinary approach can be highlighted as an important part of individual and relationship functioning. Miranda and David are a composite of the many different patients and many sexual concerns that have presented to us.

Sexual dysfunction may sometimes initially present as infertility. This case outlines a scenario of a young woman experiencing genitopelvic pain penetration dysfunction (GPPD), which became a barrier to her ability to conceive. The couple initially presented to the reproductive endocrinologist, who referred them to a fertility counselor specializing in the assessment and treatment of sexual dysfunction. The client's GPPD was treated using an interdisciplinary approach. Treatment involved an initial phase of individual cognitive-behavioral therapy (CBT) with the fertility counselor and concurrent pelvic floor physical therapy, and a second phase involving couples-based CBT. Following significant improvement in her GPPD, the client was able to have pain-free intercourse resulting in a successful pregnancy without requiring assisted reproductive technologies (ART).

Referral Summary

Miranda, 29, and her partner David, 32, presented to the fertility clinic requesting in vitro fertilization (IVF) using a gestational carrier. Miranda had had no pregnancies. Similarly, David has no children. They disclosed to the reproductive endocrinologist that they have only attempted vaginal intercourse twice and have not attempted to conceive without medical intervention. Miranda reported anxiety about sex and pregnancy. Miranda's recent pelvic examination was within normal limits with the exception of pelvic floor tightness. The reproductive endocrinologist determines there is no medical indication for involvement of a gestational carrier. It appears Miranda's sexual dysfunction is masquerading as infertility. She referred the couple to the fertility counselor, who specializes in treating sexual dysfunctions, to discuss decision-making related to family planning and assessment and treatment of sexual dysfunction.

Miranda's Initial Appointment with the Fertility Counselor

Miranda arrived alone to the appointment and appeared anxious when discussing her sexual history. Miranda reported she and David desire children. David desires a child who is biogenetically related to them, based on his family values. However, Miranda is fearful of sexual intercourse and is uncomfortable talking about sex. Her therapeutic goal is to reduce anxiety and discomfort around sexual activity and be able to engage in sexual intercourse (with hopes of achieving pregnancy). The fertility counselor gathered initial psychosocial history, medical history, psychiatric history and sexual functioning information, summarized below.

Miranda, who is Caucasian, was raised by her biologic parents in Indiana, United States (US). She has two older brothers. She described her childhood as "good." Miranda was raised within a Catholic upbringing but does not currently identify with any particular religion. However, she still adheres to many principles and beliefs informed by Catholicism. Miranda works full-time in marketing and has good social support. She described one incident of unwanted sexual touching when she was 20 years old, but denied associated distress. Miranda identifies as heterosexual and has been in a relationship with David for 4 years. They have been living together for 2 years and she described their relationship as "strong, but sometimes I can't believe he wants to be with me." Miranda had one prior dating relationship in high school, and they engaged in some sexual activity, but not intercourse.

Miranda has medical diagnoses of chronic migraines, interstitial cystitis, and irritable bowel syndrome that are well-managed. Miranda was diagnosed with generalized anxiety disorder and major depressive disorder at the age of 21 and found individual CBT and sertraline (100 mg) moderately effective. Miranda denied history of substance use. Her scores on mental health self-report measures completed at this session indicated a depression score below the clinical cut-off point and anxiety score reflective of moderate generalized anxiety.

Sexual Functioning Screen

The fertility counselor conducts a basic screen for sexual function problems, uses a ubiquity statement to help normalize the topic, and expresses appreciation for the sensitivity of the topic when it appears that Miranda is uncomfortable [1]. The fertility counselor (FC) also uses basic therapeutic rapport-building techniques (e.g., appropriate eye contact).

> FC: "Sexual function is an important part of well-being for many people and can affect fertility. I ask all my patients about their sexual functioning. You mentioned you and David have only attempted intercourse twice. You also mentioned feeling afraid of sex and pregnancy. Can you tell me more about any sexual concerns that have contributed to your avoidance of sexual intercourse or feeling fearful of sex and pregnancy?"
>
> Miranda: [averts her eye gaze and fidgets in chair] "Umm, well, this is sort of uncomfortable for me to talk about. But, yes. It just doesn't seem like sex is possible for

me, it has never worked before and I'm scared now that it's going to hurt too much. I just want to be able to have that part of our relationship actually work and I want to be able to have a baby one day. I know David really wants that, too."

FC: "I understand that talking about sex can be uncomfortable and appreciate you talking about it with me as it allows me to understand and help you. It sounds like this sexual issue has been distressing to you and your relationship. If it is okay with you, I'd like us to schedule a follow-up appointment to talk more about these concerns and about what treatment options are available to help you.

Miranda: "Okay, I think that could be helpful. I've never really talked about it with anyone."

Miranda's Follow-Up Session with the Fertility Counselor

Miranda and the fertility counselor meet 2 weeks later, for a more thorough assessment of Miranda's sexual function and sexual history, following the International Society for the Study of Women's Sexual Health (ISSWSH) process of care model [2]. In taking a sexual and reproductive history, Miranda reported she and David attempted vaginal intercourse once 2 years ago, and again 3 months ago. Miranda noted that on both occasions, when David attempted to penetrate, it was like he "hit a brick wall" and was not able to insert his penis. Miranda felt pain and tension localized to her vaginal opening when David attempted penile insertion and they stopped trying when she became tearful. They have not attempted intercourse since then. They do still engage in kissing, cuddling, and oral sex, though Miranda often prefers to wear her bra and underwear when doing so. Miranda had her first gynecological exam at age 18 and reported feeling anxious and fearful (embarrassed and not sure what to expect) during the pelvic exam. Otherwise, her pelvic exams have been normal with the exception of notable pelvic floor tension. Miranda, who reached menarche at 13, has never used a tampon. Her mother never showed her how and she was too embarrassed to ask anyone for help. She hesitantly admits to masturbation, using a vibrator monthly for clitoral stimulation, and is reliably orgasmic with it.

Assessment of Sexual Function

Using a combination of clinical interview and self-report measures, the fertility counselor assesses Miranda's functioning in all domains of female sexual response, pain and distress. A biopsychosocial perspective (incorporating information from medical chart review and initial appointment) is used to identify contributing, modifiable biological, psychological, and interpersonal factors [2]. A summary of information collected via interview is below.

Desire: Miranda experiences low spontaneous sexual desire, which has worsened over the past 2 years. She experiences responsive sexual desire on most occasions when David initiates sexual activity. She reports a desire discrepancy in their relationship, whereby David would like to engage in sexual activity at least twice per week, but Miranda feels she can "go weeks without wanting sexual activity."

Arousal: Miranda denies significant impairment in cognitive arousal (mentally feeling "turned on"), though her anxiety about penetration and pain distracts her from the arousal. She experiences genital arousal (pleasurable sexual sensations and vaginal lubrication), but if distracted by anxiety, she loses arousal, becomes dry and feels discomfort.

Orgasm: Miranda is able to orgasm on most occasions when masturbating alone using her clitoral vibrator. She does not experience orgasm with David in part because she is too self-conscious to let go and ashamed to tell David about the use of a vibrator. She feels guilty about masturbating and afraid David would view it as a sinful act if she told him.

Pain: Miranda has been experiencing persistent difficulties with vaginal penetration, including attempts at penile–vaginal penetration, pelvic exams, and use of tampons, for over 5 years, although these attempts have been infrequent. She reports tightness of her pelvic floor muscles in anticipation of, and during, these attempts at penetration. She reports significant fear and anxiety about vaginal pain in anticipation of any genital contact, which has contributed to her eventual avoidance of sexual intercourse and further attempts at penetration.

Distress: Miranda reported significant distress, particularly related to her pain, anxiety, and difficulties with penetration and sexual activity, and secondarily, her lower desire levels. She reports these sexual concerns impair her relationship functioning and family planning goals.

Self-Report Measures on Sexual Functioning

Miranda completed the *Female Sexual Function Index* [3] and her score indicated a positive screen for female sexual dysfunction. She completed the *Female Sexual Distress Scale-Desire/Arousal/Orgasm Inventory* (FSDS-DAO) [4,5], with a total score suggesting bothersome sexual distress. To elicit additional information regarding her thoughts associated with sexual pain, Miranda completed the *Vaginal Penetration Cognition Questionnaire* (VPCQ)

[6]. Her responses indicated she holds strong beliefs that her vagina is not compatible with penetration and that penetration would be catastrophic and painful (e.g., "I am afraid that the inside of my vagina will be damaged by penetration").

Partner's Interview and History

Partner sexual functioning may also affect one's sexual functioning and can help or hinder treatment. The fertility counselor invites David (with Miranda's agreement) to attend an individual session to gather information regarding his sexual functioning using a basic sexual function screen [1] and provide psychoeducation on sexual functioning and to inform treatment planning.

David, like Miranda, is Caucasian and was raised in Indiana. He reported a happy, typical childhood. He is active within the Catholic Church. He denied significant psychiatric or substance use history. However, the fertility counselor noted David exhibits some obsessive-compulsive personality traits and insecurity. The couple's sexual difficulties appear to be exacerbating his insecurity. David denies any sexual problems and reports he has engaged in "successful" sexual intercourse with a previous female partner. He is able to achieve orgasm via masturbation, but reports feelings of guilt associated with this behavior due to his religious belief that masturbation is sinful. He reports distress related to Miranda's sexual problems and avoids attempting intercourse with her, as he does not want to hurt her. Conversely, he is angry at the situation because Miranda's sexual difficulties "make [him] seem less like a man."

Treatment Plan

The fertility counselor determines Miranda meets criteria for GPPD and assesses Miranda's motivation for treatment [1,2]. Miranda expressed high motivation to address her GPPD and low desire. The fertility counselor is competent to treat the presenting sexual problems, having completed training in female sexual function through postdoctoral fellowship coursework and supervision in sexual medicine, and continuing education coursework. The following treatment plan is agreed upon:

1. Referral to a gynecologist for physical examination of vulvovaginal pain to rule out other potential physical causes of vaginal pain/discomfort. Following this appointment, a diagnosis of GPPD is confirmed and the exam was notable for significant pelvic floor tightness.

2. Referral for pelvic floor physical therapy for treatment of pelvic floor tightness and pain.
3. Weekly, individual CBT with Miranda (Phase 1), followed by couple's sensate focus therapy (Phase 2), both facilitated by the fertility counselor.

Pelvic Floor Physical Therapy

Pelvic floor physical therapy (PFPT) may include manual therapy, psychoeducation, relaxation and breathing (re) training, local tissue sensitization, electromyographic biofeedback, therapeutic exercise and instructed, progressive use of vaginal dilators [7]. For Miranda, the aim of this treatment is to reduce pelvic floor hypertonicity and pelvic pain. The physical therapist and fertility counselor maintain contact throughout Miranda's treatment for coordination of care, particularly in relation to Miranda's at-home practice with gradual exposure to situations that approximate vaginal intercourse including practice with a dilator kit.

Individual Cognitive-Behavioral Therapy with the Fertility Counselor (Phase 1)

This treatment incorporates three core aspects: (1) relaxation training along with systematic desensitization to fear of anticipated pain with penetration; (2) restructuring of maladaptive cognitions contributing to sexual dysfunction; and (3) gradual, behavioral exposure to situations that approximate vaginal penetration for Miranda to complete at home [8]. Gradual exposure will provide Miranda corrective experiences with sexual function and allow her to (re)establish a sense of control over sexual function. The fertility counselor conceptualizes Miranda's sexual dysfunction as developing as a defense mechanism, whereby her vaginal muscles constrict to protect her from anticipated or perceived discomfort and pain that she expects with penetration. Over time, her avoidance of sexual activity is reinforced and anxiety about penetration is maintained. A summary of session content is presented in Table 6.1.

Throughout treatment, the fertility counselor reminds Miranda that she has control over the exposure practice, which allows for increased self-efficacy and mastery. The fertility counselor also coordinates with the PFPT throughout treatment. During at-home exposure practice, Miranda is instructed to practice the specific hierarchy item until her anxiety/discomfort has reduced by at least 50% or she is able to successfully achieve comfortable penetration at least twice. In general, each

exposure practice takes approximately 15 minutes to complete, though she is instructed to discontinue if experiencing significant pain, fatigue or overstimulation. Miranda is also instructed not to attempt any penetration with David in order to unpair lovemaking with anticipatory anxiety and restore the focus on pleasure without pressure for both of them.

Miranda's hierarchy is shown in Table 6.2. Her self-reported anticipatory pre-exposure anxiety/distress levels increase across the items in her hierarchy as the items more closely approximate vaginal penetration, and this represents a fairly typical hierarchy in individuals with GPPD. She reported higher anxiety/distress levels with penetration involving a dilator or her partner than items involving her own hand or finger for penetration, as she feels less in control in those contexts. At session 8, her anxiety/distress levels are much lower across all items, though she does still experience some anticipatory anxiety with penetration, which is expected to continue to decrease with continued exposure practice and as she gains more pleasurable sexual experiences.

Couple's Sensate Focus Sex Therapy (Phase 2)

Using the Sensate Focus for Sex Therapy treatment manual [9], the fertility counselor works with Miranda and David on weekly sensate focus sex therapy. At the beginning, the couple is instructed to not actively attempt sexual intercourse. All sensate focus exercises are completed by the couple in their own home approximately two to three times per week. Each exercise is timed long enough to allow for the practice of mindful awareness of sensation and reduced distraction but without causing boredom, typically around 15 minutes. The series of at-home touching exercises are personalized and designed with the couple's input in a hierarchical and progressive manner [9]. Table 6.1 provides a summary of session content following the treatment manual.

Therapist Comments on Treatment

Phase 1

Miranda admitted to avoiding at-home exposure exercises for several weeks. Between sessions 4 and 5, she only engaged in one at-home practice due to her anxiety and fear of pain. The fertility counselor experienced impatience and frustration with the stalling of therapeutic progress, but used Miranda's resistance as an indication

Table 6.1 Summary of case study treatment

Session number(s)	Session content	At-home practice exercises
Phase 1[a]		
1	Education on reproductive anatomy, female and male sexual function, desire discrepancies, biopsychosocial model of sexual function	Review of resources
2	Introduction to cognitive-behavioral model and thought record form	Thought record form related to sexual function and penetration/pain
3	Review of homework and introduction to cognitive restructuring of relevant maladaptive cognitions. The fertility counselor uses Socratic Questioning techniques, practice with the thought record form to challenge maladaptive beliefs	Thought record form with practice identifying alternative cognitions
4	Introduction to relaxation training and gradual, behavioral exposure. Psychoeducation on relaxation training, role of anxiety in genitopelvic pain penetration dysfunction, and habituation to anxiety via graded exposure. Paced breathing exercise. Introduction to the behavioral exposure hierarchy form	Daily paced breathing exercises. Completion/review of exposure hierarchy. Purchase dilator kit in coordination with PFPT
5–7	Review of progress with homework, problem solving around barriers to exposure practice, continued modification of maladaptive cognitions, and continued psychoeducation	Daily at-home, in-vivo exposure exercises based on personalized exposure hierarchy (see Table 6.2)
8	Review of homework and therapeutic process and progress. Re-assessment of symptoms and completion of self-report measures	Continued completion of at-home, in-vivo exposure exercises and relaxation training
Phase 2[b]		
1	Discussion of contributing factors to the couple's sexual problems and treatment planning	Read manual handouts
2	Provision of psychoeducation regarding sensate focus, mindfulness, and instructions for at-home practice of exercises	At-home touching exercises (nongenital or sexual body parts only), with each touching the other for approximately 5–15 minutes
2	Processing of treatment progress and provision of psychoeducation	At-home touching exercises with the exclusion of breasts, chest, and genital areas
3–5	Processing of treatment progress and provision of psychoeducation	At-home touching exercises with the inclusion of breasts, chest, and genital areas is the focus, together with self-examination of anatomical structures
6–7	Processing of treatment progress and provision of psychoeducation	At-home exercises with mutual touching. Initially, exercises exclude touching of breasts, chest, and genitals and then later include such touching
8–10	Processing of treatment progress and provision of psychoeducation	At-home exercises with genital touching (initially without penetration, and later with insertion without, and then with, movement)

[a] Session content informed by ter Kuile et al. 2010 [8]
[b] Session content and handouts guided by Weiner and Avery-Clark, 2017 [9]

the hierarchy needed to be more gradual than initially designed and was respectful that Miranda's anxiety has been entrenched for years.

During the final session of Phase 1, it is determined that Miranda's GPPD has significantly improved. She is able to achieve penetration using the largest dilator size, which approximates the size of David's penis. She feels ready to initiate couples' sensate focus therapy to reach her goal of vaginal intercourse. Miranda's scores on the self-report measures (FSFI [3] and FSDS-DAO [4,5])

Table 6.2 Miranda's behavioral exposure hierarchy to guide at-home practice: anxiety/distress rating scale from 0 (no distress) to 100 (maximum distress)

Exposure item	Pre-exposure/treatment anxiety/distress rating	Post-exposure/treatment anxiety/distress rating at Phase 1, Session 8
Placing hand on vulva	30	0
Placing finger at introitus	40	0
Inserting one finger into vagina	45	5
Inserting two fingers into vagina	50	5
Partner inserting finger into vagina	60	10
Partner inserting two fingers into vagina	70	20
Inserting dilator (size 1)	60	10
Inserting dilator (size 2)	70	10
Inserting dilator (size 3)	80	20
Inserting dilator (size 4)	90	20
Inserting dilator (size 5)	100	30
Inserting dilator (size 6)	100	30
Pelvic exam	90	40
Vaginal intercourse	100	50

confirm improvement in her sexual functioning and decreased sexual distress. She also scored lower on the VPCQ [6] indicating fewer maladaptive cognitions about pain and penetration.

Phase 2

David admits that he gets frustrated when he has to relinquish control and allow Miranda to guide sensate focus exercises. David expresses disappointment that Miranda did not achieve orgasm with vaginal intercourse and expressed the negative cognition that this means "I'm not a real man and my penis is not enough to please her." The fertility counselor experiences annoyance toward David for these male ego beliefs, and is mindful to practice her own relaxation and mindful awareness of distracting cognitions ("he can be such a jerk to Miranda") during sessions. The fertility counselor assures the couple that women are more reliably orgasmic with clitoral stimulation rather than vaginal penetration and this does not reflect partner inadequacy. David also acknowledges performance anxiety about achieving intercourse for conception. The fertility counselor reminds the couple to disentangle sex (lovemaking) from procreation and purposely engage in sensate focus exercises during non-ovulatory times, and to continue this practice even after successful vaginal intercourse to keep sexuality and procreation unpaired.

The couple engages in pain-free vaginal intercourse before sessions 9 and 10. At session 10, they report significant improvement in sexual functioning and satisfaction. Miranda's scores on the self-report measures are now out of the clinical range of dysfunction. She also reports decreased endorsement of catastrophizing, control and negative self-image cognitions.

Countertransference

Throughout assessment and treatment, the fertility counselor maintains an introspective focus and honest awareness of her own attitudes, beliefs and perceptions about sexuality and her feelings about Miranda and David's beliefs and behaviors. The fertility counselor acknowledges her opinion that the couple's religious values promote submissiveness of women and unrealistic expectations regarding sexual activity (e.g., masturbation is sinful). The fertility counselor is mindful to not place negative judgment on the couple's religious beliefs and values, but rather to maximize their sexual function despite the limiting nature of them. The fertility counselor admits her own dismay for the power imbalance she observes in the relationship. David's goals and decisions dominate the relationship and Miranda often ignores her own needs in lieu of meeting David's. Furthermore, David's negative beliefs and expectations of Miranda trigger her feelings of guilt and inadequacy. The fertility counselor is aware of her own negative judgments about David, and is cautious not to impart these judgments on Miranda unnecessarily. The fertility counselor works with Miranda to gain self-awareness so that if she chooses to acquiesce it is done consciously and by her own decision, which may help reduce her frustration toward David. The fertility counselor works with David to manage his own fears of relinquishing control.

Summary/Conclusion

Miranda's GPPD was successfully treated using individual CBT, PFPT and couple's sensate focus sex therapy. At a 6-month follow-up appointment with the fertility counselor, the couple reported they were able to achieve pregnancy via timed intercourse and continue to practice mindful, pleasurable sexual activity during nonovulatory times. This case illustrates the importance of a collaborative, interdisciplinary approach to assessment and treatment of sexual dysfunction with the fertility counselor, PFPT, gynecologist and reproductive endocrinologist working together to address the couple's presenting concern. In addition, the fertility counselor was mindful of the biopsychosocial nature of sexual functioning, and addressed relationship/partner and religious factors and psychological (e.g., anxious cognitions and behaviors) factors affecting Miranda's sexual functioning.

References

1. Althof SE, Rosen RC, Perelman MA, Rubio-Aurioles E. Standard operating procedures for taking a sexual history. *J Sex Med* 2013;**10**:26–35.

2. Parish SJ, Hahn SR, Goldstein SW, et al. The International Society for the Study of Women's Sexual Health Process of Care for the identification of sexual concerns and problems in women. *Mayo Clin Proc* 2019;**94**:842–856.

3. Rosen R, Brown C, Heiman J, et al. The Female Sexual Function Index (FSFI): a multidimensional self-report instrument for the assessment of female sexual function. *J Sex Marital Ther* 2000;**26**:191–208.

4. DeRogatis L, Clayton A, Lewis-D'Agostino D, et al. Validation of the female sexual distress scale: revised for assessing distress in women with hypoactive sexual desire disorder. *J Sex Med* 2008;**5**:357–364.

5. DeRogatis LR, Edelson J, Revicki DA. Reliability and validity of the Female Sexual Distress Scale-Desire/Arousal/Orgasm instrument in a phase 2B dose-ranging study of bremelanotide. Poster session presented at: 167th Annual Meeting of the American Psychiatric Association; May 3 –7, 2014; New York.

6. Klaassen M, Ter Kuile MM. Development and initial validation of the Vaginal Penetration Cognition Questionnaire (VPCQ) in a sample of women with vaginismus and dyspareunia. *J Sex Med* 2009;**6**:1617–1627.

7. Bergeron S, Corsini-Munt S, Aerts L, et al. Female sexual pain disorders: a review of the literature on etiology and treatment. *Curr Sex Health Rep* 2015;**7**(1):59–169.

8. ter Kuile MM, Both S, van Lankveld JJDM. Cognitive behavioral therapy for sexual dysfunctions in women. *Psychiatr Clin N Am* 2010;**33**:595–610.

9. Weiner L, Avery-Clark C. *Sensate Focus in Sex Therapy: The Illustrated Manual.* New York, NY: Routledge, 2017.

CASE 7 "It's Complicated": The Intersect Between Psychiatric Illness and Infertility

Katherine Williams and Lauri Pasch

Introduction

Katherine Williams: I have been a psychiatrist for over 25 years. My commitment to the field of infertility began when there was very little recognition of what a major life stress this journey is for people. I have a Bachelor's Degree in Psychology from Stanford University, a Doctor of Medicine degree from Wake Forest University, and I completed my adult psychiatry residency at Harvard Medical School and Stanford University. My desire to understand the interaction of female reproductive hormones and mental health led me to complete a 3-year National Institute of Mental Health research fellowship at Stanford after my residency. During these fellowship years, I participated in research on premenstrual dysphoric disorder, and the central nervous system effects of infertility medications. I co-founded the Women's Wellness Clinic in the Stanford University Department of Psychiatry, and as director of this clinic, I am responsible for the education and supervision of medical students and psychiatry residents who rotate through and learn about the evaluation and treatment of a wide range of conditions affected by the female reproductive life cycle, including premenstrual dysphoric disorder, and perinatal and perimenopausal mood and anxiety disorders. As the mental health specialist for the Stanford Fertility Clinic, I provide consultations regarding the use of psychiatric medications in pregnancy, the management of complex cases including personality disorders or acute psychiatric emergencies. It is an honor to serve in this role in the fertility clinic and I love being part of a team dedicated to helping women during their challenging fertility journey.

Lauri Pasch: I have been a psychologist working in the field of reproductive health for over 25 years. I have a Bachelor's degree in Psychology from the University of Michigan. I completed my Ph.D. at the University of California Los Angeles in clinical psychology and internship in behavioral medicine at Kaiser Permanente Los Angeles. I completed fellowship training at the University of California San Francisco in psychology and medicine. My entire career has been focused on perinatal mental health, with a particular focus on the psychological consequences of infertility and its treatment. My NIH-funded research has highlighted the high rates of depression and anxiety in IVF patients and the unmet need for mental health care. I have been part of the treatment team at the UCSF Center for Reproductive Health for the last 20 years, where my focus is supporting patients facing the stress of fertility treatment and promoting healthy family-building.

The Case of Dorothy

Infertility evaluation and treatment often includes interacting with a wide variety of medical personnel, invasive procedures, such as vaginal ultrasounds and medications with potential for central nervous system side effects. Women with a previous history of psychiatric illness are at risk for psychiatric destabilization during the infertility journey.

Our goals in this chapter are to illustrate examples of clinical challenges with psychiatric patients, as discussed in the accompanying *Clinical Guide* chapter. The case presented is fictional and made up from a compilation of clients from our clinical practices. While the client in this chapter is a cisgender female in a heterosexual relationship, the struggles presented are universal for a pregnant person whether they are single or partnered with a man or a woman.

The Beginning: A "Rocky Clinic Entrance"

Dorothy (34 years old) presented to the fertility specialist after 3 years of trying for a baby naturally with her husband, who had recently left her. When she made the initial appointment by phone, she stated to the front desk staff that she was "desperate" to have a baby before her thirty-fifth birthday. The front desk receptionist, Mary, who made Dorothy's initial appointment, alerted the nurse manager of the "difficult interaction" she had with the patient. Mary said that Dorothy had been very irritable and demanding; when Mary tried to calmly explain that the next available evaluation appointment was 2 weeks away, Dorothy yelled at her, saying "You just don't want to take care of me," and hung up. The next day, Dorothy called back and left a message requesting to take the offered appointment, but Mary "forgot" to return her call.

Pre-initial visit receptionist/staff notes and paperwork can be extremely useful for early identification of patients who may be at highest risk for psychiatric disturbances during infertility evaluation and treatment. Information from front desk office staff regarding patient interactions can help clinicians learn about potential patient emotional issues and problematic personality traits/disorders. While there is no consensus regarding screening infertility patients or anxiety, depression or psychosis prior to/at evaluation visits, many clinics do utilize screening tools such as the Patient Health Questionnaire 9 (PHQ-9) which has excellent reliability and validity for depression screening [1].

Dorothy demonstrated several important "warning" signs of a "rocky clinic entrance."

Her reaction to the need to wait 2 weeks demonstrated poor frustration tolerance, and her yelling demonstrated impulsivity. Her claim that the clinic did not want to take care of her demonstrated paranoia and projection. The differential diagnosis for her irritability and demanding presentation may include severe adjustment disorder, a mood disorder, such as bipolar disorder or personality problems, such as narcissism or borderline personality disorder.

When a patient is identified early as having either a previous history of psychiatric illness, ongoing use of psychotropic medications, high scores on psychiatric screening questionnaires or disturbed early interactions with clinic staff, the fertility clinic nurse manager should be immediately notified, and mental health support staff recruited for early evaluation and treatment. Mary's "forgetting" to call Dorothy back is an example of how office staff may unconsciously act out in response to difficult patients – especially personality disordered patients. Mary's behavior was passive aggressive, her own self-protective stance in response to Dorothy's aggressive verbal assaults.

When the nurse manager learned of Dorothy's behavior on the phone, she counseled Mary to set firm limits with her if she was insulting or extremely irritable, and tell Dorothy that she could not schedule her unless she was able to hear her requests slowly and clearly. The nurse manager offered to "stand by" when another staff member called Dorothy back the next day. To everyone's surprise, Dorothy was calm, and told the receptionist "how wonderful she is" and how their clinic is "the best there is."

The nurse manager explained to Mary that such dramatic mood swings were of concern, and that now it seemed that Dorothy was idealizing them. The nurse manager made a note to herself to immediately review Dorothy's intake questionnaires and medical/psychiatric history. She also reviewed the staffing availability for the day of Dorothy's appointment, and matched her with a fertility specialist who had special interest in psychiatric patients, as well as a nurse who demonstrated exceptional clinical wisdom and patience. She made sure that no medical students or residents would be joining them in the exam, and she blocked out extra time for the visit. She also alerted their mental health consultant about the appointment, and made sure that they would be available if there were a psychiatric emergency.

On her intake paperwork, Dorothy listed multiple psychiatric medications, including lamotrigine [Lamictal] 200 mg/d, quietapine [Seroquel] 50 mg/d and fluoxetine [Prozac] 40 mg/d. On the depression screening questionnaire, the Patient Health Questionnaire Nine (PHQ-9), Dorothy scored severely depressed, and endorsed suicidal ideation every day.

The presence of a psychiatric disorder or use of psychiatric medications are not themselves contraindications to pursuing infertility evaluation and treatment. When a patient is on multiple psychiatric medications, the fertility specialist should clarify whether the patient has discussed the risks and benefits of continuing these medications in pregnancy with their treating mental health professional. If the patient does not have a mental health professional, the fertility clinic should request that they obtain a psychiatric consultation prior to fertility treatments in order to create a team approach to medication safety in pregnancy.

Each of Dorothy's medications is considered relatively safe in pregnancy; however, no studies exist of the effects on the infant of these three medications combined [2,3].

At Dorothy's first appointment she sobs and says she needs to get pregnant immediately. When asked about the sperm source, she takes out a photo of her ex-husband and says she just needs to find a sperm donor who looks like him and has the same very high IQ.

The fertility specialist and her nurse provide empathic listening as Dorothy explains that her husband left her because he said she was "too needy." They ask in a nonjudgmental and respectful way why she was taking the psychiatric medications. Dorothy immediately became defensive and said "there is no rule that I can't get pregnant taking these medications." The fertility specialist again empathizes with Dorothy's distress. She explains that she is not trying to put up "roadblocks" to her goal of getting pregnant immediately, but that she was asking because she wanted the healthiest pregnancy for Dorothy and her baby.

Patients with primitive psychological defenses frequently use splitting and projection. In splitting, the patient may devalue a person who they find threatening, and idealize another person [4]. Dorothy had demonstrated this tendency in the initial phone calls, so the staff were prepared for a difficult interaction, and had learned that empathic listening and responses, as well as kind limit setting, are helpful interventions with such patients.

The fertility specialist clarified in her intake interview that Dorothy did have both a psychiatrist who prescribed her medications, and a therapist with whom she was doing Dialectical Behavior Therapy (DBT). Both professionals were new, as she had "fired" her previous psychiatrist when he hospitalized her involuntarily to a psychiatric hospital 8 weeks ago due to suicidal ideation after her husband left her.

Within a few minutes of meeting Dorothy, the fertility specialist identified Dorothy as a high-risk psychiatric patient. The specialist's immediate goals are to (1) assess for current safety; (2) clarify and recruit the patient's current mental health team; and (3) begin the process of reasonable and realistic fertility treatment planning, which includes managing Dorothy's expectations for immediate fertility treatment. Dorothy will need psychiatric evaluation and treatment prior to initiation of fertility treatments, and the fertility specialist will need to build an integrated psychiatric–fertility treatment team and program.

The fertility specialist reviewed Dorothy's PHQ-9 and asked her about her suicidality. Dorothy stated that she had no current plans to harm or kill herself, stating "I am trying for a baby – why would I kill myself?" The physician reviewed with her that she had answered that she had thoughts of killing herself daily, and Dorothy said "If I don't get pregnant, that's how I would feel. I don't feel that way today because I have confidence that you will help me."

The fertility specialist told Dorothy, in her most empathic and kind manner, that she could only imagine how difficult it has been for her to have her husband leave her on the eve of her thirty-fifth birthday when she has been wanting a child for so long. She told her that she wanted to help her bring a child into the world in the safest and healthiest way, and to do so she will need to partner with Dorothy's current mental health professionals. The specialist explained that she has experience helping women taking psychiatric medications who have struggled with emotional issues and that when there is a team approach, the fertility treatment is most successful. She emphasizes that she really hears Dorothy that she wants to have a baby by her thirty-fifth birthday, and she will do all she can to help her achieve her goal, within safe parameters and that "slow and steady wins the race." She emphasized that she hopes that Dorothy will partner with her and her team and sign a consent for her to work with Dorothy's mental health professionals.

The fertility specialist also identified other support people in Dorothy's life. Dorothy shared that her older sister, Meg, was her "shoulder to cry on," and that Meg, a nurse, was "always there for me." The fertility specialist learned that Meg lived nearby, and the specialist obtained written permission to talk with Meg if needed as well. She encouraged Dorothy to bring Meg to the next appointment, which would include a vaginal ultrasound and treatment planning once Dorothy's blood work was complete.

The fertility specialist also spent time discussing the sperm donor next steps and methods with Dorothy. She provided information about sperm banks, and told Dorothy that she would need to meet with the clinics' fertility counselor to discuss the emotional aspects of donor-assisted reproductive technologies.

Dorothy became angry and said she was being "prejudiced against" because she was a single parent. The fertility specialist again responded with empathy and said how she understood how difficult this all is, but that all third-party reproduction patients, whether single or partnered, are recommended via ASRM guidelines to meet with a fertility counselor [5].

Dorothy settled down again once she learned she was not being singled out. She agreed to meet with the counselor, as well as to signing consents for the fertility specialist to speak with her current psychiatrist and DBT therapist, as well as her sister Meg.

The fertility specialist and her team faced significant early challenges with Dorothy. "Safety first" is always the first goal in patient care, and once they reviewed the PHQ-9, they needed to clarify whether Dorothy was acutely suicidal. On examination, she was not acutely psychotic, she denied active substance use, and was future oriented. She had a treatment team and a follow-up appointment later that afternoon with her psychiatrist. Dorothy agreed to the fertility specialist calling her psychiatrist to discuss her medical care. Dorothy was in agreement with consultation with the fertility counselor and set up an appointment with her for later in the week, and she signed a release for the team to speak with her sister Meg.

Middle Phase: A Team Approach of "Slow and Steady"

The fertility specialist sent written consent and called Dorothy's psychiatrist, DBT therapist and her sister Meg. All of them spoke with the fertility specialist and said that Dorothy had a history of mood instability. Some psychiatrists had given her the diagnosis of Bipolar II Disorder, but after the most recent hospitalization, the current agreement was that she suffered mainly from her longstanding borderline personality traits.

Meg's sister explained that she and Dorothy had had a chaotic childhood and that Dorothy had suffered sexual abuse by an uncle. She says that Dorothy was always an extremely bright student, but that the trauma had left her with "emotional scars" that included unstable relationships, chronic depression, and passive suicidal ideation when under extreme stress. She said that Dorothy had been doing very well overall for the past 10 years, but that the marriage had been suffering in the past 5 years as her husband had had an affair, which destabilized Dorothy. Meg said that Dorothy's husband, a well-known executive, had never wanted children, and he had become increasingly distanced from Dorothy when she began to push for children. Meg, who was happily married with two late-teenage children of her own, said she knew that Dorothy had always wanted children, so these recent events with her husband had been devastating. She said that Dorothy had never made a suicide attempt, and that she had been "surprised" that she had been involuntarily hospitalized. She said that the involuntary hold was dropped after 72 hours, but that Dorothy had chosen to stay hospitalized voluntarily in order to engage in treatment as she had found the DBT skills training "life changing."

The fertility specialist spoke with Dorothy's psychiatrist and confirmed that she would be seeing Dorothy that day, as well as her therapist. Both reported that Dorothy had been extremely collaborative and compliant with treatment. The psychiatrist said that she did not think that Dorothy met past or current criteria for Bipolar II disorder. She said that she had been considering tapering Dorothy off the Seroquel since Dorothy was sleeping well now and that the other two medications were useful for the depression she had recently experienced, but that she was not convinced that either the higher dose of Prozac was needed, nor the Lamictal. She said that she was planning to "serially assess" Dorothy and collaborate with her to decrease her medications now that she was in DBT. The psychiatrist emphasized that Dorothy had not been suicidal while under her care, and that she was not clear whether the involuntary hospitalization was entirely justified.

The DBT therapist confirmed that Dorothy had been dedicated to learning skills and that the therapist would be able to continue to work with her indefinitely and be available for coaching at all times of day. She too confirmed that Dorothy had not been suicidal in their 6 weeks of working together.

Besides confirming Dorothy's immediate safety, an urgent concern for the fertility specialist is whether this patient should be immediately disqualified from further fertility evaluation and potential fertility treatment. Since Dorothy denied active suicidal ideation, and this was corroborated by her psychiatrist, therapist and sister Meg, who appeared to be a very mature and knowledgeable historian and health professional, this patient was not immediately disqualified.

In our opinion, other immediate disqualifiers for fertility treatment include active substance abuse, ongoing domestic violence and psychosis, and none of these were a problem for Dorothy. Her recent marital collapse seemed to have destabilized an ongoing problem with mood dysregulation, fears of abandonment and tendency to use primitive psychological defenses such as projection, splitting and idealization. While Dorothy had been given a presumptive diagnosis of borderline personality disorder, she demonstrated a willingness to work with the fertility team and no active self-harm activities. Fertility evaluation and treatment are stressful, and when combined with such recent stresses, it further increases the risk for mood instability. Please see Table 7.1 for a list of when to delay or discontinue fertility treatment.

The goal of the next phase of treatment for Dorothy was to try to help her to "slow down" the urgency to become pregnant in order to: (1) continue to maximize her coping skills and support; (2) clarify her need for multiple medications and trial lower doses and medication tapers; and (3) help her realistically evaluate and approach sperm donation.

Dorothy did not meet criteria for the treatment team to say that she could not continue her evaluation for

Table 7.1 When to recommend delaying or discontinuing fertility treatments

1. Current psychosis
2. Acute suicidal ideation
3. Severe vegetative symptoms of depression
4. Mania
5. Ongoing substance abuse/dependence
6. Borderline personality disorder, with acute emotional dysregulation leading to inability to work with treatment team; active self-harm activities
7. PTSD with active dissociation, severe and disabling symptoms
8. Current severe panic attacks
9. Severe and disabling OCD
10. Active domestic violence

fertility treatment. Nevertheless, there were several "red flags" that led her fertility team to emphasize the need to "slow down." The empathic response to her situation helped Dorothy settle down her urgency and agree to a "team approach." The goal of the middle phase of treatment for Dorothy was to build a responsive, responsible treatment team to help her make decisions about her desire for a child as a single parent, her ability to parent without her husband, and clarify her diagnosis and what medications were truly needed during pregnancy and postpartum.

Dorothy completed all her lab work which revealed a normal FSH, AMH and no indication that she was in danger of infertility. She was relieved, and the knowledge that "there is nothing wrong" settled her down. The fertility specialist called her to give her the results, and explained that the goal was to "go slow and steady for the healthiest pregnancy" and that given these results, there was no rush to ovarian stimulation.

Dorothy met with the fertility counselor and discussed her sperm donation plans. The counselor provided feedback to Dorothy about how to evaluate sperm donors, and the potential psychological adjustments for both mother and child to sperm donation. Dorothy was very appreciative of the counseling session, and asked for extra meetings so that her sister Meg could join them. During these sessions, the counselor learned that Meg, who was 10 years older than Dorothy, was excited to help Dorothy raise a child, as her own children were heading to college soon. The counselor was impressed with the emotional bond between the sisters, and the maturity and psychological stability of Meg. Dorothy asked Meg's husband to join them for a session as well, and Meg's husband confirmed his long-term commitment to Meg and that he supported her support of her sister. Meg's husband revealed his disappointment with Dorothy's husband for his affair and provided collateral information that Dorothy had never been so emotionally unstable as the weeks after he left her. He emphasized that Dorothy had never been acutely suicidal as far as he was aware, and that she had never been hospitalized.

The fertility counselor provided feedback to the treatment team that Dorothy had indeed "slowed down" and that she had stopped being obsessed with finding a donor who matched her ex-husband's characteristics. During their counseling sessions, Dorothy began to explore the characteristics and traits that were important to her, and ultimately chose a sperm donor who she felt would fit in well with her family. The counselor was impressed with Dorothy's realistic appreciation for the process, that while she may "choose" a donor, she has no idea what the child will be like. The counselor was confident that Dorothy was

able and willing to support and love a child with special needs, or a child "different" than her expectations.

Realistic expectations are crucial for parenting, and an especially integral process for third-party reproduction. Assessment of realistic expectations is especially important in the case of a patient with a history of probable borderline personality traits/disorder. The goal of this middle phase of "slow and steady" was to further evaluate Dorothy's ability to self-observe and not immediately engage in splitting behavior. The counselor, over the serial visits, was increasingly impressed by Dorothy's ability to self-reflect, her appreciation of the role of trauma in her development and her genuine commitment to helping a future child have a "different life." The counselor's only lasting concerns were regarding Dorothy's determination to never have her child sexually abused. The counselor, over time, was not impressed with the previous diagnosis of borderline personality disorder. Instead, the counselor was aware of how Dorothy had seemed to have acutely decompensated when her husband had an affair, and that in fact for most of her life she had been self-regulated and without signs or symptoms of personality disorder. Dorothy had Meg join many of the appointments, and the fertility counselor appreciated the corroboration of Meg with her own impressions of Dorothy.

Dorothy met every 2 weeks with her psychiatrist, who had discussed her history at length with her previous psychiatrist. Both agreed that the onset of Dorothy's mood instability coincided with her husband's affair. Prior to this, she had never had significant mood instability, had never been suicidal, and never seen a psychiatrist. Her prior psychiatrist reflected that Dorothy had a history of premenstrual mood disturbance and that he had started her on Prozac at that time. He explained that as the marital instability escalated, he was very worried about her mood instability while taking Clomid in order to get pregnant. He began the Lamictal empirically in order to improve her mood stability, and increased her Prozac. He explained that the increase in Prozac led to more insomnia, which increased when her husband left her for his affair partner.

The previous psychiatrist acknowledged that Dorothy had never had a manic episode and that there was no family history of bipolar disorder. During the time that they worked together, Dorothy had not been in psychotherapy, and he had been working with her as "medication management" only. In retrospect, the psychiatrist acknowledged the complexity of Dorothy's situation, and that he was not familiar with the potential central nervous system effects of Clomid or the enormous emotional stress of fertility treatments. He admitted that Dorothy's passive suicidal ideation had been of great concern as "he did not know her that well" and that he felt given the stress she was under, and her suicidal ideation, that the safest course of action was an involuntary hospitalization for evaluation and treatment.

Final Phase: The Road to a "New Life"

Dorothy tapered her Lamictal and Seroquel over the next 12 months, under the care of her new psychiatrist. She continued DBT with her therapist. She explored sperm donation options and began to reconsider her "obsession" with having a child immediately. As she approached her thirty-fifth birthday, Dorothy decided to pursue ovarian stimulation and egg freezing. She reflected to all of her mental health professionals, who agreed, that she had been stable and doing well for over a year. She decided that if she froze her eggs, she could "take it slow and steady" and date and see if she found a partner who she wanted to have children with.

Dorothy completed ovarian stimulation protocol while taking Prozac 20 mg/d only. She reported that the cycle definitely increased her feelings of mood lability, but she did not have suicidal ideation or severe anxiety or depression. She froze her eggs and the fertility treatment team said goodbye to Dorothy with feelings of affection and respect.

Dorothy's case reflects the challenging intersection of mental health and infertility evaluation and treatment.

The complexity of Dorothy's history and presentation required patience and investment on the part of the fertility specialist. First, her safety needed to be evaluated. Next, her differential diagnosis needed to be clarified, and the decision regarding whether "to treat or not to treat" needed to addressed. The psychiatric fluency of the fertility specialist is crucial. Without the ability to empathize with the patient and engage them, no treatment planning can occur. Dorothy's case illustrates the complex, important intersection of psychiatric and fertility treatments.

References

1. Maroufizadeh S, Omani-Samani R, Almasi-Hashiani A, Amini P, Sepidarkish M. The reliability and validity of the Patient Health Questionnaire-9 (PHQ-9) and PHQ-2 in patients with infertility. *Reprod Health* 2019;**16**(1):137.

2. Clark CT, Wisner KL. Treatment of peripartum bipolar disorder. *Obstet Gynecol Clin North Am* 2018;**45**(3):403–417.

3. Raffi ER, Nonacs R, Cohen LS. Safety of psychotropic medications during pregnancy. *Clin Perinatol* 2019;**46**(2):215–234.

4. Zanarini MC, Weingeroff JL, Frankenburg FR. Defense mechanisms associated with borderline personality disorder. *J Personality Disord* 2009;**23**(2):113–121.

5. Practice Committee of the American Society for Reproductive Medicine and the Practice Committee for the Society for Assisted Reproductive Technology. Guidance regarding gamete and embryo donation. *Fertil Steril* 2021;**115**(6):1395–1410.

"Be Fruitful and Multiply": Addressing Spirituality in Fertility Counseling

Megan Flood and Eileen Dombo

Introduction

Megan Flood: I am a Clinical Social Worker in private practice in Washington, D.C. For more than 20 years, I have worked with individuals and couples navigating the, often difficult, pathway to parenthood. In addition to my clinical work, I have taught at The Catholic University America's National Catholic School of Social Service. I am currently on the faculties of The Washington School of Psychiatry and the Center for Existential Studies and Psychotherapy. Like many who choose to work with issues related to infertility, I navigated my own difficult journey in family building.

Eileen Dombo: It is my pleasure to reconnect with Sharon Covington and Megan Flood in updating this essential text in working with clients who are navigating the vicissitudes of fertility. In addition to over 25 years of clinical work with individuals and couples, I am an Associate Professor, Assistant Dean and Chair of the Ph.D. Program at The Catholic University of America's National Catholic School of Social Service, where my teaching and research focus on trauma and spirituality in clinical practice. I have also taught at The Washington School of Psychiatry, and am the Editor-in-Chief of the *Journal of Religion and Spirituality in Social Work: Social Thought*. In the community, I serve as the Chairperson for the Archdiocese of Washington Child Protection Board. My interest in working with this population stems from my lifelong personal and professional commitment to advocating for women, especially those in underserved populations.

In this chapter, we will share case material from our practices that highlight examples of interventions from Chapter 8 in the *Clinical Guide*. All identifying information has been removed. Most cases are an amalgamation of clinical material.

Spiritual Bypassing

As discussed in Chapter 8 of the *Clinical Guide*, spiritual bypassing, the term created by John Welwood in 1984, refers to the use of spiritual ideas, practices and rituals to sidestep more psychologically painful work that may be necessary to face unresolved emotional issues. This is often an unconscious process, and can be a delicate matter to raise in counseling with clients. It is important to address this in an empathic and caring manner, not wanting to discount the client's religious practices, but focusing on disentangling the emotional and psychological from the religious and spiritual; often parts that are deeply intertwined.

Tran and Jake, a gay couple in their late thirties, present for treatment to address a crisis in their partnership. Although neither partner is currently religious, Jake, who had been raised Catholic, begins to feel uncomfortable with pursuing egg donation and a gestational carrier to create their family, because of the Church's prohibition against assisted reproductive technology (ART). Tran's attempts to persuade Jake by listing all of the other parts of their lives that the Church does not endorse (most notably their same-sex relationship), are met with greater and greater resistance from Jake, who seems to become more devout at every session.

The fertility counselor, Peter, a Catholic himself, identifies Jake's stridency as possible spiritual bypassing, in part because of his strong countertransference experience that something is being omitted. In supervision, Peter wonders if the couple might be ambivalent about moving forward with becoming parents, for some reason. As he continues to work with the couple, issues of fear related to becoming biological parents emerge in the work. Both Jake and Tran have serious genetic illnesses in their families of origin, and each is fearful of raising his concerns with the other. Jake engages in spiritual bypassing by unconsciously halting the process of fertility treatments with his sudden religiosity, thus protecting both partners from facing doubts about their capacities and desires to have a biological child. As the therapy progresses, Tran and Jake are better able to articulate their hesitations, and ultimately agree to pursue adoption. This allows Jake to work toward making peace with his internal conflicts with his religion.

Fertility Counselor Stance of Informed Not-Knowing

We are strong proponents of remaining current about matters that are pertinent to the populations we serve, and believe that use of our own personal experiences with spirituality and infertility, as well as our countertransference reactions, can often enhance our work with clients. However, we firmly believe that it is most essential to remain in a stance of informed not-knowing in clinical work. As we explained in Chapter 8 of the *Clinical Guide*, we consider what we bring to the clinical encounter a sketch or outline, that may provide some structure to help clients tell *their* version of the story. The fertility counselor brings knowledge, training, and personal experiences with infertility and spirituality, but the client is the expert about their own experiences, beliefs and feelings.

> *Melinda and her clients Dav and Miriam are members of the same Orthodox Jewish community (although they worship at different synagogues). Melinda has extensive professional and personal experience with infertility; she used a donor embryo to become pregnant with her only daughter, and feels no conflict between her religious beliefs and her own treatment choice. As she works with Miriam and Dav, she finds herself feeling frustrated by what she sees as Miriam's dogmatic interpretation of Orthodox Jewish beliefs regarding ART. Melinda is aware of some countertransference emerging in her work with this couple, specifically, her feeling that were Miriam and Dav to proceed with using a donor egg, or to undergo an adoption process that resulted in adding a child to their family, Miriam would change her mind about the importance of being biologically related to the child. Melinda views her countertransference of frustration as a signal that there is something she is not understanding about her clients' experience; her awareness of the differences between her viewpoint and that of her clients reminds her to adopt a stance of informed not-knowing in her work with them.*

Melinda's religious background is important in her work with Miriam and Dav; in fact, the couple was referred to her because of her connections in the Jewish community. Her familiarity with the couple's religious beliefs strengthens their work together, to the degree that they all "speak the same language." At the same time, Melinda's awareness of maintaining a position of informed not-knowing helps her appreciate how the couple's understandings and experiences differ from her own. In spite of the similarities in their backgrounds, informed not-knowing helps Melinda tune into her clients' unique interpretations and experiences.

Telling the Story

One of the most healing aspects of therapy for clients struggling with infertility is the opportunity to tell the story of their family-building journey to a neutral, caring and unrelated individual who is familiar with matters related to infertility, yet who does not advocate any specific religious or spiritual opinions about choices or intervention options. Therapy with a fertility counselor who is both experienced in working with infertility and open to understanding the client's spiritual orientation can provide an opportunity for the client to organize experiences, feelings and beliefs into his or her own unique story, without having to edit details for a particular audience. See Chapter 8 in the *Clinical Guide* for further discussion of Jaffe & Diamond's notion of the Reproductive Story.

> *Saily begins therapy for depression after her sister-in-law gives birth to a baby boy, the first grandchild in the family. She is puzzled by her feelings of apathy towards her nephew, who is a source of great pride to the family. The priest in Saily's Hindu temple holds a ceremony for the entire community to celebrate the auspicious date of the baby's birth. Saily, the baby's godmother and only aunt, plays a special role in the ceremony. Although Saily's family and many members of her temple are aware of her history of infertility, no one, including Saily, considers that her depression and her infertility might be related. On the contrary, the community and Saily consider her position as godmother an enviable one because of her special relationship to the baby and to God. Furthermore, they view her childlessness as karma and express their belief that Saily's role is to serve others. Saily's depression seems incongruent with her community's and her own spiritual expectations of herself.*

Saily's presenting problem of depression seems inexplicable to her in the spiritual context of events in her life. She feels ashamed of her self-perception as unloving and unappreciative of her family's good fortune. Her fertility counselor, Eden, who is a single woman, desiring of children, with a different but also significant religious orientation, has a strong concordant countertransference reaction. Eden's identification with Saily helps her be curious with Saily about whether Saily's feelings related to her infertility experience might be relevant. Together, they begin to understand Saily's current reactions as a piece of a larger story of her life. In therapy, Saily constructs a narrative that makes sense of her depression; she is not an unappreciative godmother, unwilling to fulfil her karmic duties. Instead, she is a mother, grieving the losses of her own babies. Her lack of enthusiasm about her nephew is a logical part of a larger story, and makes sense when considered in the context of her life. Saily becomes able to see herself as worthy of empathy, which alleviates feelings of guilt about her ambivalence toward her nephew.

Naming the Losses

As you will recall from Chapter 8 in the *Clinical Guide*, clients experiencing infertility usually feel an acute sense of grief, but may not have labeled their experiences as such, because of the intangibility of the losses. In addition to losing previously held assumptions about fertility, good health, success, masculinity, femininity and, the future, clients may also feel the loss of connection with faith, higher powers, and spiritual communities. It is the fertility counselor's task to help their clients name these losses as worthy of grieving.

Karim and his wife Laila have suffered six miscarriages over the last 4 years and are contemplating pursuing IVF at the recommendation of Laila's obstetrician. Laila is eager to begin treatment; Karim is supportive but cautious about the financial and emotional investment of conceiving via ART. Karim and Laila are Muslim, but neither he nor his wife is outwardly religious. Karim notes that until his experience with infertility, he considered his Islamic faith to be an internal source of comfort and support. He describes his earlier belief that he had an ongoing internal conversation with Allah, but now he feels as though he is talking only to himself; Allah isn't listening, and maybe isn't even there. Just as Karim's assumption that he would easily become a father is being challenged by his infertility, so too is his former assumption of a loving God shaken.

As she listens to Karim's story, Wendy, Karim's fertility counselor, is aware of her powerful counter-transference feeling of sadness. He describes feeling uncertain how to characterize the miscarriages; after all, he says, in a very matter of fact tone, it's not as though he and Laila lost an "actual child." Still, he describes feeling as though he has suffered several deaths. Like many clients, Karim is reluctant to identify the miscarriages in the same category as other less ambiguous losses. Wendy's willingness to identify Karim and Laila's miscarriages as losses worthy of grieving lends legitimacy to Karim's experience of this very thing. Conceiving of the miscarriages as losses allows Karim to consider that he may be grieving other related losses, too, such as the ability to achieve pregnancy via lovemaking, and the financial stress of IVF. As they work together, Karim and Wendy realize that Karim is also wrestling with the profound existential loss of his faith in God. Any one of these losses, alone, would be difficult to endure; for clients experiencing multiple losses simultaneously, feelings of grief are intensified.

In helping clients name all of the losses related to infertility, including those having to do with a shift in faith, fertility counselors like Wendy validate the intensity of the feelings and create space for grieving previously unnamed, ambiguous losses.

Speaking the Unspeakable

As we discussed in Chapter 8 in the *Clinical Guide*, clients dealing with infertility commonly experience feelings of envy, rage, hatred, frustration, fear and doubt, many of which may be discouraged by members of their faith communities as unkind, inappropriate and, even, blasphemous. Fertility counselors working with this population are tolerant, accepting, and may even be encouraging when clients express these feelings, which clients often are both appreciative of, and may be somewhat alarmed by. It is important both to allow space for expression of these feelings, and to attend to the experience of saying out loud and feeling in session frightening and forbidden material.

Leah is an active member of a Christian Evangelical church. She and her husband were raised in the tradition, met each other at church, and identify their faith as central to their lives. When Leah suffers a late miscarriage, church members organize a meal-delivery schedule and an extra prayer service to provide support to Leah and her husband. Leah feels grateful for the support, but also finds herself feeling envy and rage towards church families with infants and small children, many of whom visit Leah during her recovery. She finds herself bristling when well-intentioned friends tell her the loss is "God's plan," although she herself might have agreed with this sentiment before the miscarriage. Leah recounts with regret an incident with a pregnant friend who tells Leah that she feels blessed to be expecting a child. Leah's angry response, "Well, then, I guess I'm cursed!" is met by her friend's shock and judgment; Leah feels exposed, ashamed, and misunderstood.

Fertility counselors working with clients like Leah are accustomed to hearing such stories. In addition to painful feelings of loss about the miscarriage, Leah is aware of her "unchristian" feelings of jealousy and rage, but notes that she does not believe she should have them, let alone, express them. Richard, Leah's fertility counselor, feels his stomach turn a bit as Leah is talking, and uses this countertransference to understand how awful Leah herself is feeling. His suggestion that she can say anything at all in the privacy of therapy at first feels foreign to her. However, as Leah begins to experience Richard as receptive to hearing all of her feelings, even those she considers most unspeakable, Leah begins to feel more tolerant of these feelings in herself. This tolerance allows Leah to examine the "bad" feelings and decide how to manage them if they arise again. Moreover, by sharing these feelings with a supportive fertility counselor, Leah finds that she is also more freely able to experience loving and concerned feelings toward her pregnant friend.

Grieving the Losses

As we explained in Chapter 8 of the *Clinical Guide*, as clients are able to identify their infertility-related losses, including those having to do with issues of faith, and articulate the unspeakable feelings related to these losses, the task of treatment becomes helping clients engage in the grieving process. In addition to expressing feelings of grief in their own time (there is no rush, and no time limit), some clients will find it helpful to include the practice of a ritual, which may or may not be connected to formal religious rituals. Spiritually sensitive fertility counselors are attuned to ways in which clients' spirituality or religiosity may serve as a source of support in the grieving process.

Melia and Lou suffer a late-term stillbirth when Melia is 36 weeks pregnant with a baby girl they named Lydia. The couple had prepared a nursery and had a collection of ultrasound images of the baby taken throughout their problem-free pregnancy. There is also a photograph taken of Melia holding Lydia after the delivery, which Melia reports to the fertility counselor after several sessions. Nina, the fertility counselor, is aware of a strong countertransference reaction of desire to see the picture, and takes a risk in asking if Melia and Lou want to share it. The couple readily agree, and say they didn't think anyone would want to see the picture. They proudly bring the photograph and other items such as infant clothing and stuffed animals to subsequent sessions. Nina's expression of interest, admiration, and sadness provide space and permission for the couple to begin the work of grieving the loss of Lydia. The couple subsequently decide to hold a memorial service for Lydia in their garden, and invite close family and friends to share memories of the pregnancy, reflections about the photograph, and wishes and dreams for the couple.

Nina's interest in seeing the photograph of Lydia communicates her willingness to see and hear every part of Melia and Lou's experience, and honors them in their role as parents to Lydia. The couple's work with Nina helps them construct a ritual to recognize Lydia as a part of their family, and to include important people in their lives in their grieving process. Couples may ritualize any part of the infertility process; for example, attending religious services before IVF, saving ultrasound images of embryos or planting seeds in the ground after a miscarriage.

Identifying Options

Once clients have spent time in therapy exploring their feelings about infertility, parenthood and their dreams of how their future family might look, they may feel eager to identify solutions that will put an end to a stressful and disappointing life phase, as we discussed in Chapter 8 of the *Clinical Guide*. If clients are spiritual, the fertility counselor can help them clarify how their beliefs may inform decisions about parenthood, moving forward.

After several years of infertility, including five rounds of IVF, and nine months of individual therapy, Jessica informs Pat, her fertility counselor, that she would like to consider other medical interventions to achieve pregnancy. As a devout Mormon, Jessica is aware that her church does not approve of third-party sperm, egg or embryo donations. It is important to Jessica to adhere to the teachings of her church, but she is also aware of her very strong desire to be pregnant, and feels that she will deeply grieve the loss of that experience in her life. Pat, who became pregnant via donor egg, is aware of a strong countertransference desire for Jessica to forsake her religious beliefs. Together, Jessica and Pat explore how it might feel for Jessica to go against the teachings of her faith in order to achieve pregnancy using donor gametes or embryos. Ultimately, Jessica decides to pursue adoption, but agrees with her husband to keep trying to conceive each month without medical assistance. This compromise helps Jessica feel that she is not giving up her dream of experiencing pregnancy, while also remaining adherent to the religious guidelines that are important to her.

In therapy, Jessica is given permission to imagine a variety of options. She is able to acknowledge that she has a choice in how she will proceed, and finds that her choice includes adhering to the teachings of her church. Fortunately, Pat's awareness of her countertransference helps her to avoid adding undue influence to Jessica's decision-making. Jessica's ultimate decision to pursue adoption while continuing to try to conceive naturally accommodates the three desires that are most important to her: her faith, becoming a parent and trying to achieve pregnancy.

Spirituality as a Source of Strength

It is critical for fertility counselors to encourage clients to identify and draw upon spiritual or religious beliefs and communities, if they are a source of comfort and support.

Leslie and Jack are devout Catholics who have been unable to conceive after 3 years of trying. The couple is committed to adhering to church guidelines regarding treatment for infertility and have decided to continue their attempts without medical assistance. In therapy, Leslie and Jack acknowledge the emotional pain of this decision. Although their struggle is painful, they find the weekly ritual of Communion reaffirming of God's presence in their lives; the miracle of Communion reminds them of God's power. Biblical stories of suffering and modern examples of Saints such as Mother Theresa help the couple endure their infertility, and experience their own suffering as a legitimate response to their situation. They are close to the parish priest, and often meet with him privately to pray. Leslie and Jack volunteer to teach Sunday school, and have developed relationships with many of the children and families in the parish. Both Leslie and Jack believe that God will decide how children will be part of their lives, and they feel comforted knowing that if they are unable to have children of their own, God will provide other opportunities for them to have meaningful relationships with youngsters.

For Leslie and Jack, their Catholic faith is paramount to their identities. Their desire to become parents is fueled by their faith tradition. While they grieve the pain of infertility in therapy, they feel their decision not to pursue medical intervention aligns with their Catholic identities. Their fertility counselor provides space to honor that while being supportive of their work with a priest; this is seen as a fruitful opportunity for collaboration with a faith leader in accordance with the couple's wishes. As this case illustrates, the fertility counselor must be mindful of their role with regards to religion and fertility and seek collaborative alliances when appropriate.

Julia receives devastating news at a 26-week ultrasound. She is informed that the baby has a heart defect that will likely result in stillbirth or a medically compromised, shortened life for the infant. Julia's doctor gives her the option to terminate the pregnancy for medical reasons. Her fertility counselor, Michael, who is not religious or spiritual, is aware of his countertransference reaction of alarm, and finds himself feeling strongly that Julia should end the pregnancy to spare herself further heartbreak. He gently explores this option with her, but Julia chooses to keep the pregnancy. Raised in the Southern Baptist African American church, Julia is a firm believer in the power of prayer. She feels comforted by her relationship with God through daily prayer, Bible study, and attending services every Sunday, and knows that whatever the outcome, God is with her. Several weeks later, another ultrasound reveals that the baby is developing normally, and, after a full-term pregnancy, Julia delivers a healthy baby boy.

Although Michael is skeptical about religion, personally, his experience with Julia demonstrates the power of faith for some clients, and is a humbling reminder to him of the potential dangers of minimizing this and of conveying his own reactions and opinions to clients.

Nonreligious clients may also engage in spiritual rituals that provide a sense of meaning and connection during the, often lonely, experience of infertility. As we discussed in Chapter 8 of the *Clinical Guide*, fertility counselors can help these clients identify or create such rituals.

While traveling abroad after Lisa's failed IVF cycle using Laura's egg and donor sperm, the couple learn of a religious shrine in Greece for childless women at the top of a steep mountain with many steps. At the top, pilgrims light candles and pray to Greek goddesses and the Virgin Mary to become pregnant. Although Lisa and Laura are not religious and do not identify as believers in a traditional sense, they are moved by the idea that they are not alone in their sadness, and decide to climb the mountain to feel a part of a timeless community of people yearning to become parents. The experience is profound for the couple, and they now remember it when they feel alone in their struggle.

While this couple might not have identified this experience as religious or spiritual, their fertility counselor, Saundra, understands that it is meaningful and that it helps Lisa and Laura feel connected to something greater than their infertility. It is not necessary to label such an experience as spiritual or religious to the client if the client does not consider it as such. Nevertheless, the fertility counselor may consider clients' search for meaning, purpose and connection to something greater than their own experience in the same vein as other more traditional expressions of spirituality or religiosity.

Conclusion

The case studies presented in this chapter are designed to give fertility counselors a sense of how themes of spirituality can be present with clients experiencing infertility, and to outline some concrete interventions. The case illustrations demonstrate the ways in which a thorough assessment of the client's spirituality can be vital to understanding the meaning made of infertility. It is also critical for the fertility counselor to pay attention to countertransference when providing counseling for infertility with clients who raise themes around spirituality. In order to meet clients where they are, and be most effective in helping them reach family building decisions that are best for them, fertility counselors must attend to the spiritual dimensions they present.

CASE 9 Counseling Recipients of Nonidentified Donor Gametes

Carol Toll and Patricia Sachs

Introduction

How did we come to do this work? Our stories are remarkably similar. We are both social workers in a private counseling practice, embedded in a fertility clinic that has grown substantially over the years. We have each been in practice for over 30 years, working with individuals, couples and groups. Our early training and experience included insight-oriented psychodynamic psychotherapy as well as cognitive-behavioral therapy, and we practice using a range of approaches. Being flexible and comfortable using an array of tools is essential in this work with fertility patients.

We each have also experienced our own struggles with fertility, journeys that led us to specialize in fertility counseling. Knowing you have "walked in their shoes" or "been on the other side" can be comforting to patients, who then feel that you can truly empathize and "get" what they are going through. We are grateful to share a sliver of our 30 years of experience with fertility patients. We hope our chapter will be a support to your current and future work in fertility counseling.

In the beginning of our journey into fertility counseling, the recipients were frequently heterosexual/opposite sex couples using either a nonidentified egg or sperm donor, typically due to issues related to egg or sperm quality and/or quantity. The concerns we addressed were mainly around the couple's grief from losing the genetic connection to a potential child: had they dealt with the loss of their "fantasy" child in a way to support bonding with their donor-conceived child?

We also wondered with them how they would select their donor. We assumed in general that recipients would want to choose a donor who physically resembled them, if possible, so as to protect privacy and enable the child to "fit in" with the family look. Knowing that research was indicating that openness with a child about the use of donation led to better overall adjustment and family functioning [1], we wondered whether they would plan to disclose the donor origins to their child? We typically had one required counseling session, one opportunity to try to cover many issues and hopefully educate about the current thinking on creating and raising a donor-conceived child.

Thirty years (and a pandemic) later, recipient counseling has expanded to include many types of families being formed through gamete donation: single women and single men, same sex couples and trans people. Their options include the same as opposite sex couples: donor sperm, donor egg, donor embryo, as well as gestational surrogacy; but their journey is much different, as it is a highly intentional process and often not related to infertility.

Our approach to counseling has expanded as well. We have grown to ask ourselves: What do we hope that the recipients will leave with? And, what do we, as fertility counselors hope to get out of the session? Though we still typically have but one opportunity to meet with recipients, our approach has expanded to placing greater emphasis on making a connection rather than to cover every topic from all angles. We try to be open to the idea that there can be many paths to a happy family, not just one. We now measure a "good outcome" as one where the recipients feel that the session clarified issues and bolstered their confidence to make informed decisions with life-long implications. Our goal is to begin a relationship whereby recipients will return to us for follow-up, if needed, in the future. We now view this step in their journey not just as the creation of a child, but rather of a donor-conceived family.

In our view, recipient counseling involves attending to the process of a session as well as the content covered. We have had to adapt to abrupt changes during the COVID-19 pandemic by learning to conduct counseling virtually. There have been benefits as well as detractions with the use of this technology. No doubt future counseling will include a hybrid/mixture of in-person and remote sessions.

Case Experiences: The Quilt

Through these cases, we have tried to illustrate the often-fragile nature of the work we do.

Recipients may come in to the office with their personal defenses already in place. They may also have their pre-conceived ideas about what the counseling session will be like. They most likely come to the session with a history of loss, grief and disappointments, and worry that we are yet another step in their process of being "judged." They therefore may be defensive, and reluctant to open up, to be vulnerable, and to show us their true selves and feelings. Part of our job is to help lower their defenses by explaining why we do what we do. For example, explaining that we are going to ask about the race, cultural, and/or sexual/gender background that they identify with, as a means of exploring whether this is important to them in donor selection, can help us to align with, rather than, offend them (see "Patchwork Square 2" below). Rather than persisting in addressing all the issues on our "checklist," we also try to personalize the session by enlisting their ideas about what they hope to cover or get out of it. We feel that we have accomplished something when/if recipients say at the end: "This turned out to be more than a check-off on our list. It was a useful learning experience and now it is clear why it is part of the process and we are glad we did it. We learned something."

The cases we have chosen are a compilation of some of the more salient issues we have encountered in our experience of recipient counseling over three decades and are, thus, fictitious. They reflect some of the issues we have struggled with and from which we have tried to learn. What has been especially helpful to us has been to be part of a team of fertility counselors with whom we have shared cases, and from whom we continue to learn.

We also chose the following cases within the framework of "families come together in lots of different ways." This is increasingly true of the recipients we counsel during their fertility journey. We listen, learn, assess, counsel, educate and provide tools for their future family. As we have said, we hope the connection formed in the session will bring them back to consult with us should the need arise.

Each session is as a "patchwork square," which when pieced together over time creates a rich "quilt" of experience we can draw from and offer to those we counsel. While we cannot spread out the whole quilt here, we have chosen these cases as our "patchwork squares," offering examples of challenging and frequently encountered issues.

Patchwork Square 1: "Too Many Embryos, Too Many Decisions"

Jorge, a single, gay man in his forties, from a Latin American background, comes for his recipient counseling session for egg donation, the first step in a process in which he will, also, ultimately need a gestational carrier. He had only recently come out to his family as being gay, in the context of telling them that he was pursuing having a baby as well. Despite his very close bonds with his parents, he had always feared rejection if he told them he was gay, as they are quite traditional. Fortunately, his fears proved unfounded, and his parents were accepting and supportive, telling him that they "just want him to be happy." I wondered if he had worried about me in that way, as well. That is, would I judge him, as a single, gay man, in terms of his fitness for parenthood? Having seen several other single men, both gay and straight, for recipient counseling sessions in the past, I felt fairly well prepared to address the unique issues that might arise in this specific situation. This, and his warm and relaxed demeanor, helped us to make a good immediate connection. We focused on what he was looking for in an egg donor. He said he wished to find "the best possible donor" in terms of health and education, though not necessarily someone from his same cultural background. We explored his thoughts about how he would handle disclosure with his potential child and we briefly discussed issues relating to gestational carrier selection. Since he was working with an agency, they would be helping him to find a "match." I fully expected not to hear from him again until his gestational carrier had been evaluated and it was time for a group counseling session with him, the carrier (and spouse/partner, if she had one), and me, in order to complete the consultation.

I was surprised when, several months after our initial counseling session, he contacted me for a follow-up, stating that he needed to talk urgently about the outcome of the donor egg cycle. A high number of embryos had been created, but to his surprise, they were mostly female, and the male ones were of lesser quality. He wanted to first know my reaction to this news, as he thought it must be an extremely unusual situation. He seemed to be feeling unprepared and panicked about this outcome, and I felt like he needed my reassurance that this was, in fact, not a typical situation and that he was justified in his reaction. I told him that indeed, it did seem to me to be an unusual imbalance of male/female embryos, though I couldn't say for sure. He appeared overwhelmed by the amount of information he had been given, all at once: how many embryos had been created, and what was their gender and quality. His mind started spinning to all the possibilities: would he transfer a male embryo first, since it might be his only attempt at fatherhood, and perhaps it would be easier to parent a son first? Would he then want to transfer a female embryo in the future, since he always had imagined having two children? As a single parent, he did not want to transfer two at a time, risking multiples. And what if he never had a son? Coming from a culture of 'machismo', there was a certain pressure to continue the male line, which he felt was very important in his family, though this was not his only reason. He knew that in his heart, he would feel sad if he never had the opportunity to at least try to have a son.

My goal with him was to help him to clarify and separate out what he wanted, as opposed to what his family might want for him. I also wanted to help slow things down; I could empathize with how overwhelmed he felt facing so many decisions, but I wanted him to see that not all of them had to be made right now. Though surprised by the outcome of the cycle, he did not have to feel panicked and out of control. He could begin to think about things, but the reality was that he had some time, since he had not even identified a gestational carrier yet. He could imagine several scenarios, but ultimately there would be some things that could just not be guaranteed or controlled, despite his careful efforts. I hoped that in time, and through the long process ahead, he would gain confidence in his ability to become a father, no matter what the gender of his child(ren). I felt gratified that he had trusted and connected with me enough in our first session to reach out again when he was clearly in distress about all the decisions he was facing.

I do not know what the outcome of his case was, and, as I write this, he may still be in the process of identifying a gestational carrier. Will he choose to transfer a male embryo, despite its poorer quality, as his only chance for a son, and will the treatment be successful? If it fails, will he try again, with another male embryo? Or if he is successful in having a son, will he try for a second child, this time a daughter? What will he tell his family, if anything, about the dilemmas he faced?

We see people at the beginning of their reproductive journey and often wonder how things will turn out, especially if we feel a deeper connection and their story touches us in some poignant way. We become invested in their progress and hope for "good outcomes" for them, making it hard to let go. But realizing that they, and not we, are the best judges of how the story ends, makes it a bit easier. And yet, in this work, it is always hard for us to not know the end of the story.

Patchwork Square 2: "Talking About Race and Culture Through a Screen"

We write this chapter at a time of social change, with heightened awareness of diversity and inclusion. We struggle with the most appropriate language to use when addressing these issues with recipients so as to be respectful, accurate, and sensitive. Achieving this, while at the same time finding a "way in" to the issues around donor selection, can feel delicate and challenging. These complexities can be magnified with the growing use of virtual counseling.

As fertility counselors, we are seeing a growing number of recipients from diverse cultural backgrounds. It is important to realize that, as a counselor, simply being from a different background from the recipients can raise issues, and it is essential that we increase sensitivity and cultural awareness. How does diversity impact donor selection? One approach is to individualize our care by exploring what is important to particular recipients with regard to characteristics they are looking for in a donor, or *not,* as the case may be. Perhaps the racial, ethnic and cultural background of a donor is important to them and their family; perhaps not. Rather than making assumptions, we need to ask and understand.

The following is a case example of a single woman who was seen for her required recipient counseling session. As a backdrop to the session, we are noticing that more single women appear to be creating families with the use of nonidentified sperm donation. Perhaps the COVID-19 pandemic has created a new sense of urgency in trying to reach one's life goals, or there has been more time to pursue them. Societal changes, as well, have normalized many different types of family arrangements.

Alexandra, a single woman in her early thirties, was seen virtually for her required counseling session as a nonidentified donor sperm recipient. Viewing her through the screen, she appeared to be biracial (African American/White) or perhaps Latina. She seemed a bit guarded or reserved from the start, sitting a bit back from the computer screen with her body turned slightly away from it. I didn't know why this might be, so could only guess: Was she disappointed to open the screen and find that I was not from her same racial/ethnic background? Or that I was older? Perhaps she was approaching the counseling session as simply one more appointment to check off her list, one more obstacle before she could proceed with treatment, rather than something that might be helpful. Perhaps I should have asked how she was feeling about "having to do" this consult, as a means to lowering her defenses.

A short while into the session, I asked her where she "was from," intending to gain some information about her family's cultural/ethnic origins. This question seemed to cause her to become even more defensive, as she replied that she was "from Florida." I felt frustrated, but I realized that I may have offended her by the manner in which I asked this question, and that she also didn't know where I was going with it. It was only when I then explained that I was asking in the context of exploring whether the cultural background of a potential sperm donor would be important to her or not, that she seemed to understand and be more open to addressing the issue of donor selection. What also might have helped ease the tension in this situation would have been for me to ask directly, right when I sensed she was pulling back and becoming defensive, whether I had said something to offend her, creating a "microaggression," or whether there was something I could say to make things better or make her feel more comfortable. When a potential mistake is made, it needs to be addressed right then in the session, in order to repair the break and try to re-establish rapport.

In addition, the fact that the counseling session was done virtually may have also complicated our interaction in this case. Had I been in the same room with Alexandra, I may have gotten more clues about her (and she, about me), and might not have had to ask. Or if we had been able to meet in a waiting room, chat on the way back to the office, and begin to build some rapport, we might have "warmed up" to each other prior to the session's start, leading her to be a bit more open.

We disclose a lot about ourselves from the moment we enter a session: our approximate age, our gender, our marital status (if we are wearing a ring), and at least something about our racial and cultural background. It is important to have an awareness of how these visible aspects of ourselves may impact clients, in order to address and understand these issues if they arise in the counseling session. It is also important to understand that the same is true for our clients, as we can make assumptions (conscious or unconscious) based on appearance, first impressions, or while gathering initial data. The landscape of interpersonal interactions during these consultations can be full of rocky terrain which must be navigated mindfully and carefully.

Patchwork Square 3: The Perfect Donor – Accepting It Is "Not Me"

In this case, Sarah and John, an opposite-sex married couple, are being seen to discuss the prospect of using an egg donor to build their family. Their history involves many life experiences, but for Sarah, completing her graduate degree, and for John, establishing his own business, have collided with their current plan to become parents. Their individual investments in establishing their careers left them little time or energy for finding partners. The fortieth birthday milestone was a wake-up moment for each of them and they soon put their attention to exploring relationships. This happily brought about their meeting, marriage, and desire to start a family. Sarah and John tried on their own without success and turned to a fertility clinic for help and, after IVF cycles were also unsuccessful, egg donation was presented as the next option. Sarah was initially resistant and grieving, while John, although saddened, was more accepting and turned to the task of finding a donor. They begin to look at donor profiles of frozen eggs, fresh eggs, agency eggs and just don't see "their" donor. In our session, John discusses donor characteristics such as his desire for her to have an excellent education. Additionally, she must be young, smart and athletic. Sarah seems to be less specific in her descriptions and, in fact, seems to be somewhat embarrassed by John's tone, putting her head down and her hand on his, to slow down the outpouring of must haves.

This case reflects how hard it is to give up one's own genetic contribution to the imagined or dream-child for both partners. Having done all the "right things" has not helped Sarah and John in this situation, which might be their first setback, as hard work usually gets them what they want. When meeting this couple in a session, there is much for me to understand about their sense of loss and frustration, while I also want to help them become more realistic about the idea of the donor. I aim to acknowledge but not judge their loss. I say, "it is hard to find a donor when you are looking for yourself, and you are not on the list," while also empowering them by adding "this will be your child by the choices that you make and you will be the only parents, as a donor is not a parent of your child." By using empowering language, I support their desire to maintain control, while nudging them to develop a more realistic, but not "less than" frame of mind.

Establishing rapport from the outset is so important in these sessions. I start to walk the tightrope with Sarah and John, balancing expressing empathy with their dilemma by saying "most people have not done this before and it can be overwhelming at first" with introducing the realities "you may have to be somewhat flexible, as donors are real people, not lists of characteristics." Sensing I am being prodded by John to prove myself as the "expert," I start feeling exhausted. I realize, however, that what I am experiencing is more a reflection of their exhaustion. Sarah's low-key reactions and desire to "turn down the heat" in the session, also signal the strain on her. Near the end of the session, I feel maybe I have done my part after all, when I start to hear a change in their tone. John begins to make eye contact and listen more and challenge less, while visibly relaxing. Sarah sits up and raises her gaze, even smiling at times. I sense a shift, that Sarah and John are opening up and willing to at least start to explore a path leading to "their" donor.

As a fertility counselor, I need to stay open and fresh, to listen closely and not be misled by the similarities or repetitions from many previous sessions. I may have heard this before, but it is never the same story. The accumulated experiences of these individual sessions add to our patchwork quilt and richness of the work. My hope is that being able to pass along some of the patchwork squares of wisdom to Sarah and John will help them to feel less alone with the challenge of finding "their" donor.

Conclusion

We have learned that an important goal of counseling is to empower recipients to make their own decisions about what will work best for their future family, enabling them to "own their family." Our role is to help explore with them, but ultimately their job is to decide what will be best for them. Over time, we have come to value even more the ideas of self-determination and autonomy; the families being created belong to the recipients, not to us. And, unsure whether we would have had the same fortitude, we admire their resilience in pursuit of their family.

References

1. Illioi E, Blake L, Vasanti J, et al. The role of age of disclosure of biological origins in the psychological well-being of adolescents conceived by reproductive donation: a longitudinal study from age 1 to age 14. *J Child Psychol Psychiatry* 2017;**58**(3):315–324.

CASE 10 Counseling Nonidentified Gamete Donors

Laura Josephs and Uschi Van den Broeck

There is nothing more beautiful than someone who goes out of their way to make life beautiful for others.
— *Mandy Hale*

Introduction

Laura Josephs (LJ): I'm a psychologist, and for several decades I've spent much of my time immersed in the world of people working very hard to create their families. I've personally benefited from assisted reproductive technology to create my own family. For many years, I've been part of a very active donor egg team at the Center for Reproductive Medicine at Weill Cornell in New York City and, thus, have in my mind the pressing need of our donor recipients to move forward with building their families. Having consulted with so many prospective egg donors over the years, who are truly giving of themselves, I am also mindful of their feelings and their experiences. Ideally, gamete donation is a positive situation for donor and recipient, and part of the fertility counselor's role is to aim to get it as close to that ideal as possible.

Uschi Van den Broeck (UV): I started working as a young psychologist 15 years ago at a university fertility center and Ob/Gyn unit. What it means to wish for a child, the hopes, the dreams and the big and small losses along the way have always drawn me into the stories of couples, men and women trying to build or expand their families. My training as a family therapist inspired me to learn more about the family dynamics of third-party reproduction and listen closely to my patients as they explored what it means to be mothers, fathers and a family together. As I became a mother myself, yet again a new perspective was opened and challenged me toward more growth as a person and as a professional. Holding together all of these different perspectives (prospective parents, children, doctors, society . . .) and making it work for all of them is at the core of being a fertility counselor for me.

In what follows, we will present four clinical cases where the fertility counselor is left with questions or concerns regarding a potential gamete donor. Identifying details of the cases have been deeply disguised to protect the privacy of these individuals.

Concerns About Gamete Donation in Regard to Psychological Issues with the Donor

Sara

Sara was a 26-year-old single woman who worked as a manager in a clothing store. She had completed almost 2 years of college and had worked in a variety of jobs since high school. She said that she had several friends. Her relationship history was limited. She'd had a romantic relationship with a young man 2 years earlier. She stated that they were together for 4 months but then he abruptly stopped calling her. Sara had lived independently at various points but was currently living with her mother. Sara's dad had passed away when she was in middle school. She had no siblings.

Sara denied serious psychological problems. She said that she briefly went for therapy following her father's death. She denied use of psychiatric medication, alcohol and substance abuse, past and present psychotic symptoms, and psychiatric hospitalization. Clinically, there was no evidence of overt psychopathology. Her clinical presentation was notable for a certain blandness. She had difficulty describing herself as a child. When asked about the high and low points of her life, she was unable to name a low point, despite having lost her father. When probed about certain key life experiences, she tended to describe her responses in general rather than more specific terms – for example, when asked about her father's death, she finally said simply, "it was hard." At the same time, she had a rather definitive response to the question about whether she would be open to identity-release as a donor – allowing the prospective child to be given identifying information of the donor when the child reaches the age of 18. "That's not good for the child," she stated.

The clinical interview suggested the possibility that there was low reflective functioning, a diminished ability to recognize and understand her own emotional experiences [1]. Of course, there is always the possibility that the prospective donor is anxious in the evaluative situation, and that situational anxiety may be inhibiting her from fully revealing her thoughts and feelings to the counselor.

Psychological testing could help to better understand the underpinnings of Sara's self-presentation. However, the results (PAI) were concerning and problematic, with a suggestion of mood instability and volatile relationships, and a question raised about suicidal ideation. Diagnostic considerations included borderline personality disorder, persistent depressive disorder and generalized anxiety disorder.

The multidisciplinary team was supportive of the recommendation that Sara not be used as an egg donor. Possible emotional fragility meant that physically going through the egg donation process, including hormonal medication and, psychologically, dealing with the long-term implications of egg donation – feelings about one's genetic material being utilized in order for someone else to have a baby – might be destabilizing. In addition, a risk of passing on psychopathological tendencies to a donor-conceived child could not be ruled out.

When Sara was informed of the team's decision to not move forward due to the psychological evaluation, she was very upset and stated that she was having "a lot of problems" at her job and was worried about losing her job. She said she had been "very stressed out" lately. Also, her job insecurity was making her highly interested in the donor compensation. She asked if she could retake the psychological test. The fertility counselor then went on to speak with her about some of the test findings, including the question of suicidal thoughts. Sara acknowledged that she sometimes struggled with passive suicidal ideation but denied a wish to die and denied any intention or plan to harm herself. She was in fact open to referral for psychotherapy, and referrals were provided.

In this case, Sara's clinical presentation, her psychological testing and even her responses to the team's decision to not use her as an egg donor were all consistent with someone with a degree of psychological fragility and possible significant psychopathology. Moreover, psychological testing results in donor evaluation carry a slightly different weight than testing results in the context of psychotherapy. While it is customary in a therapy setting that one's clinical evaluation should take precedence over psychological testing results, in the setting of gamete donor evaluation, the subject is actively working to present well. For example, in her donor evaluation, Sara had not mentioned any difficulties at work; this only emerged when she was trying to explain her problematic test results. When there is a motivation on the subject's part to procure a positive evaluation, clinical findings are more likely to tilt in a direction that appears less pathological. This is the notion of "faking good," or social desirability [2]. In such situations, we may want to give greater weight to psychological testing results, which are less susceptible to faking good or impression management. Notably, here was a case where the fertility counselor (LJ) felt that rejecting this prospective donor was ultimately a good decision in terms of both this young woman herself and any potential recipients. However, it was clear that in the short term, the rejection was indeed felt as such by the prospective donor, in addition to being an economic blow for her in terms of the money that she was counting on. As mental health professionals, our sensibilities and training center around helping others and enabling them to achieve life goals. Even with our therapy patients, we may sometimes give feedback or advice that they don't like, but we're rarely standing in the way of what they're pursuing. Countertransferentially, it is uncomfortable to be a "gatekeeper" who is psychologically consulting with a person only to literally block their path.

Sophie

Sophie was a 26-year-old woman who worked as an elementary school teacher. Sophie's evaluation took place in 2020 in NYC, during the COVID-19 pandemic, and we sat with each other virtually, via videoconferencing. Telehealth for psychological consultation became a necessity during the pandemic, and mental health professionals were put in a position where we would need to make the best of this situation, which was new and unfamiliar for many of us. How might that affect my (LJ) ability to pick up on nonverbal cues, my ability to "read" this young woman's affect?

Despite the new and unfamiliar way of doing consultation, Sophie appeared to be open and forthcoming with the fertility counselor. Notable in Sophie's life history was the loss of her mother during childhood, at the age of 6. Her father remarried when Sophie was 11, and Sophie reported a good relationship with both her father and her stepmother. Unlike Sara, Sophie was able to speak pointedly and specifically about the loss of her mother, remembering that in the year after her mother's death, when she went to a friend's house for a playdate, she would hope that the friend's babysitter – not the mom – would be present. "It was too hard to be reminded of what I didn't have," she stated.

When asked to describe herself as a child, Sophie recalled that she had been "quiet and reserved" but always had at least a few friends. She stated that she was "still reserved around new people." In the clinical interview, Sophie presented as well-related, if a bit reserved – as she noted – and on the serious side. Sophie had occasionally pursued psychotherapy. She denied significant psychological problems, she denied psychiatric medication usage, and she denied alcohol/substance abuse.

Sophie's psychological testing (MMPI-2) raised concerns about "low mood," and "tendencies toward depression." When the fertility counselor called Sophie to let her know of the test findings, Sophie expressed surprise. She said that she was not aware of a low mood nor of feeling depressed. However, she acknowledged that the past half year, during the pandemic, had been difficult for her. Her young students were coping with family illness and even loss of family members, along with significant challenges to their ability to learn in the context of frequent stints of remote learning. This discussion was consistent with what she had talked about during her donor evaluation. Sophie was encouraged to discuss her state of mind and any psychological symptoms with her psychotherapist. The fertility counselor and the donor egg team were comfortable with her re-taking the psychological test in a year, and with her reapplying to the program, if she desired.

Taylor

Taylor was a prospective donor where some psychological findings emerged which suggested somatic reactivity when under stress, raising the possibility that the donation process could be unduly stressful for this young woman. This concern was discussed with the donor egg team and also with the donor, and ultimately the decision was made to use the donor and work with her.

Taylor, age 28, worked for a nonprofit organization which focused on helping residents of low-income communities. Though she acknowledged that the donor compensation would help her to pay off student loans, her wish to be an egg donor appeared to be consistent with important core values of altruism and service to others.

Taylor was on a low dose of an SSRI, which she began taking 2 years prior, for anxiety. The medication, along with regular psychotherapy, was described as very helpful and Taylor functioned very well in her work life and her personal life. She denied other significant psychological history or psychopathology, and there was no psychopathology evident in her clinical presentation. She denied alcohol/ substance abuse. She described close relationships with family members and friends. Taylor was single;

a long-term relationship ended about 1 year ago. She felt that she would like to be married someday but did not want to have children herself. She expressed that she could see amongst some of her friends "such a wish to have children – they want a kid so badly." Several were experiencing fertility problems and having a very hard time of it. This was part of what prompted her to donate her eggs.

Taylor's psychological testing (MMPI-2) showed that she potentially had tendencies to experience somatic symptoms when under stress, and the psychological profile generated by the test suggested the possibility of a somatization disorder. Taylor had appeared very forthcoming during the clinical interview, consistent with her approach to the MMPI-2, which was open and cooperative. No significant psychopathology was apparent during the interview nor in her description of her life. The fertility counselor presented Taylor's case to the donor egg team. This case was less about what tendencies toward psychopathology could be passed down genetically to the prospective genetic offspring, in terms of Taylor's reported history of anxiety. (It should be noted, of course, the recipient patients would always be informed of any current or historical psychological difficulties.) The psychological concern was more that in putting Taylor through a donation cycle – ovarian stimulation and egg retrieval – we would be introducing some bodily discomfort. Might this physical discomfort be potentially stressful for this donor, and might it then trigger further somatic symptoms?

The fertility counselor discussed the risk of egg donation being unduly psychologically stressful or destabilizing with Taylor in a follow-up phone call. She was not surprised by the MMPI-2 results. She told the fertility counselor that when she began medication and psychotherapy for anxiety, one of the stressors at that time was a viral illness, and in the aftermath of that illness she experienced lingering somatic symptoms. Anti-anxiety medication ameliorated these symptoms. She felt confident that she could comfortably go through the donor cycle. Taylor and the fertility counselor agreed that they would maintain some contact during the cycle and immediately afterwards. In fact, Taylor's self-assessment proved to be correct. She handled the physical and psychological aspects of the egg donation cycle very well. She did not experience increased anxiety nor any symptoms suggestive of somatization. In addition, she said that being an oocyte donor felt very rewarding; if anything, she became more keenly aware of the value of what she was providing to patients in need of these eggs.

The fertility counselor was glad and of course relieved that Taylor came through her donation without psychological incident. This particular donor evaluation brought into acute focus the responsibility we bear each time we approve a donor. We are putting the weight of our psychological authority behind the decision to "pass" a donor; we are assuring her and the donor egg team that she will likely be able to tolerate the stresses inherent in egg donation.

Concerns About Gamete Donation in Regard to Donor Motivation and Implications of Donation

John

John, aged 35, had been in a stable relationship for 4 years and the couple has 2 sons - 1 and 3 years old. He explained that the idea of donating sperm had been in his thoughts for a number of years as he wanted plenty of offspring. Ideally he wanted a big family as he himself grew up in a large, boisterous and happy household. However, his partner, Jenny, has always been very outspoken about not wanting more than two children. The arrival of their son, Jason, made it all the more clear in their family that two children would be more than enough. John described a sort of existential aching which he had become more aware of in recent months. Donating sperm brought a comfort in knowing he would have more offspring than the ones he would be fathering. He wasn't looking to parent but he was looking for a way to procreate in a safe way that didn't interfere with his daily life. He deliberately hadn't spoken to anyone about his plan to donate sperm because he feared their negative reactions. When prompted about these thoughts he admitted he was convinced his partner wouldn't understand or agree with sperm donation. John specifically chose to donate his sperm in a fertility center far removed from his home town. This suited his purpose as it would allow him to keep his donation hidden from his partner and children while still fulfilling his need to have more genetic offspring. He had thought of a plan to explain his absence from home for periodic donations as he planned them as business trips.

The fertility counselor (UV) explained the implications of anonymity (legal system at the time) and challenged John's assumptions that anonymity would mean complete privacy in light of recent advances in direct-to-consumer genetic testing. Furthermore, the fertility counselor stimulated reflection about his donation from multiple positions such as his own position as a man and a father, the possible meaning of donation for his partner and their relationship, as well as for his children and potential donor offspring. The focus was on exploring his views and anticipating the future rather than eliciting "right or wrong" answers. In this way, the fertility counselor shifted from a screening role to a supportive and guiding role that helped to clarify John's motivation and his decision-making process [3].

During the session with John, I (UV) felt unease about the lengths to which John went to keep his donation hidden from his partner and the possibility of this being very destructive for his relationship if the truth of it ever did come out. Taking the perspective of his partner, I could imagine feeling deeply betrayed and hurt by John's actions. However, listening to his narrative I could also understand his deep longing for more offspring. For John, donation made sense on an existential level. I questioned my own position and that of the team in denying him the opportunity to donate if he was aware of all risks and implications. The guiding question in the back of my mind: "Is the choice to donate for John acceptable at this point in time with the information he has now?" "Would he be able to deal with the many unknowns about future (legislative, societal, technological) issues and adapt to a possible changing culture and practice in sperm donation?"

In the multidisciplinary team meeting, the fertility counselor voiced concerns about John's donation which were based on his personal motives for procreation, how these would fit into the current practice of limitations to anonymity and in relation to his current relationship and family life. Despite the team's recommendation for transparency (about his donation to his partner) and reservations about his decision, John was allowed to choose and move forward as a sperm donor and not inform his partner, as partner consent is not obligatory. However, the counseling session helped John to become aware of the meaning of his donation in light of his own values and personal wishes that superseded being honest with his partner. Finally, the counseling session furthered John's understanding of the possible complexities for the future as a donor. Though he felt comfortable donating in an anonymous system, he was also able to take a new perspective on what this could mean for his own future as well as that of his family and offspring. I (UV) felt reassured that the implication counseling provided John with enough reflection to make an informed and balanced decision.

Final Reflections

Counseling a gamete donor and finding him/her to be an appropriate candidate feels like a "win-win" for the fertility counselor, the fertility team, the donor and the recipients. For the fertility counselors writing this chapter, and likely for most fertility counselors working in the area of egg and sperm donation, telling a donor that he/she has been "turned down" by the gamete donation program for psychological reasons is one of the most difficult aspects of the job. For the most part, the donor applicants are sincere individuals who genuinely want to help. Also, being rejected for psychological reasons feels very personal, like one's personhood, one's individuality has been negatively judged. It might even bring questions forward about their own suitability to be parents themselves. So the fertility counselor must remain mindful of both internal and external pressures to "pass" a gamete donor, and must be aware of and willing to go against these intrapersonal and interpersonal pressures.

Fertility counselors are often ideally placed to listen to and be in touch with the many "voices" that are speaking: the donors, the recipients, donor offspring, the fertility team, the counselor, society and so on. How are the "voices" and needs of all these stakeholders explicated and taken into account in our decision-making process to continue with a gamete donor? We need to have a proactive approach to clarify sometimes sensitive issues in order to be able to have a constructive and clear working alliance with potential donors. We also need to be aware and vigilant concerning the effects of our own personal values and experiences on our clinical practice. Furthermore, we need to fluidly take on different roles – screening, counseling or supporting – in the counseling working relationship and be aware of our position in the fertility team where multiple perspectives

(medical, psychological, ethical, cultural . . .) come together to make a balanced, ethically supported decision that represents the whole team, while upholding our professional integrity [3].

Finally, whatever its counter-transferential stresses, participating in the donor evaluation process can be very gratifying, and even put one in touch with some of the better aspects of human nature. As fertility counselors, it can be humbling to witness this particular kind of altruism – either as compassion for those confronted with infertility or as social engagement for nontraditional family building – and how it can make sense on a deeper level, making meaning in gamete donors' personal lives. Rarely is compensation or payment the sole driving force of a gamete donor, and our professional attunement often signals a warning "yuck" factor when the gamete donor's narrative and motivations are imbalanced. As fertility counselors, we not only have the privilege to witness these intrinsic human thoughts and behaviors but we owe it to potential donors (and donor families) to make explicit their motivations, challenge their assumptions and support them in making sure that gamete donation leaves a lasting positive imprint in their lives.

References

1. Katznelson H. Reflective functioning: a review. *Clin Psychol Rev* 2015;**34**(2):107–117.

2. Edwards AL. The relationship between the judged desirability of a trait and the probability that the trait will be endorsed. *J Appl Psychol* 1953;**37**(2):90–93.

3. Braverman AM. Mental health counseling in third-party reproduction in the United States: evaluation, psychoeducation, or ethical gatekeeping? *Fertil Steril* 2015;**104**(3):501–506.

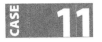
Maya Grobel and Elaine Gordon

Introduction

Elaine Gordon: I am a licensed clinical psychologist with 30-plus years working with reproductive patients and healthcare professionals. I have dedicated my career to providing patients with the tools to make informed family-building decisions. The ethics of third-party family building has always been my passion, motivated by witnessing the unique evolution of reproductive policies and patient care. As a reproductive practitioner, I utilize various treatment modalities in my practice including psychodynamic theory, cognitive-behavioral therapy, crisis intervention and more.

Maya Grobel: I am a licensed clinical social worker in private practice. After many years as a fertility patient, I became a proud parent through embryo donation, and shifted my practice to working in reproductive medicine. I take an eclectic and solution-focused approach to treatment, helping fertility patients and those building a family in alternative ways. My professional and personal experience, coupled with my desire to increase awareness and make embryo donation more accessible, prompted me to co-found EM•POWER donation, an educational organization dedicated to embryo donation.

As fertility counselors we are called upon to support both embryo donors and recipients at different stages of their journey, as well as patients who are considering various embryo donation relationship arrangements. Helping patients understand their options and the implications of them for themselves and their collective children is essential.

Most recipients and donors have struggled to conceive; however, while a potential donor has achieved success, the recipients remain in the midst of their struggle. Most embryo donors did not anticipate becoming donors and are now faced with an unanticipated dilemma – choosing among often unappealing disposition options.

Disposition options include: (1) store for future family building; (2) discard; (3) donate to science; (4) compassionate transfer; (5) donate to another for family building.

Clinics vary in their recommended counseling protocols for embryo donation arrangements. They run from no required counseling at all, to counseling throughout the journey. Counselors can be invaluable assets and provide much-needed guidance and support throughout these complex relationships. The following case illustrates many of the intricacies and issues discussed in the *Clinical Guide*, Chapter 11. The patients presented are fictional and represent a composite of common situations we have seen in our clinical practice. The case of Liz and Mike donating their excess embryos involves a number of parts in their journey which illustrate the complexities of embryo donation.

Case of Liz and Mike: Part 1

Liz and Mike went through 4 years of fertility treatments before having their twin girls via an unknown egg donor and IVF. Liz had a history of multiple pregnancy losses, a challenging pregnancy, delivered at 32 weeks via emergency cesarean section, and required a hysterectomy immediately afterwards.

The twins remained in the NICU for several weeks and Liz suffered from mild postpartum depression. After several months, the family was doing well. Just after the twins' third birthday, Liz became consumed with thinking about disposition of their remaining nine embryos (five male, four female). Prior to the start of treatment, Liz and Mike had elected to donate their embryos to science. But now, Liz couldn't fathom the prospect of destroying or donating them to science, as she now viewed them as potential children, genetic siblings to her children. Liz always dreamed of having a son and experienced despair over her inability to carry another child although, with the twins, she believed her family was complete. The more she considered the option to donate their remaining embryos to another, the more comfortable she became with the idea.

The egg donor they worked with had consented to re-donation in the initial contract but was not amenable to contact. Mike initially had other thoughts, stating he would prefer donating to science. He was uncomfortable with the idea of his genetic children being raised by other parents.

When Liz inquired about embryo donation at her clinic, she was told they only offer an "anonymous" nonidentified arrangement. The embryos would be relinquished to the clinic and distributed to multiple recipients with a one pregnancy limit, and she would have no information about the outcomes.

Unsatisfied with that option, Liz began to explore ways to donate that would give her more control. She was adamant about her daughters having access to any genetic siblings, preferring an open/known arrangement, and became overwhelmed trying to navigate the process. Her clinic nurse referred her to a fertility counselor.

Counseling Embryo Donors

Patients are asked to make an embryo disposition decision at the onset of treatment, when their focus is on family building, making it difficult to fully process the implications of donation. However, once their family is complete, and they are faced with storage fees, or storage time limits for their remaining embryos, they are forced to confront these options. Several studies have highlighted the distress this causes for patients, citing the frequency of patients changing their minds from their initial elected disposition choice [1]. This supports the need for education and counseling as it pertains to the remaining embryo decision-making dilemma [2].

Exploring the Decision to Donate

Counseling around disposition options offers potential donors the space, time and support to make an informed decision regarding their embryos. Liz and Mike needed to find a way to process their differing feelings about the remaining embryos and come to an agreement. For Liz and Mike, one of their biggest challenges appeared to be how they conceptualized their embryos, one of the most significant issues regarding disposition [3]. Liz viewed her remaining embryos as potential children, full genetic siblings to her daughters. As such, she felt a responsibility for them and their fate, a common feeling [4].

Mike was previously comfortable with donating to science or for lab training, as he did not see their embryos as potential children. But his conceptualization had shifted after becoming a father, as he now understood the potential the embryos had. Now he had difficulty imagining his genetic child(ren) being raised by other parents. The counselor had to dissect Mike's feelings about his genetic tie to them, as it seemed to play into his reluctance to donate, as opposed to Liz being more inclined to do so, a common issue for couples where only one shares a genetic link to off-spring.

Motivations for donating or not donating remaining embryos needed to be explored with the couple. In addition, the discussion included expectations of any donation arrangement, such as grief and loss around genetic relations, as well as the needs and rights of the collective

children [4]. Other topics discussed were Liz's challenging pregnancy and delivery, her fantasy about having a son, and how this might impact her relationship with potential recipients. Liz expressed interest in how other embryo donors handled these issues, and was referred to a 6-week support group to meet others in a similar situation.

Embryo Donor Support Groups

Support groups can be an effective modality for patients [3]. When facilitated by a fertility counselor, there is an opportunity to highlight the stages of decision-making, the commonality when partners are not in agreement, and multitudes of feelings, excitement and fears they may have while building community and decreasing isolation.

Case of Liz and Mike: Part 2

Liz and Mike were at a crossroads and decided to pay for another year of storage. After some time and lots of discussion, they agreed to donate their embryos in a known/directed way. Mike didn't want to participate much in the process, feeling this was more "her thing," which left Liz with little support from him.

The couple decided to put the embryo donation conversation aside for a bit and take a trip to attend Liz's twenty-fifth anniversary high school reunion. There, Liz ran into a former boyfriend, Dan, and his wife, Ella. Liz and Ella hit it off, and Ella opened up about the fertility struggles she and Dan were having. Liz's immediate reaction was to offer some of their embryos to them. Liz mentioned it to Mike on the way home, and they agreed to first meet with their fertility counselor.

Supporting the Donation Decision Process

The fertility counselor will need to pay attention not only to what is said in the room, but how the couple interacts with each other when exploring how they each feel about this arrangement, especially given that Liz and Dan had a previous romantic relationship. The counselor can highlight that Mike needs to feel comfortable with these recipients and not just agree to end the dilemma. Considering that Liz and Mike will have an open and ongoing relationship with the recipient family shows the importance of having a cohesive arrangement and an agreed-upon narrative that will support the needs of both families.

The session with the counselor focused on how they will manage ongoing relationships, the meaning of genetic relatedness, what constitutes family and the necessity of relinquishing control [5]. The counselor also helped Mike and Liz identify any deal-breakers, anticipate future challenges, and decide how many embryos they would like to donate to Ella and Dan, if they plan on having multiple recipients, and the sequential donation process for any remaining embryos.

Case of Liz and Mike: Part 3

Liz and Mike agreed to donate five embryos to Dan and Ella. They worked out the logistics for the transfer and decided that Ella and Dan would travel for the transfer since they were only a few hours away. Each couple retained their legal counsel, with Liz and Mike's attorney writing the contract. Dan and Ella met for a recipient consultation with the same fertility counselor as Mike and Liz. Ella was very excited, but Dan appeared to have some residual feelings about losing his genetic contribution to their potential child. The couple shared a long history of multiple miscarriages and rounds of IVF. They had been saving up for an egg donor cycle but knew they were at least a year away from being able to afford it.

Counseling Embryo Recipients

Recipients come to embryo donation for various reasons, though there is often a history of reproductive challenges and trauma. Fertility counselors can support patients in processing their fertility history and exploring how they will embrace nongenetic parenting. Encouraging honest communication between recipients and donors, both individually and jointly, can help set up ways to handle any conflicts that may emerge down the line.

Exploring the Fertility Journey and Embracing Becoming a Parent Through Embryo Donation

While Dan and Ella both expressed gratitude and excitement, they also had feelings of grief and loss that needed to be processed. They met with the fertility counselor a few more times, and Dan met with her individually to discuss his disappointment in postponing their original egg donation plan. Genetic loss is a common theme in donor conception arrangements and patients will need to make peace with their current situation and embrace nongenetic parenting. Of the four parties, Dan is the only one who will have no gestational or genetic tie to the child he will parent. Helping patients identify their expectations and concerns and hopes as they relate to parenting a nongenetic child can help them increase confidence in themselves as parents and begin to conceptualize this unique family-building choice.

The Joint Consultation

When a donor and recipient have matched, the fertility counselor becomes an integral part of supporting the group in discussing expectations, boundaries and communication regarding their relationship.

Helping Patients Navigate the Donor–Recipient Relationship

It is important to discuss any past relationship history as well as relationship expectations into the future. How and when to discuss their respective family-building stories with the children should also be determined. These stories will hopefully complement one another and form a cohesive narrative for both parties. In addition, different parenting styles or child-rearing philosophies should be shared and respected.

Making room for everyone's voice will be necessary as the children grow. The children must be able to express their needs and desires in the future, as there is no way to predict how these children will feel about one another and their level of interest in having an ongoing relationship

At various times, the two couples' fertility histories might impact their relationship. Knowing Liz had numerous miscarriages and a challenging pregnancy, and Ella also experienced repeated losses, may prove to be an important point of discussion. The fertility counselor may pay extra attention to potential relationship disruptions that could occur when donating within a family or to a friend. There may be a sense of added responsibility on both sides if the outcome is not successful. There may be an additional sense of loss within the relationship and the hopes that the match had for their extended "family" unit.

It's also important to note that Ella and Dan may desire some space to establish themselves as parents, and may be unsure how to best navigate the relationship with the donors. They may want to express their gratitude but need some distance to feel as though the pregnancy is their own. Addressing some of these potential feelings and concerns can help validate and normalize them for the participants. If and when things come up, they can better manage them together and communicate adaptively around difficult topics.

Case of Liz and Mike: Part 4

The consultation went well, and they proceeded with plans for the first transfer. Ella became pregnant on the first try with one of the male embryos and delivered a healthy, full-term

baby boy. Liz was happy for them but struggled with some unexpected emotions. When she shared her feelings with Mike, he became frustrated, saying, "This was your thing! Now you're regretful? It's too late!"

Liz was upset, knowing that the donation process had taken a toll on their marriage. They were busy with their twin toddlers and full-time jobs. Liz did not regret her decision but was surprised to have such mixed emotions. She scheduled a few sessions with her fertility counselor to process her unresolved feelings. Liz was able to work through her mixed emotions and felt good about the donation.

Ella and Dan did another transfer a year later and had a daughter. All the children got together at least once a month and knew each other as "special siblings." Because Liz and Mike still had four embryos ready to donate and three remaining from Ella and Dan's cycle, Liz continued to casually engage with the embryo donation Facebook page.

Liz never envisioned her fertility journey going on for so long. She decided to donate the remaining embryos so she could achieve closure and move on without having to think about embryos. She decided to post on Facebook and was flooded with inquiries from potential recipients, each with their own heartbreaking fertility story. After communicating with a number of candidates, she connected with a single woman, Ann, age 44. She was a family medicine doctor who always wanted to be a mother but never found a suitable partner. Ann appeared to be smart, thoughtful, and financially stable but lived across the country from Liz and Mike. While Liz always hoped to find recipients nearby, she felt a connection with Ann.

They scheduled a video chat during which Liz discovered that Ann is of Japanese descent, a different ethnicity than Liz and Mike, and Dan and Ella, who are all Caucasian. Liz had no issues donating to someone of a different race but wasn't sure how to talk about the apparent fact that the child would not resemble Ann in any way; she worried about how that might feel for the child. Liz also wasn't sure what to make of the fact that Ann referred to the process as embryo adoption, not donation, which raised some questions for Liz. Liz didn't know how to discuss these issues with Ann and scheduled a consultation with the fertility counselor.

A Donation Journey with a High Number of Embryos and Multiple Recipients

When there is a large batch of remaining embryos, embryo donors will often donate to multiple recipients. What this process looks like may vary depending on the individual situation, how the embryo donor is matching with recipients, and if the original donors include the first set of recipients in subsequent donations.

Matching Options

Donor and recipient matches can be made through family or friends, the clinic, a matching platform or agency, or through social media.

Embryo and Family Conceptualization Factors: Adoption or Donation

Another consideration often found in embryo donation is the different conceptualizations of the embryo and the family. Ann believed she was entering into an adoption arrangement whereas Liz was proposing a donation agreement. The American Society for Reproductive Medicine (ASRM) states that embryos have special significance compared with gametes, but should not have the same legal or moral status as persons [6]. While embryo donation is different from adoption from a legal, scientific and relational standpoint, it is not uncommon for patients to view embryo donation as an adoption and interchange the two terms. There are also several agencies that do in fact treat embryo donation as an adoption. The fertility counselor can help the parties discuss a cohesive narrative, even if there are some differences between the families.

Role of Culture, Race, Religion

A frank discussion about how culture, race and religion impact various family constellations might be relevant. Inequities continue to exist in assisted reproductive practices where there is a shortage of embryos to meet the needs of diverse populations. Because Liz expressed curiosity about how ethnic differences between Ann and the potential child will be addressed, it is important for the fertility counselor to address these issues with an emphasis on considering the potential perspective of the child.

Underserved Populations

Single people, people of color and the LGBTQIA+ communities have historically been underrepresented in embryo donation arrangements, as some embryo adoption agencies have and continue to pose limitations on who has access. Ann may feel she has a decreased chance of finding a match as a Japanese single woman and may need support from a counselor to help her ensure she is making the best choice for herself.

Multiple Recipient Dynamic

Because Ann was the second recipient, and had a different relationship history than the first couple, she may feel like an outsider, or be hesitant to get "too involved" until she knows if the pregnancy is successful. Depending on the arrangement, it may be important to incorporate and connect the different recipients and the donors. In multiple recipient arrangements, there also needs to be a point person, often the donor, who works to facilitate both the logistics as well as ongoing communication between the groups.

Case of Liz and Mike: Part 5

After Liz and Mike had several counseling sessions, they ultimately decided to donate their remaining embryos to Ann. Once the necessary psychological consultations and legal contracts were completed, the embryos were shipped to Ann's clinic for transfer.

Over several months, Ann did multiple embryo transfers with no success. With only one embryo remaining, Ann asked if Liz and Mike would be open to sending the remaining three embryos from Dan and Ella's batch, if Dan and Ella felt they wouldn't need them.

Liz had a lot of emotions to process and was hesitant to give Ann any additional embryos. Liz felt a sense of guilt that the transfers hadn't worked but also felt upset that the embryos had been "wasted," and was concerned that Ann may never successfully carry a pregnancy.

Ann met with her fertility counselor and shared how guilty she felt that none of the embryos worked and said she felt "at the end of her rope" with her family-building process. She was about to turn 45 and felt a deep sense of grief about how her life was turning out. She was afraid to tell Liz how she felt and purposefully withdrew from the relationship, feeling hopeless and depressed. Ann decided to possibly try the last transfer with a surrogate, her younger sister, who had offered to carry for her, but that had not been included in their legal contract and needed to be discussed.

Both Ann and Liz's fertility counselor suggested another joint session to help Ann and Liz reconnect and decide how they would best move forward. Just before the joint session, Liz learned that Ella and Dan's first child wasn't meeting developmental milestones. The child had been assessed at the regional center and needed further evaluation, but there appeared to be speech and language delays and some behavioral concerns. Liz brought this up in the joint session, and Ann became highly anxious.

Unexpected Challenges

Fertility counselors often provide support to clients when matches hit unexpected challenges. Both donors and recipients can feel stress at any stage of the process, whether it be a miscarriage, an interpersonal conflict, or working to integrate new genetic health information.

In this case, Ann was feeling hopeless and needed some time to explore the possibility of her sister as her carrier. Liz and Mike were feeling unsure about a surrogate being added to the mix. The additional health information known about Ella and Dan's son was a concern for all about what, if any, genetic risks the children or embryos might carry. A referral to a genetic counselor can provide additional information to Ann as well as to any other potential recipients for Liz and Mike's embryos.

Long-Term Family Support

Fertility counselors may meet a client (donor/recipient/children) years after they have either donated their embryos or have become parents through embryo donation. There are several reasons for this: they may be seeking support with how to disclose to older children, they may have initially made a decision to have an unknown arrangement and are now navigating connecting to genetic relatives, or perhaps they simply want to discuss ongoing relationship issues between parties. Children may also have different emotional needs and require professional counseling.

Reflections from the Fertility Counselor: Transference–Countertransference

In embryo donation cases, there are a number of areas where transference–countertransference issues may arise and could potentially impact the therapeutic relationship. Transference occurs when clients direct their feelings onto the clinician. Generally they are unaware they are doing so. Countertransference is when the clinician projects his/her beliefs onto the client [7]. An awareness of these potential issues must be addressed for successful, unbiased counseling.

Some fertility counselors may come to this work after having their own fertility challenges or an alternative path to parenthood. This could mean a potential for them to have personal experience with embryo donation in the form of having their own remaining embryos they are faced with having to make decisions about, or as one considering embryo donation as a family-building choice.

They may also have personal experience with gamete donation in known/directed or unknown/nonidentified arrangements, and have personal feelings about issues such as disclosure, number of genetic siblings raised in different homes, diversity in families, an adoption narrative for embryo donation, and embryo conceptualization and disposition.

Additionally, counselors who have decided to live childfree after a fertility journey may bring their own specific perspective. The distance counselors have from their own fertility journey may also play a factor, as some who have been in practice for a significant amount of time may have developed a different perspective than a clinician newer to the field with less distance from their own journey. This could manifest, for example, in a seasoned counselor having a more patient approach in supporting clients, believing that things will work out for the best in the end, while a newer counselor may feel a sense of urgency to help the clients make a decision so they can move forward in their process. It is beneficial for counselors to be keenly aware of their own fertility-related history and how it might impact their therapeutic work. It is also important to note that some therapists have no personal experience with fertility struggles or alternative family building at all, and that may factor into the therapeutic work as well.

One specific consideration that fertility counselors need to explore is their conceptualization of an embryo. Religious, spiritual, moral and ethical values may impact their feelings about embryos, and consequently their work with clients. They may have feelings about the number of excess embryos a couple creates or about how many genetic siblings raised in different homes feels appropriate to them. They may have personal beliefs about discarding or donating excess embryos to science or lab training. They may also have firm beliefs about disclosure to children and embryo donation facilitated in an "anonymous" or nondirected way without much fore-thought into the potential needs of children, and may not agree or share views with their embryo donation patients in terms of what they think is in the best interest of the client's child/family. They may have feelings about patients who seek an embryo of a different race or ethnicity without intention of exposing the child to his/her culture, and may have their own feelings about an adoption narrative in embryo donation, as many counselors are taught that the term embryo adoption is misleading and not an appropriate term, even though it is very commonly used by patients. Counselors should also note any countertransference or feelings of alignment with one party during the joint consultation, as a counselor may be facilitating a consultation in which the donors and recipients may have competing interests.

Having honest dialogue with clients and providing psychoeducation that includes best practices for children can help educate clients so they can navigate their own decision-making in a way that feels best to them. Being able to separate oneself from the decision-making process of a client is imperative for an adaptive therapeutic alliance. Seeking supervision is essential if/when these issues arise.

References

1. Klock SC, Sheinin S, Kazer RR. The disposition of unused frozen embryos. *N Engl J Med* 2001;**345**(1):69–70.

2. Christianson MS, Stern JE, Fangbai S, et al. Embryo cryopreservation and utilization in the United States from 2004–2013. *Fertil Steril* 2020;**1**(2):71–77.

3. Nachtigall RD, Becker G, Friese C, Butler A, MacDougall K. Parents' conceptualization of their frozen embryos complicates the disposition decision. *Fertil Steril* 2005;**84**(2):431–434.

4. Goedeke S, Daniels K. We wanted to choose us: how embryo donors choose recipients for their surplus embryos. *J Reprod Infant Psychol* 2018;**36**(2):132–143.

5. McMahon C, Saunders D. Attitudes of couples with stored frozen embryos toward conditional embryo donation. *In Vitro Fertilization* 2009;**91**(1):140–147.

6. Ethics Committee of the American Society for Reproductive Medicine. Defining embryo donation: an Ethics Committee opinion. *Fertil Steril* 2016;**106**(1):15–282.

7. Parth K, Datz F, Seidman C, Löffler-Stastka H. Transference and countertransference: a review. *Bull Menninger Clin* 2017;**81**(2):167–211.

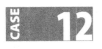

Special Considerations in Gestational Surrogacy Assessments and Arrangements

Mary Riddle and Tara Simpson

Introduction

Mary Riddle (MR): As I was working toward my doctorate in Clinical Health Psychology at Yeshiva University, I had my own struggles with infertility. My husband, Dan, and I were undergoing fertility treatments at New York Hospital with Dr. Zev Rosenwaks, who holds a very special place in our hearts given that he helped bring two of my three beautiful children into the world. I was also fortunate enough to have been counseled and supported by Dr. Laura Josephs, to whom I am also very grateful. We have three amazing children (Lilly, Nolan and Ned). Two of them were "high tech" and the third, as my husband likes to say, was "free"! I promised myself that, if I ever got through the hell that was infertility, I would devote my career to helping others along their journey.

After moving from New York to Pennsylvania, I was asked to consult on a surrogacy case that had gone awry, and that case marked the beginning of what would become the primary focus of my work in reproductive medicine. It wasn't the direction I thought my professional life would go, but as is often the case in life, we can't always predict where we will end up. My own practice as a psychologist has led me to conduct research into the questions that were raised in clinical practice – most notably in the assessment of gestational carriers (GCs), which remains a research interest.

Tara Simpson (TS): It was while finishing my coursework toward my Doctorate in Psychology that my husband and I began to try to have a baby and I found myself struggling emotionally as we transitioned into treatment. In retrospect, I realize that my journey to motherhood was shorter and less intensive than many of the clients I have met with over the course of my career, but at the time, and still upon reflection, it was the most difficult time in my life. The experience impacted me so personally that it shifted the trajectory of my professional life. I often say I would not be able to do this work if I did not go on to conceive my daughter, Lilly, and eventually complete our family with my son, Nathaniel.

While the process was difficult, I had great support from the weekly support group I attended through Resolve. Later, I would go on to be mentored, trained, collaborate and work with the editor of this book, as well as many of the authors. My own personal struggle became my own professional strength. I started a private practice, as well as became a consultant to a fertility center. As the daughter of a nurse midwife, I have grown up seeing my mother assist other women during the pregnancy and delivery of several thousand babies. It has been in the fabric of my life to see how another person can transform and assist individuals and couples in achieving a family. It is still striking, yet humbling, to find myself in a similar role.

In this chapter, we present a series of cases that encompass a number of the issues covered in our *Clinical Guide* chapter. Between us, we have conducted hundreds of gestational surrogacy arrangements (GSAs). In preparing this chapter, we have collaborated, and include compilations of cases where identifiers have been removed. The cases correspond with clinical chapter topics including the role and competence of the fertility counselor in a GSA, their role and competence in psychological testing, and representations of what we consider to be common challenges that we have faced in regard to relationships, expectations and vulnerabilities. These cases represent de-identified elements of cases that we have worked on but represent no case in its entirety. We tried to pick elements that we have struggled with and learned from and hope that you find these professionally valuable.

Role and Competence of Fertility Counselors in Gestational Surrogacy Arrangements

TS: Several years ago, I was pulled into a case that had gotten extremely complicated. The history of the case that I inherited was as follows: a therapist, who did not specialize in fertility counseling, had been asked to evaluate a potential GC and conduct the intended parent (IP) meeting. The therapist met with the potential GC and the content of the interview centered on the GC's past and present psychological functioning only. In the end, the therapist submitted a one-page report, omitting any recommendation as to if the arrangement should move forward or not. The fertility doctor, seeking more information than what was provided before moving forward with the arrangement, referred the couple and their GC to me. The IP patient, frustrated about having to undergo (and pay for) the evaluation again, stated "why do any of you get to decide if we can be parents?"

As a fertility counselor, any GSA evaluation is complex. My inheritance of a case that had been conducted by an unqualified practitioner, combined with a defensive IP, made it more challenging. The situation made me uncomfortable and frustrated, yet I was anchored in my confidence that I could competently assess this arrangement. The damage that can be done if one is not well trained during any component of GSA is significant and being tasked with "cleaning it up" is even more difficult.

A fertility counselor has a responsibility of making a recommendation based on their expertise and the data obtained from all participants. Professionals may be uncomfortable stating their opinion, particularly if it delays or negates an arrangement, due to worries of upsetting patients or disrupting the plans of an agency, attorney or fertility center. While not stating a decision is problematic, one of the most challenging aspects of the GSA arrangement is the perception by others that a fertility counselor serves only as a gatekeeper to another person's pursuit of parenthood. When I find myself starting to believe the narrative that I am "squashing someone's dreams to be a parent or GC" I will remind myself that I have many other roles in this scenario.

When I am challenged on the purpose of the evaluation by patients, I will reply that the IPs can eventually become a family, but the necessary time has to be put in to have the crucial conversations about how they envision achieving this goal. I will also remind the clients that I have the training and skill set to help them become a family in the best possible way- not that my role is to decide who gets to become a family. When a case is not recommended to move forward, it isn't always a "no," but is often "not this way." I remind myself, as well as the IPs, "This is the start of your child's story . . . let's make it the best one it can be."

In this particular case, I spent a great deal of time aligning with the IPs' resistance and reflecting their feelings of frustration, lack of control, fear, and disappointment at the additional time and expense that was perceived to be occurring. It was also important to continue to educate the IPs on the purpose and importance of all aspects of the GSA evaluation process. It was essential that I clarified and reiterated that it was not my job to decide who could be parents but to help all parties enter into an arrangement that will be positive for all.

Once the IPs were able to acknowledge that the goal of a competent evaluation is to protect participants, they were much more open to the process. I met with all parties, conducted all aspects of the evaluation, and recommended that the arrangement move forward based on the thorough review and exploration of the necessary content and considerations inherent in the GSA standard of care. I was grateful that some important and powerful conversations stemmed from the evaluation, which several members of the arrangement had not carefully considered in the previous evaluation. The participants were now ultimately able to be fully discuss all pertinent aspects of a GSA leading to a solid informed consent of all parties as well as deeper communication as they moved forward.

Role and Competence of Fertility Counselors in Psychological Testing

MR: I was asked to facilitate a group meeting for some IPs and a GC. As is my usual practice, I asked the fertility counselor, who had done the psychological assessment, to send over her report. This was a fertility counselor who was new to the field and I didn't know her very well. In the report, the testing results were noted to be within normal limits and unremarkable. When I met with all the parties, I was struck by the interpersonal style of the GC, whom I found to be abrasive and difficult. I became concerned about the interpersonal dynamics of the group. The GC and IPs had already met and "loved" each other, and everyone was ready to check this last component off the list and be on their way.

I decided to review the raw test data and I was told that the fertility counselor had "cleared" the GC based only on the computerized summary and had never really looked at the data separately. She told me that because the protocol was "valid" and that there were no clinical elevations, she had no reservations. I scored the GC's PAI myself and, when I made my own interpretations, it appeared that, while the PAI was "technically" within normal limits, there was scale suppression due to positive impression management (PIM) and the scales that appeared to be suppressed were DOM (Dominance), BOR (Borderline), and PAR (Paranoid). I felt that this was not a GC I would have "cleared" but wasn't sure what I could do this late in the process. I felt intense frustration at the fact that, despite all the work that has been done to educate newcomers to the field about the importance of competence in testing, this fertility counselor had not done her due diligence in terms of interpreting the results and now the arrangement was in big trouble.

I voiced my concerns to all parties, including the fertility clinic. The IPs insisted on using this GC and moved forward with the transfer. The GC became pregnant and, initially, things went smoothly. Sadly, the arrangement fell apart over time and, although the GC delivered a healthy baby, the parties did not speak to each other for the majority of the pregnancy due to a falling out over miscommunication and the GC's perception that the IPs were somehow "out to get her." The perceived incident was quite trivial, but the warning signs were in the testing.

Common Challenges in Gestational Surrogacy Arrangement Participant Management

TS: I was contacted by an IP of a GSA that I had cleared 4 years prior. The IPs were moving forward again with the same GC who had given birth to their daughter, although they would be working with a different fertility center. The IP requested that my previous report be forwarded to the fertility center to satisfy their "clearance" for the upcoming cycle. I let the IPs know that I would need to meet with all parties again to update the evaluation. The IP informed me that they were in a rush, since the GC and IP mother had both started medication for the cycle and the transfer was scheduled. At the time of the inquiry for the report, my schedule was booked out a few weeks and I would not be able to accommodate all of the appointments in the time frame they were requesting. Exasperated with the difficulty in scheduling and having to be reassessed, the IPs informed me that the GC had moved out of state, therefore requesting to have all the sessions completed via telehealth since "that can be scheduled anytime."

When clients request components of the evaluation to be omitted, rushed, or outside the standard practice for my profession, it pulls up feelings of frustration and guilt. The request to "cut corners" may lead to feeling defensive and thinking as if my work is not valued. At the same time, I will catch myself sympathizing with the clients and questioning the fee (is it too high?), the time (is it too much time?), and the formality of the consults (is it necessary?). When I begin to doubt the boundaries and the protocol, I run the risk of aligning with the client's skepticism regarding the entire process. In addition, discomfort about being perceived as "the bad guy" may also materialize, which in actuality feels like the antithesis to my intent to be in the field in the first place.

In this case, despite the fact that the participants know each other and had a great prior experience, it does not signify their current readiness to embark on the process again. I framed updating the evaluation as an opportunity to revisit what worked, what they would change, and what they learned. An anchor to my work is one of protection of all parties and if you set boundaries with that goal in mind it helps the participants feel secure in the purpose of the assessment. Ultimately, I utilized the existing relationship that I had with all participants and their trust in my ability to help them navigate their previous surrogacy journey by stating that the second arrangement needs just as much care as the first. In addition, I emphasized that although this arrangement involved all the same participants, that this journey is during a different time, and with a different proximity to one another following the move of the GC. Once I set the boundary for the participants, they were much more open to taking the time to talk about their visions for this second pregnancy. Despite the initial rush and hesitancy to talk again, all parties were enthusiastic and open to the process, which resulted in great discussion and confirmation that all parties were ready to move forward – just as much as they were the first time.

Relationships, Expectations, Vulnerabilities

MR: I was contacted by an agency and asked if I would be able to provide several sessions of psychotherapy to a GC whom I had not assessed, but who was struggling after her delivery. The GC told me that, going into the arrangement, she had wanted more children, but wasn't ready for them yet. The GC entered the GSA both with high expectations about this adventure and trust in the relationship with the IPs. The GC became pregnant with twins and initially the IPs were very attentive. The GC went into labor early, required an emergency cesarean section, and because of complications, an emergency hysterectomy post-birth. The hospital couldn't contact the IPs because they had gone out of town and, because this hospital had never had a GC birth before, told the GC that they couldn't honor the birth plan and she never saw the babies. The hospital discharged the GC and she went home devastated and confused. She finally heard from her agency that the IPs had ultimately shown up 3 days after the birth to take the babies home. The GC never heard from them again. It was no surprise that she was slipping into a clinical depression.

This case represents everything I worry about going into a GSA assessment. There was clearly a number of issues that hadn't been addressed prior to the outset of this GSA: the GC's desire for more children; provision of education in order for the GC to provide fully informed consent and weigh the risks of a pregnancy on her future family plans; expectations on both sides for communication and future contact; and confirmation that a birth plan was in place. I was coming in at a point where it was too late to do any of these things and I had to work to set aside my assessment hat and focus on the task at hand, damage control and helping the GC process the many layers of grief inherent in this arrangement. This included the grief of the loss of the idealized vision of this pregnancy, the loss of the relationship with the IPs, as well as the loss of her uterus and hopes to expand her own family. It was also important to help the GC process the inevitable anger over feeling used and manipulated, as well as the anger she felt that neither she nor her own children ever got to see the babies. This case stays with me and reminds me of how important it is for all of us to hold each other accountable for competent ethical practice in this field.

MR: I was called by another fertility counselor to provide consultation on a case in which the family of a GC was struggling. The fertility counselor had evaluated a GSA and, having no concerns, "cleared" the arrangement to move forward. Per ASRM guidelines, the fertility counselor had interviewed the GC, made sure to ask about the GC's own children, and that the GC and her partner had considered their own children in their decision. The GC assured the fertility counselor that she had spoken to her children and that they "loved" the idea of their mother being a GC. She and her partner stated that they had had open conversations with their children, and that they would continue to talk with them moving forward, answering questions in an age-appropriate way.

Several months later, the fertility counselor learned that the GC was in a panic because her child's school called her and told her that her son (who was a first grader) had started to exhibit signs of anxiety and had developed a nervous tic. When the GC went to talk with the little boy, he burst into tears and asked her if she was going to give him away if he was bad. She tried to assure him that, no, of course she wouldn't do that, but he was inconsolable. The fertility counselor met with the GC and her husband, and carefully asked about the process by which they had shared the news of the surrogacy with their son. It turned out that the GC had not told her son about it until after her pregnancy was showing and simply told him she was "having a baby and giving it to some nice people."

In consultation, we talked about the lack of focus in our field on families of GC's and the limited amount of research we have to guide our discussions with GCs about the impact of surrogacy on their families. My own research has shown me that there is a tendency toward idealization of the process and even that GCs sometimes over-estimate the degree to which their own children feel positively about their mother being a surrogate. The fertility counselor had become very anxious about the case and worried that she did something "wrong" and that she would get a bad reputation and lose work. We talked about the fact that our role is multi-faceted and, rather than panic about her future referrals, she needed to focus on helping this family through this crisis. The fertility counselor met with the GC and her husband and provided counseling with the family to help prepare the little boy on what he could expect through the process. The fertility counselor also began to provide GCs with articles and literature to help facilitate these conversations and encouraged parents to have discussions often and early about their plans for surrogacy as well as to involve their children, if possible.

Gestational Surrogacy Arrangements: Specific Dilemmas

TS: A matched GC has been treated for depression symptoms with an antidepressant medication for 5 years. She has been stable and reports overall positive well-being. The GC stated during the consult with me that she plans to wean off her medication in preparation for the upcoming cycle "because it is the right thing to do. I took it with my two pregnancies, but I can't do that for this couple . . . they have waited too long for a baby." The IPs state, "We don't care if she stays on her medicine since is there really any harm? We have waited so long for a good match."

It is often the disagreements and conflict that arises that serve as "red flags" in a GSA assessment. However, it is also in the agreeability and the compromises that each stakeholder attempts, where potential problems may also occur. This case was a challenge since each party was trying to "please" the other party, but in actuality the acquiescing can highlight blind spots or introduce other potential complexities the parties are working to avoid in the first place. Each stakeholder needs to have informed consent about any of the decisions that are to be made by the other. I found myself in a position of wanting to protect each of the parties in this scenario. More specifically, I wanted to make sure the GC was emotionally healthy to embark on this new type of pregnancy, and to be aware of what would be her baseline emotions after she stopped taking medication. I wanted the IPs to speak to their OB so that they have full informed consent of what antidepressant medication can impact a fetus and baby. Often parties feel the demand to be gratifying to the other and, in the attempt to be agreeable, it can actually result in different and difficult problems.

Ultimately, the GCs and IPs did their research and both parties felt comfortable with the GC tapering off medication. The stipulation of this was that I, along with the GC's psychiatrist, wanted her to be off of the medicine for 6 months before moving forward with the arrangement, and with the stipulation that she would resume medicine (and have therapy options) if any mood issues surfaced during pregnancy or postpartum. All parties thought that the well-being of the GC and the arrangement were worth the extra time and the GSA eventually did move forward with all parties' well-being, right to information, and mutual preservation of the relationship intact.

MR: An agency called and told me that a GC, who had been matched to a gay couple, was having cold feet and wanted to pull out of a GSA because her family disapproved of gay marriage and homosexuality in general. The agency asked if I could "talk to her." My sense was that this agency wanted me to convince the GC to move forward so that the arrangement would not fall apart. I saw the need to clarify my role and told the agency that I was willing to meet with the GC so that she would have space to talk through her feelings, but that I had no agenda and that my role was not to "convince" her of anything. I made it clear that my role was not to provide input that would influence any of the parties' decisions. I made an appointment with the GC and her husband. I gave her space to talk about her feelings and she felt certain she could not proceed because she felt she would have to lie to her friends and family about carrying a baby for a gay couple.

We arranged a group meeting with my expectation being that the GC would tell the IPs she could not move forward with the arrangement. As the conversation went on, I was really struck by the compassion and respect that the IPs had for her and the depth of their understanding at her predicament, particularly in light of the fact that the sole reason she didn't want to move forward was because they were gay. She felt she would have to lie to her family and didn't feel that she could tolerate that. The IPs then said that they understood what it was like to live a lie (prior to coming out) and that they would never ask anyone else to do that. I was deeply touched by the conversation. I am Catholic and know that my own church doesn't recognize surrogacy as a valid family-building option, which is something I have had to reconcile within myself. I have my own feelings and beliefs about the rights of gay couples to build families. The IPs were devastated by the fact that they might lose their surrogate, but also were not going to push her into doing something that she felt any discomfort with. I found myself holding back my desire to tell her she would be lucky to work with this couple and I tried to sit still in my role of holding space for this conversation. The arrangement ultimately moved forward with positive outcomes all around. My feelings are that the opportunity to come together for the purpose of open and honest communication played a key role in the success of this arrangement.

Conclusion

We present these cases not to frighten or discourage practitioners who want to do this work, but to present the very real and complex nature of these evaluations. They are fraught with legal and ethical pitfalls, and clinicians should not jump into these types of assessment without a great deal of knowledge, training, experience, consultation and supervision. We must hold each other to the highest standards of our field and recognize the vulnerabilities of all parties: GCs who have a deep desire to help someone build their family and IPs who may have suffered great losses on their fertility journey. Coupled with that are the professional pressures clinicians face from agencies, lawyers, physicians and sometimes even the parties themselves. Stakes are high in these types of evaluations and, in our opinion, they pose the greatest liability risks in our field. We hope our past experiences and challenges will help and guide you in your professional pursuits.

DNA and the End of Anonymity: Disclosure, Donor-Linkage and Fertility Counseling

Kate Bourne

Introduction

I am a social worker who has worked in the fertility field in Melbourne, Australia since 1991. I was attracted to this area as my parents had struggled to conceive. I initially worked at IVF units where I developed a particular interest in donor conception issues. I became particularly interested in donor linking so moved to the Victorian Assisted Reproductive Treatment Authority (VARTA) to develop expertise in this area. As the manager of the Donor Register Services, I led a team of counselors who supported and connected donor-conceived people, parents and donors. I am a member and past Chair of the Australian and New Zealand Infertility Counsellors Association and participated in the development of donor-linking guidelines for professional practice. I now work privately, specializing in working with clients who have had direct-to-consumer DNA testing and the implications for them.

In the following case study, all names used are fictitious and are loosely based on real life scenarios. All identifying information has been changed and does not represent any one person but rather common issues. I will be using the term *donor siblings* to refer to people who are conceived by the same donor but raised in different recipient families. They are usually genetic half-siblings unless donor embryos were used. The term *"siblings" or "sisters/brothers"* will be used to refer to people raised in the same recipient family. They may be full genetic siblings or genetic half-siblings if a different donor was used.

Deborah: The Discovery of Being Donor-Conceived

Deborah, a 42-year-old cisgender Caucasian female, who is married with three children, contacted a fertility counselor after learning that her father couldn't possibly be her biological dad. She had taken a direct-to-consumer DNA test which had been given to her as a birthday present by a friend. She grew up knowing her dad, who had died 5 years ago, and was proud of his Scottish and Greek heritage. However, the DNA test came back with no Scottish or Greek connection, but a strong Danish link. Deborah asked her 74-year-old mother to explain the results, but she wouldn't discuss it and said that the DNA testing was bunkum.

Deborah naturally felt quite confused. Had her mother had an affair? Was she adopted or perhaps donor-conceived? She has a younger brother, David. Where did he fit in? Deborah enlisted the help of a 'DNA Search Angel' to delve deeper. Search angels are people who understand the intricacies of DNA testing results and who volunteer to assist people to understand DNA results and/or to help them to identify genetic relatives. They do this by analyzing DNA results from matches identified (even if they are matches to distant cousins), analyzing family trees posted on the DNA sites and then cross referencing this with publicly available information on social media etc.

The Search Angel was able to:

- Find a genetic half-sister, Judy (37 years), whose father was likely to have been a sperm donor and that Deborah was one of his donor offspring.
- Identify and locate Robert, who was also a genetic half-brother and was likely to have been conceived by the same donor.
- Confirm that her brother, David was likely to have been conceived by a different donor as there were no links for David to the matches she had.

Deborah turned to the fertility counselor feeling a deep sadness and rage that her mother hadn't told her about her conception, either growing up, or again when she was asked directly. This issue, however, was almost subsumed by the broader implications of the new information.

Issues to Examine in Counseling Following Discovery

Identity – Who Am I?

The fertility counselor helped Deborah to process this new information and unpack what this meant for her, allowing her to vent her anger and frustration. Deborah was experiencing a typical grief reaction; however, this was a messy, complex, intangible grief with the added difficulty of not being able to discuss it with her parents. It was as if the person she thought she was had altered fundamentally, since the foundations of who she thought she was had been undermined. Who was she now if her late father was no longer her biological parent, as she had believed? Who was her "real" dad? It felt like nothing, yet everything, had changed. It also affected her sense of belonging and cultural identity, as she had a totally different cultural heritage than what she had assumed.

The counselor advised her that she was likely to experience a range of feelings including numbness, disbelief, anger and sadness. The counselor provided a safe space that allowed Deborah to express her feelings of frustration and betrayal, while reassuring her that what she was experiencing was normal.

What Makes a Parent?

The fertility counselor explored with Deborah themes of "nature versus nurture," and "what makes a family." She reassured Deborah that her dad was still her dad as he was the one who loved and raised her and had done the "dadding." Her donor was her biological father but hadn't nurtured her. He was, however, very significant as she was likely to have inherited some physical and other characteristics. She was a product of both her dad's nurturing and her donor's genetics. This was a complex synthesis for Deborah to process, especially as she wasn't able to talk to her dad. She was encouraged to perhaps visit his grave, write a letter (or journal her feelings) and tell him that she loved him regardless.

The new information began to feel more comfortable and make more sense to Deborah as she recalled strangers had previously asked whether she had Scandinavian heritage. She also was taller than anyone else in the family, had blue eyes, and was more academic. She also felt she was quite dissimilar to her brother in appearance, interests and personality. Perhaps this was partly explained by their different donors?

Deborah grappled with the issue of what her relationship with her dad's family would be now, given that they weren't genetically connected? Would they continue to love her and want to see her? Did they know? Did she want them to find out? Deborah acknowledged that if her cousins had been conceived by a donor, she would still consider them family and want to continue to have contact and would prefer to know.

Peer Support

To feel less alone and isolated, the counselor suggested she consider reaching out for peer support, for example, join a Facebook or Reddit group for donor-conceived people. Others in the group were likely to have had very similar experiences and could support and mentor her [2,3].

Historical Context of Past Donor Conception Practice

The counselor explained the history and context of donor conception treatment so Deborah could appreciate what her parents were likely to have experienced at the time they had treatment. They were probably advised by their doctor not to tell her about her conception. And her dad may have feared that if she knew, she might distance herself from him. Many mothers also kept the secret in order to protect their husbands. This information was provided to give context around the decision not to tell rather than to excuse or support that decision.

Immediate Family Relationships: Who Knows What About Whom?

While Deborah acknowledged the possible reasons and circumstances for not being informed, she continued to feel too angry to speak to her mother. The counselor suggested she write and explain:

- She was now aware she was conceived by a donor as a result of the DNA testing;
- She understood her parents' decision to have donor treatment but was finding it difficult to accept that they had not told her;
- She continued to love her mother;
- Her dad would always be her dad;
- She needed her mother's support and understanding, and to be able to talk with her;
- It was important for her brother to be told;
- That she was aware that he had been conceived by a different donor;
- They meet to talk soon; and
- Her mother see her fertility counselor or another fertility counselor, either alone or with Deborah.

Parental Issues

After receiving the email, Dianne, Deborah's mother, contacted the fertility counselor. Dianne was devasted that Deborah had discovered her conception status. She felt guilty that she had inadvertently caused her distress. She felt angry and betrayed because the clinic had assured her and her husband that their children would never find out and that the same donor had been used for both children. It also triggered feelings of grief over her husband's death and sterility diagnosis. She felt protective of his memory and concerned he would be "turning in his grave" if he knew that Deborah was aware of their secret.

The couple hadn't discussed the issue since her pregnancy and decided never to tell anyone …. Their daughter's discovery reactivated feelings which hadn't been dealt with since treatment. Talking now about this sensitive issue was extremely challenging.

These uncomfortable emotions and renewed grief needed to be explored and worked through. The counselor helped to reframe Dianne's feelings of shame and stigma into the courage, commitment and love which had enabled them to decide to have their children another way. Dianne's feelings of guilt over unintentionally hurting her daughter were channelled to what she could do now to support her.

Disclosure

Dianne was initially reluctant to tell David. Only after the issues were unpacked, did the counselor explore talking to David including:

- *Why tell?* – It was now impossible to keep the secret, as David could make the same discovery if he had DNA testing, or Deborah might decide to tell him. Also, the importance of David knowing the truth was discussed, as this was *his* information.
- *When to tell?* – Choosing a time when David had privacy.
- *Who?* Should David's partner be present? Should Deborah?
- *Where to talk?* – Considering where David would feel most relaxed.
- *What to say?* What words to use and how to convey the story as clearly, gently and succinctly as possible.
- *Resources:* Dianne was encouraged to contact the clinic to try to get David's donor profile information and given educational resources for both she and David [3,4].
- *Support:* Provide David with the contact details of fertility counselors and peer support.

Dianne had at times found keeping the pact was a burden as it was not in her nature to be dishonest, and it had felt like lying. It may be a relief to tell the truth and it was impossible to keep the pact she had made to her husband.

Dianne was very concerned about her children having contact with the donor or other donor-offspring. The fertility counselor gently challenged her that it was time to pass the baton on. She and her husband had made a decision that felt right for them; her children now needed to make the decisions that were appropriate for them. Being conceived by a donor had implications that they may need to explore. Also, if her children chose to find out more about their donors in the future, this was not because she or her husband had failed in any way as

parents, but instead a natural and normal curiosity. It was important that she support them in whatever they chose to do.

Dianne then decided to tell David. He in turn contacted the fertility counselor to help him come to terms with processing this new information. The two siblings had very different reactions to finding out. Perhaps because his mother had told him in a loving, supportive way, David was less angry than Deborah. David however struggled to come to terms with the fact that he and Deborah were not full genetic siblings. Whilst they loved each other, they were very different and had a history of some sibling conflict.

The fertility counselor had family sessions with Deborah, Dianne and David and, given the contact with all three individually and in family sessions, it was important to:

- Remain neutral;
- Maintain strict confidentiality with each family member; and
- Be clear about the boundaries of the counseling contact.

Curiosity About the Donor and Donor Siblings

As time went on, Deborah became increasingly interested to know more about the two donor relatives that she had matched with on the DNA testing site: Robert (donor-brother) and Judy (donor's daughter). She was also curious to learn more about her donor. Were there medical issues she should be concerned about? Were they alike in any way? Why did he donate? Does he ever think about the people he helped create? She was conflicted however, since her brother and mother had concerns about her making contact. She wondered how her dad might feel if he were alive. She found the Facebook/Reddit groups helpful to ask others about this and learned of possible outcomes of contact, both positive and negative. She also learned from the fertility counselor that she may have many more donor siblings if her donor's donation had been used many times. This was most unsettling for her.

David, however, had no desire whatsoever to find out more about his donor or any donor siblings he may have, or to contact them. He also chose not to contact the peer support groups. Indeed, he felt this was inappropriate and couldn't understand Deborah's interest in doing so.

The fertility counselor assured both Deborah and David that each was entitled to make choices that were right for them and to not impose their personal decision or views on the other. She tried to reassure Deborah that it was important she do what she needed to do. Any contact or relationship that she might potentially have with donor relatives would be entirely different from the relationship she had built up over a lifetime with her dad and brother. It was likely to be challenging to contact them, however, as she didn't know whether Robert knew he was donor-conceived nor whether Judy knew her dad was a donor. Were they already in contact with each other? What if she was the one to inform them whilst at the same time, she was a genetic relative? Could this negatively impact on the chance of a positive connection?

Donor Linking: Assisting to Contact Donor Relatives

Half-Siblings

The fertility counselor discussed with Deborah the potential implications and outcomes of contacting Robert and Judy and teased out what ideally Deborah wanted to occur in the short and long term. The counselor encouraged her to contact one person at a time rather than simultaneously as the latter may feel overwhelming. She suggested Deborah first contact the person she was most interested in talking to. Deborah decided that she may potentially have more in common with Robert. If Robert wasn't already in contact with Judy, then perhaps he may be interested in contacting her together. Contacting the donor was also discussed, but Deborah was more interested in genetic half-siblings at this stage.

Deborah welcomed assistance from the fertility counselor in crafting a message for Robert explaining she had matched with him on the DNA site and asking him if he knew how they may be related. As it turned out, Robert had been raised by a single mother and knew early on that he was donor-conceived. He was an only child, so the news of a genetic sibling was exciting to learn, especially as this was the first contact he had with a donor-related peer. He reached out to Deborah, and both started an intense message exchange. They found many similarities in personality and appearance.

The Donor's Daughter

Coincidentally, Judy reached out to Deborah simultaneously. She was unaware how they may be related. Deborah suggested she talk to her dad. He denied any knowledge of how they could be connected. Deborah then gently told Judy she thought her dad had been a sperm donor. Judy subsequently put this idea to her dad, who grudgingly confirmed that he had donated

when he was a university student. Deborah also put Judy in contact with Robert. Like Deborah and Robert, Judy felt potentially overwhelmed at the prospect of having many donor siblings who may have been conceived from her dad's donation. Nevertheless, Judy found the contact positive, since she and Robert had some similar interests, personality traits and looked alike.

Deborah and Robert were very interested to know more about their biological father. They preferred contacting him directly, rather than via Judy, as they didn't want to put her in a difficult position. Robert wanted to reach out as soon as possible, whilst Deborah was more conflicted, as her mother and brother still weren't supportive of this contact. They decided to ask the fertility counselor for guidance.

Contacting the Donor

The fertility counselor prepared Deborah and Robert for all possible outcomes and helped them to manage their expectations. Given the donor's previous reluctance to explain the DNA match to his daughter, he may not be open to sharing information with them. If the donor was potentially open to information exchange/contact, what ideally would they like to achieve? They were advised to go slowly and carefully, proceeding at the pace of Deborah, the slower of the pair.

She suggested they send a registered letter marked *private and confidential*, so it could be tracked, and they would know whether it was delivered. Or, if they preferred to email the donor, she recommended they request a delivery receipt. The fertility counselor also provided emotional support, as it takes courage to reach out.

With the counselor's help, they drafted a letter to include the following:

- How the donor-siblings had verified their connection and the donor's identity;
- Acknowledging that the donor donated anonymously, so may not be expecting to be contacted;
- Awareness of the potential implications for him and his family;
- Clarification that they don't perceive him as a dad;
- Reassurance that they were respectful of him and his privacy;
- The offer to have DNA testing to confirm their genetic relationship; and
- The offer of confidential support from their fertility counselor.

Personal letters of introduction written by Deborah and Robert, with photos of each, were put in separate envelopes so the donor had control over if/when to look at them. In the individual letters they were encouraged by the fertility counselor to:

- Give a brief introduction including their age, interests, personality, occupation, and brief overview of their life and family situation;
- Use their own voice and write informally;
- Be clear about what information they would like to know;
- Explain how they would prefer to communicate initially, and what they would like to occur in the longer term if the donor was potentially interested in contact.

For examples of letters to donors, see reference [5].

Donor Issues

After receiving the letters, the donor and his partner contacted the fertility counselor. They raised the following concerns:

- Possible claims on their estate;
- The donor-conceived siblings may be needy, unduly intrusive or have a serious mental illness;
- Where does the donor's partner fit in?
- Telling their other children about the donation; and
- Concerns about the potential emotional impact on their family.

The fertility counselor was able to explore their concerns, assure them that donor-conceived people don't have a claim to a donor's estate. She assured them that Deborah and Robert were respectful, sensitive to their feelings, were not seeking inappropriate levels of contact, were psychologically healthy, and that curiosity was normal, healthy and to be expected. She also supported the donor's partner and reassured her that it was important that she and her husband face this together as it impacted their family. Her partner had donated before he met her, so he hadn't been unfaithful or deceitful. He would of course have a different relationship with donor-offspring than he would with the children they had had together. The counselor helped prepare them to talk to their two other adult children. The counselor also suggested that they and their children may potentially enjoy contact, as donor offspring are often "chips off the old block" with similarities in personality and interests.

The donor, with the help and support of his wife, eventually wrote a warm and friendly reply. All parties were supported by the fertility counselor in the early stages of connecting. They chose to initially communicate via email, then have phone contact, then video chats, before eventually meeting. The couple also told their two other children. They, like Judy, took the news well, with one choosing to have contact.

The donor was aware that other donor offspring may contact him in the future, however he was unaware of how many people had been conceived from his donation. He was very positive about the contact with Deborah and Robert but what if future contact with others wasn't as good? How would he manage multiple people contacting him? What if he had dementia or had died before they tried to get in touch with him? Whilst he felt a sense of responsibility to them, he was unsure how he could practically manage many contacts. He was encouraged by the fertility counselor to put together a folder of information that was likely to be of interest including medical information, family tree, photos, and a personal letter explaining why he had donated and describing his life, personality and interests. It was also suggested he may like to make a short video so his offspring could hear his voice and see his mannerisms. He was also encouraged to recontact the counselor if he needed support or if any exchanges were not going as he hoped.

Time Will Tell . . .

Deborah continued to need support from the fertility counselor, especially in the early stages of donor linkage as she explored the meaning of these new genetic relatives and their place in her life. The counselor was able to support her to go at her own pace and to not feel pressured to do anything which made her feel uncomfortable. As contact is currently in the initial phase, this will be an ongoing process over time. Deborah may need ongoing counseling to continue to process the implications of being donor-conceived, with potential contact with many genetic relatives. It is quite likely that she may feel closer to some more than others. She may change her mind about future connections if she finds it too time consuming or emotionally complex to have contact. Time will tell whether she decides to have continued communication with either her donor, his children and her donor siblings and whether she will regard them as friends, family or clan or a combination of each. Ultimately this will depend on whether they like each other and want to spend time together.

References

1. Australian and New Zealand Infertility Counsellors Association. ANZICA Guidelines for Professional Standards of Practice: Donor Linking Counselling. Available at: www.fertilitysociety.com.au/pr

ofessional-groups-anzica-australia-new-zealand/ [last accessed June 19, 2022].

2. Donor Conception and IVF: Books for Children. Blog written by Patricia Sarles MA, MLS, MSEd. Available at: http://book sfordonoroffspring.blogspot.com/2009/04/sometimes-it-takes-three-to-make-baby.html [last accessed June 19, 2022].

3. We are Donor Conceived Facebook Group, 2.4 k members. Available at: www.facebook.com/groups/wearedonorcon ceived [last accessed June 19, 2022].

4. Reddit Group. Donor conceived: a place for those conceived through gamete donation. 1.7 k members. Available at: www .reddit.com/r/donorconceived/ [last accessed June 19, 2022].

5. Donor Conception Network. Available at: www .dcnetwork.org/products/product/telling-and-talking-17-yrs [last accessed June 19, 2022].

6. Donor Conception Network. Available at: www .dcnetwork.org/who-are-you/donor-conceived-person/que stions [last accessed June 19, 2022].

7. We Are Donor Conceived. Available at: www .wearedonorconceived.com/personal-stories/dear-donor/ [last accessed June 19, 2022].

CASE 14 Family Life After Donor Conception

Jane Ellis, Marilyn Crawshaw and Astrid Indekeu

Introduction

Jane Ellis: I trained as a social worker and have worked in child protection, fostering, adoption and post-adoption services. As a parent to two children through donor conception, I joined Donor Conception Network (DCN) at its formation in 1993. I served as a Trustee for a number of years and have been DCN's Workshop Manager since 2011, developing the content of a range of workshops for those considering donor conception (DC), parents of donor-conceived children and professionals working in the fertility field. I also co-authored a DCN publication *Continuing the Conversation* for parents of older children. I hold a related counseling qualification and, from 2003, have worked as a counselor for both UK Registers supporting DC adults and donors.

Marilyn Crawshaw: Now an Honorary Fellow at University of York, UK, I have had an interest in the lifespan effects of DC and surrogacy since the 1980s, variously as a social worker, social work academic, researcher, policy adviser and lay Human Fertilisation & Embryology Authority (HFEA) inspector. I have related experience in maternity, children's, adoption and post-adoption services. From 2003 to 2013, I was national adviser to UK DonorLink, a government-funded DNA-based voluntary Register for adults genetically related through DC (now the DC Register). I chair PROGAR (www.basw.co.uk/progar/) which comprises UK organizations and individuals with shared relevant interests. In this capacity, I have regular contact with DCN (and contribute to their "Preparation for Parenthood" workshops), parents and donors, as well as DC adults.

Astrid Indekeu: After working for a decade as a clinical psychologist with children and their families on (academic) pediatric wards, and an internship in an academic fertility clinic for a Masters in Sexology, I was drawn into the field of donor conception in 2008. Since then, I have been active as a qualitative researcher exploring the experiences of intending parents, donor-conceived people and donors in different legal systems and cultures. As a clinical psychologist/researcher, I always seek to transfer and integrate research results into clinical practice.

With grateful thanks to Olivia Montuschi for her valuable contribution to this chapter.

I am currently active as an independent researcher and clinical psychologist with a private practice specialized in questions regarding donor conception. I also chair POINT, the Belgian–Dutch fertility counselors organization and work closely with the Belgian donor conception families consumer group.

Background

This chapter focuses on two forms of assistance – workshops and one-to-one support – offered by the Donor Conception Network (DCN) that many parents find helpful as they form and grow their families through donor conception (DC). These approaches aim to strengthen parental confidence and help parents develop skills for supporting their children, as views and understanding of DC unfold over the years. The interplay between professional and peer support is key to the success of these interventions. Case presentations are fictitious, representative of common issues and concerns in counseling, and do not represent any actual person. Any statements were made anonymously by participants and thus are nonidentifiable.

The DCN is a UK charity founded in 1993 by a group of parents through sperm donation. They aimed to challenge the prevalent view of the medical establishment that it was best to keep DC a secret from all, including the children. DCN's current membership is 2,000+ individuals and families. It produces a wide variety of resources to support parents, families and professionals.

Workshops

The DCN has been running two types of workshops since 2007, open to all regardless of where in the world that treatment might take/took place. "Preparation for Parenthood" workshops are for those considering whether DC is right for them (for more information see [1,2]). "Telling and Talking" workshops, featured in this chapter, are for parents of younger children, while written materials are available for all ages including adults [3]. Numbers are kept small and the facilitators are DCN members with professional skills in group work and adult learning, who also have older DC children. Confidentiality and respect are emphasized to ensure the workshops are safe spaces for voicing questions, doubts and fears as well as hopes for their future. Table 14.1 outlines the workshop program.

Table 14.1 Donor conception network workshop program

	Program "Telling and Talking" Workshop 0–7 years
9:30	Coffee & Registration
9.45	Welcome & Ground Rules for the Day
9.55	Aims of the Day & Introductions Exercise
10.40	What We Know & What We Are Learning Setting the Scene. A Summary of the Packs
10.55	Refreshment Break
11.10	Hopes, Anxieties & Difficult Feelings – An Opportunity to Think About What We Hope for and Dread About "Telling."
11.40	"A Different Story" Video
12:05	Discussion About the Video
12:30	Looking Back & Looking Forward What Kind of Parent Do I Want to Be?
1:15pm	Lunch Break
2:00	Practical Skills – The "How" Rather than the "Why" of Telling in Different Scenarios.
3:15	Refreshment Break
3:30	Reflections and the Future Next Steps
3.50	Feedback Sheets
4:00	Conclusion
4:15	Close

Hazel and David had twins following egg donation treatment in Spain, through an arrangement with the UK clinic where they had spent a year trying to conceive with their own gametes. They vaguely remember the UK clinic counselor talking (amongst many other things) about the importance of being open with their children about DC. In the hurly-burly of family life they have given little thought to it, but it has nagged at the back of Hazel's mind. Now the twins are four she knows they need to address this. She and David agree on the importance of honesty with the children, but she realizes now that this is complicated, including deciding who else in their family and community should know. She remembers feeling anxious before the twins were born about whether she would bond with them, but her fears disappeared once they arrived. Now she begins to worry anew about this once the twins understand about egg donation. David digs out a leaflet the counselor had given them advertising DCN's "Telling and Talking Workshops," and persuades Hazel that these might help.

Issues Brought by "Telling and Talking" Participants

Many attendees are already aware that openness is considered highly desirable for raising emotionally healthy children, and that starting conversations very early is recommended by UK law. The regulator, HFEA, states that this should always be discussed with patients [4]. In reality, many parents are not only at a loss as to how to go about this, but are hindered by a resurgence of emotions about DC that prevent them moving forward. The workshops encourage voicing and sharing of feelings, and then consider handling strategies. The aim is to help parents identify their own reactions while remaining emotionally available to their children.

Having signed up for a Telling & Talking workshop, Hazel and David realize that their first hurdle is to decide what to say to David's mother, who is caring for the twins for the day. They were private about their fertility journey to protect themselves during their many failed treatments. They tell her the workshop is about parenting.

The pre-workshop survey sent to each participant enables facilitators to be aware of particular issues and circumstances. Questions start with asking how participants are feeling about DC and what they want to explore in the workshop. Completing the survey online can allow for a depth of emotion and honesty to emerge. For example, some worry about how their child will interpret their decision to go overseas for treatment with an anonymous/unknown donor, given that UK clinics can only use identity-release donors. One said recently: "I feel ashamed and upset for my child that I have used an anonymous donor."

Fears are often expressed as anxiety or sadness at having a family that is perceived as different from the norm, or as re-surfacing grief at the loss of their initial preference for having a child connected genetically to both (if a heterosexual couple), or finding a partner with whom to have a family (if a single person). Often people speak uneasily about the contribution of the donor(s). They fear that one day their child will find and prefer their genetic parent, perhaps rejecting the nongenetic parent with such comments as "You're not my real mum/dad." One single parent, asked how she felt about the "telling process," replied: "A bit anxious. Unsure how it will be taken up. Issues related to the unconventionality of my approach. Fear that I'll be judged, criticized, rejected by my child when he is older, that he won't understand my actions."

One parent expressed conflicted feelings about possible consequences of her children being open with others: "... I don't want them to feel embarrassed or ashamed that they are donor conceived but, as they're five, they could just come out with it to anyone. It's the fear I have as their parent of how other people could react and treat them ... it's how to prepare them for the outside world while at the same time not making them feel like they're different and this is a dirty secret ... I'm not sure how open I want to be with people who aren't close friends because I feel to some extent that this is personal to them and don't want this to be what defines them."

Hazel and David complete their pre-course surveys independently. They are surprised at how liberating it is simply to write down the issues that concern them most – Hazel writes about her resurfaced fears that the children won't see her as their real mother. David is concerned about not having told his parents, who hold traditional views and who he has assumed will be shocked. Will it affect how they interact with the twins?

The session entitled "Hopes, Fears and Difficult Feelings" allows participants to share their feelings and a process of normalizing to begin. Heterosexual couples are divided into men's and women's groups to facilitate the disclosure of feelings about which they have been trying to protect their partner. In workshops for single women, the division is between those who used sperm donation and those who used double donation (the latter is increasing in number as more older women turn to DC).

David finds this session revelatory; the opportunity to talk with other men about his feelings and fears is not something he's had experience of. Those who are genetically related to their children are concerned about supporting their partners so the male facilitator encourages them to share their own hopes and anxieties. Hazel becomes emotional in her group, realizing that other women have similar anxieties to hers.

Those who have not started talking to their child or to others about DC frequently use "daunting," "scary" or "nervous" to describe how they feel about the prospect. Those who have started may now find themselves stymied by their child's questions: "Started when she was two with 'Our Story' book, read it a few times a week to her and continued till now, I got more confidence as time went on but get stumped at the donor part and she asks me what's his name?"

The program moves on to encouraging parents to consider the longer-term, when their children will decide for themselves how they feel about being donor-conceived. The final part offers the chance to practise choice of language when talking to children or to family and friends. In the post-workshop feedback one person observed: "The exercise when we practised 'talking' was very useful – it's one thing discussing this in theory but very useful saying the words out loud." Another expressed their realization that "... we tend to think the child will put more focus/weight on their origin story when in reality they'll most likely be accepting and not think of it as a 'big thing.'" Some people are nervous that they will be forced to explain about sex to their young child, whereas in reality a simple story to the effect of "a baby begins to grow when a seed from a man meets an egg in a woman's tummy" is enough.

As the workshop progresses, Hazel discovers that hearing from one of the facilitators, who has an older child through egg donation, plus watching a video of DC parents and their children, has reassured her much more powerfully than reading about it could ever do. She begins to think about it from the children's viewpoint; for them, she is simply their mummy. Although she is taken aback by the idea that "telling" is a process, not a one-off event, she is also now aware that DCN will remain a support for her and David in the long-term. David realizes that explaining about DC matter of factly, but confidently, to his parents could be effective, accepting that they might need time to come to terms with it. Many questions remain for Hazel and David, not least that their donor is anonymous, but they now know many parents are in the same position. They draw confidence from knowing they can access DCN's written resources, opportunities to get together with other parents and one-to-one help where needed.

Workshops are supported by information packs on UK law, identity and resilience, child development, DNA testing, books and resources, various literature (including research), and a video featuring DC families and young adults. These also promote awareness of how children's understanding will develop over time and the importance of seeing DC from their point of view. DCN also produces "telling and talking" booklets and a range of story books for parents to read with their children [3].

Reflections

Some participants find the workshops challenge their previous assumptions. They may remember a clinic counselor explaining the importance of openness but now understand this cannot be the "one-off" event they imagined. The realization that it is a process of keeping conversations going, ebbing and flowing as a child's understanding matures, can feel difficult for parents who want their family to be like everyone else's. As one put it post-workshop: "I still feel I'll struggle with language but today was a help with how to tackle some subjects. Honestly, I wish this whole thing would go away. But it's a fact of life and I need to deal with it in order for my children to be best equipped with questions etc."

It can be painful, too, for parents to imagine their child as an adult who might want to find out more about – and possibly contact – those to whom they are genetically connected. Instead of a short list of nonidentifying information handed to them by their clinic, it can be a reminder that the donor is an actual person, and that there may be other families to whom their child is genetically related, but not them.

At every workshop questions indicate that the strength of feelings of isolation and shame felt by some parents should not be under-estimated. The power of meeting with others in a confidential and sympathetic group cannot be over-stated, and is mentioned by almost every participant:

> I greatly benefitted from hearing from all participants and the facilitators, who are further down the line than us, was incredibly helpful. Their knowledge, experience, friendliness, acceptance, warmth and understanding, just what is needed.
>
> I think it has given me the confidence to open up. It has pushed me to talk about the donor a little bit more with my child. It has helped me understand the cognitive recognition that children go through as they got older. It has put my mind at ease a lot . . .

The desires of parents to "do the right thing" are universal. Intentions to "tell" are often not enough; active support and encouragement are also needed [5].

Workshops are designed to provide a safe and confidential atmosphere to enable participants to access and share emotions and anxieties, knowing that facilitators will be able to contain strong feelings within the group. They can also evoke strong memories for facilitators of their own experiences. Facilitators also often share relevant parts of their own fertility journeys and family life when they consider this appropriate; the line between professional and personal has to be finely judged.

After each workshop, facilitators write a debrief, informal in style, that includes their assessment of what went well, what not so well, and any suggestions for improvement. These are shared with all workshop facilitators to contribute to overall continuing learning. This is also intended to help facilitators reflexively process their own thoughts and feelings. In addition, facilitators are encouraged to talk with others directly, including DCN staff, if they wish and DCN holds an annual review meeting for all involved.

One-to-One Support

The DCN workshops, webinars or chat groups are vital forms of support for many prospective and actual parents. They can provide answers to questions and lead to long-term supportive friendships. However, some parents nevertheless struggle to answer "difficult" questions as their children get older and some couples clash over differing views about sharing information with their children and others. For these families, DCN offers an individualized service with counselors attached or affiliated to the DCN team. Beth and Jason are an example of such a couple, as related by the counselor;

> Jason telephoned the DCN office wanting to talk to someone about difficulties between himself and his soon to be ex-wife in deciding whether and how to tell their 10-year-old boy/girl twins about being sperm-donor conceived. I spoke to Jason on the phone a few days later; he said they had agreed at the time of the twins' conception that they would not be open with them. The clinic counselor had been clear that "telling" was the right thing to do but Jason had found it impossible to contemplate other people knowing about his infertility and also thought that being open would confuse a child. He reported that Beth agreed with him.

Beth and Jason's feelings about "telling," particularly before having a child, are not unusual. They had tried for many years to conceive a child. It took two years for Jason to agree to have his sperm tested, not being able to believe that he could not give his wife a baby. When he was diagnosed azoospermia, it was devastating. He believed that Beth felt shame herself at having to use sperm from another man to have the child she so wanted. Their complicated and unshared feelings prevented them from properly talking to each other about how they felt. They were unable to even begin to think about what being donor conceived might mean for their children. It has become clear to DCN over the years that those who find difficulty in addressing their "here-and-now adult" issues often find moving on to consider the perspective of the child almost impossible. The counselor picks up the story:

> The poor communication in Beth and Jason's marriage, plus the pressures of parenting, had eventually led to the

couple separating. Jason felt guilty that he had not allowed himself to get too close to the children and Beth resented having most of the parenting responsibilities left to her. Beth started divorce proceedings. Relationships between the couple became distant and because they could not agree on childcare arrangements, the courts became involved. On learning that the children were donor conceived, the judge directed the parents to reach an agreement about how and when the children should be told. Contact with the Child and Family Court and Advisory Support Service led Jason to both DCN and individual counseling; he was finding the latter helpful in untangling his feelings about his infertility. He said he now understood why the children should be told of their origins but Beth was opposed as apparently she dreaded having to tell her parents, with whom she and the children were now living. Could we help please?

In DCN's experience, it is hard to predict in cases of parental disagreement about "telling" the children as to whether it will be the genetic or nongenetic parent who does not want to be open. As is to be expected, DCN has a number of divorced couples amongst its members. The key to continuing strong parent–child relationships, as with all separated families, lies in the willingness of each parent to put the interests of their child(ren) first.

Continuing to talk to Jason, I discovered that he had resisted becoming too emotionally involved with the children because he feared their future rejection if they learnt he was not their biological father. He realized now that his unresolved fears and shame about being infertile had deprived them all of the intimacy of a father/child relationship. We talked through his feelings about the children now, what he was doing to repair their relationship and how he imagined a "time of telling" might work out. He was keen to take the lead as the nongenetic parent but feared that Beth would oppose this as she was still doing most of the day-to-day parenting. I asked Jason if he thought Beth might agree to speak to one of the DCN team and he agreed to ask her.

A week later, Beth telephoned the DCN office and spoke to one of my colleagues, who had been alerted that she might be in touch and made clear that she herself had not spoken to Jason. Over the course of the next hour, she acknowledged Beth's pain on discovery of Jason's diagnosis, the pressure she felt the clinic put them under to "move on" to donor sperm and her mixed feelings about agreeing not to tell anyone. It emerged that she was not as fearful of telling her parents as Jason had thought, but was actually slightly enjoying opposing something that Jason now wanted. Beth could now see that this attitude was not in the children's best interests and spent the rest of the session talking through the emotional and practical implications of

telling the children, taking into account their age and the imminent divorce. Beth and my colleague agreed that a joint session between the four of us might be very helpful.

Hearing both sides of the story is very useful in considering how best to help. It is important to take into account the age of the children and other factors in the family's life when planning to share information about DC. Beyond the age of around seven or eight, "telling" children becomes a "sit down moment" rather than the slow building block process of sharing the family creation story from early years that means children have always known. Of course, "telling" at any age is always a process that will carry on over many years but if done with care and support, children in middle childhood are beginning to be capable of fairly sophisticated understanding. Even so, research suggests that a fuller grasp of understanding nongenetic connections is not likely until at least the early teenage years. Importantly, being aware of their origins before puberty/adolescence allows the information to be absorbed ahead of the potentially destabilizing impact of teenage years. It almost goes without saying that the start of the openness process should, wherever possible, never coincide with times of heightened emotions in the family due to other concerns [6,7].

Following further individual sessions with Jason and Beth to explore their willingness to acknowledge their own part in the current situation and to work together, at least with regard to DC issues, a joint meeting was set up. As preparation, they were encouraged to read our booklet "Telling and Talking 8–11." By this time the divorce had taken place but arrangements for "telling" were not yet settled.

My colleague and I first established ground rules that the focus should be solely on matters to do with Jason's infertility diagnosis, the decision to use DC, whether to share this information with the twins (in the past and currently) and their future well-being. It was further agreed that the conversations should be conducted with each person talking about their own feelings and not accusing the other. We then invited Jason and Beth to speak individually about their feelings over the years. Jason was surprised to learn that Beth had supported his wish not to "tell" because she wanted to protect him but did not feel strongly about it herself. Beth was surprised to learn that Jason was now able to acknowledge his remoteness as a parent and lack of support for her during the twins' early years. She found it difficult to accept that Jason was willing to change in the future and Jason voiced doubts about Beth's willingness to share the children's care equally. It was challenging for us to keep their focus on DC matters, but with reminders and guidance the point was reached where each partner was able to talk about working together in the interests of the children and agreeing that they should be "told" soon. Beth and Jason agreed that they should do the "telling" together and Beth slightly reluctantly agreed that Jason should take the lead. We concluded the session by supporting them in thinking through what language they would use and an agreement that both parents would ensure they were available to their children for further and future questions.

Reflections

Both counselors were very much aware of their limitations when undertaking this consultation as their expertise lies in sharing family origins information and not in disputes between partners/parents. However, in order for the parents to come to an agreement (as ordered by the court and, of course, best for the children) about "telling," they felt that they needed to be able to acknowledge past mistakes and understand more about each other's feelings. The individual sessions were able to establish this was likely possible.

The counselors found it was helpful to have two of them working with this couple. Their relationship had become so strained that otherwise each may have suspected the other was unduly influencing a sole counselor. Sharing the different accounts heard in the individual sessions was helpful for maintaining the balance in the joint session. In cases of separated parents where trust between the couple has been present, DCN counselors have found it possible to manage as a sole counselor.

References

1. Crawshaw M, Montuschi O. It 'did what it said on the tin': participants' views of the content and process of Donor Conception Parenthood Preparation Workshops. *Hum Fertil (Camb)* 2014;**17**(1):11–20.

2. Fine K, Mitchell T. Donor conception: family of choice. In: Fine K (Ed.), *Donor Conception for Life*. London: Karnac Books, 2015, pp. 69–93

3. Donor Conception Network. Telling and Talking series, including Continuing the Conversation and Mixed Blessings. Available at: www.dcnetwork.org/catalog [last accessed June 19, 2022].

4. HFEA. *Code of Practice (9th ed.)*. Available at: https://portal.hfea.gov.uk/knowledge-base/read-the-code-of-practice/ [last accessed June 19, 2022].

5. Rupnow JM. *Three Makes Baby*. Dallas, TX: Rupnow and Associates Publishing, 2018.

6. Daniels K. *Building a Family with the Assistance of Donor Insemination*. Wellington, NZ: Dunmore Press Ltd., 2004.

7. Saransohn Glazer E, Weidman E. *Having Your Baby Through Egg Donation* (2nd ed.). London: Jessica Kingsley, 2013.

CASE 15 The Male Experience with Fertility and Counseling

William Petok and Brennan Peterson

Introduction

William Petok: I have been a psychologist, primarily in private practice in Baltimore, Maryland, since 1980. I am also a Clinical Associate Professor of Obstetrics and Gynecology at the Sidney Kimmel Medical College of Thomas Jefferson University in Philadelphia, Pennsylvania. My graduate training at the University of Maryland, College Park emphasized a behavioral approach to problems. I did a subsequent post-doctoral year at the Family Therapy Institute of Washington where I learned to approach people's problems from a systemic and strategic perspective. I was "invited" to work with fertility patients by my brother-in-law, Bill Schlaff, then in his REI fellowship at Johns Hopkins. He explained that he was developing skills at helping couples achieve a pregnancy but did not know how to help them with the psychosocial issues that accompanied their fertility challenges. With my training in family therapy and the understanding that these problems implied a family crisis, I willingly stepped into the void. I have never been sorry that I did!

Brennan Peterson: As a professor of marriage and family therapy, researching the mental health implications of infertility has been one of the most rewarding experiences I have had. I began researching infertility as a graduate student and was drawn to this topic because of the real-world psychological implications of those experiencing fertility struggles. As a mental health professional, I realized the demand for fertility counselors far outweighed the number of counselors available. Because socialization of masculinity causes a conflict that many men can't resolve on their own, it has been a privilege to work with men as a fertility counselor. I have great compassion for those whose lives have been so unexpectedly disrupted by the multitude of stresses that accompany an infertility diagnosis. It has been an honor to witness, firsthand, the courage it takes to face the emotional suffering and psychological distress that is so common for men during this experience.

The case presented here reflects the male experience with infertility. It is a fictional representation of common issues seen when the diagnosis is a result of male-factor infertility and raised in the *Clinical Guide* chapter.

Glen and Louise

Glen was 36 when he entered couples therapy with his 34-year-old wife, Louise. They had been married 2 years and had already completed one unsuccessful round of IVF. Glen was azoospermic, from an as yet undetermined cause, and Louise was closing in on 35, when her ovarian supply would statistically begin depleting, adding to their reproductive challenges. It is my usual practice to inquire about surgeries a man has had in case a problem with conception could be attributed to the procedure. This would be especially true for surgeries anywhere near the genital region. Glen had had a double hernia operation at 4 years of age but there was no report of damage to his penis or scrotum.

Both Glen and Louise said they focused on their careers and were selective in dating, which led to a delayed marriage for each of them. After meeting on an online dating site, they dated for 6 months and were engaged for another 6 months before the wedding. Two years later, they experienced marital and work stresses related to differing approaches to their relationship. In addition, they began having struggles conceiving, which increased this distress. Louise indicated, indirectly, that if Glen had been more attentive to his reproductive health, he would have known about his azoospermia earlier. She blamed him for their infertility struggles and as a result, Glen became defensive, trying to avoid the issue and finding fault with her. At this point Glen was willing to use a sperm donor but Louise wavered on an egg donor. She was used to being successful and the thought of "failing" by using a donor was an insult to her sense of self. Glen, a sports enthusiast, was comfortable with "bringing in a relief pitcher." In his view, this would

The addenda referred to in this chapter are available for download at www.cambridge.org/covington-case-studies

be a team victory no matter which players were on the field.

After 2 months in therapy that centered on improving their relationship, Glen told me privately that if they did not have a child, he felt the marriage would not last. While he had never said that to Louise and asked me to keep it in confidence, he told me that a child would provide a focal point on which they could agree. He hated the idea of failure but realized that the marriage might not work out. It was too painful for him to be around friends who all had children. At the same time, he said that starting over with dating, given his azoospermia, was more than he could bear.

Eight months into their therapy, Glen noted that there were two things they could not talk about: where to live and children. A month later, while Louise was on a business trip, Glen told a friend about his fertility issues. He told me it was one of the most difficult discussions he had ever had. He had not shared his azoospermia with anyone. His condition was antithetical to the image he had of a sports-loving guy who was a hard charger in business. He was wrapped up in projecting himself as a very masculine man and the fertility issue was emasculating to him.

About 1 month later, Glen and Louise acknowledged that the vast majority of their disagreements were infertility related. They disagreed if they should proceed with sperm and egg donation. Glen was unhappy and scared. In the next month, he attended her sister's wedding where "lots of little kids" were present. It was incredibly difficult for him. At the same time, he noted that his anger at the situation, often directed at Louise, was almost instantaneous.

In the middle of counseling, they decided to move to better accommodate Louise's employment and took a hiatus from therapy.

Six months later Glen came in for a visit. He told me they redoubled their efforts at family building after realizing that their arguing and discontent had been worsened because they had avoided the critical decisions about donor egg and sperm. Once they "made that leap of faith" they forged ahead. Louise came to view carrying a child as the success and validation she needed and was willing to use an egg donor. At the time of our meeting, Louise was 8.5 weeks pregnant with a child conceived from donor sperm and donor egg. It seemed that our discussions earlier in their therapy regarding a sound marriage being based on friendship and mutual support had an impact on their thinking, and more importantly, their behavior

toward one another. We had also talked about what constitutes becoming a parent, is it genetics or something more than that. Both wanted to *raise* a child, something that can get lost in the pursuit of *creating* a child.

Counseling Points to Consider

Fertility Awareness Is Limited in Men

Glen was surprised when he and Louise had difficulty conceiving. At the advice of their treatment team, he had had a physical workup and semen analysis as well as genetic testing. The results identified he had Klinefelter's syndrome (KS), a genetic disorder expressed as XXY. Because XXY males typically do not appear different from other men and because they may not have any symptoms, XXY males often do not know they have KS. Because he was unwilling to discuss this in counseling, I could not help him understand the implications. I suspected this had to do with his lack of knowledge about fertility for men and elected not to press him, not wishing to deteriorate the therapeutic relationship. I decided to take it up at a later time when our relationship was well established, and Glen felt safe enough to discuss the implications of his genetic diagnosis.

I knew that unlike women, who upon reaching puberty become aware of reproductive health, young men do not receive medical information or attention to that aspect of their lives. This circumstance is global [1]. In addition, similar to many who delay family creation until education and career goals are achieved, Glen had a combination of factors hitting him at once. This included Glen and Louise's selective approach to choosing dating partners, so it was not surprising that they experienced a great deal of regret, sadness and irritability with one another. I had to focus on that aspect of their relationship if we were going to make any headway. It seemed to me that a better friendship in their marriage would help them. Knowing they "had each other's back" was a goal. To that end, I employed techniques recommended by both John Gottman and Richard Stuart for improving the positives in their relationship and strengthening their friendship [2,3]. Their brief relationship prior to marriage really had not allowed those things to develop more deeply.

Language as a Therapeutic Tool

An essential consideration for me as a fertility counselor is to normalize a man's lack of fertility awareness, removing the "blame game" from the couple's discourse and from his own internal dialogue. This allows the couple to focus on the team effort required to have the baby they want. Glen and Louise were truly in this together, as both had medical factors which contributed to their fertility status. Both had valid reasons for delaying creating a family with potential adverse consequences.

Getting them to view their circumstance as a shared "responsibility" rather than blaming one another was a key to having Glen and Louise move forward. For men, language which enhances ideas such as "team," "collaboration" and "partnership" is desirable and leads to cooperation. Language that suggests blame will create defensiveness, particularly if he is feeling identified in some way as the source of their trouble. Phrases such as "this is all your fault" or "if it weren't for you this wouldn't be happening" can crop up, as they had here. A fertility counselor must be on guard and reframe these statements. This situation allowed me to talk about both of their bodies not doing what they expected, creating a "shared responsibility" for their predicament.

As it happened in this case, Glen was an avid sports fan, played in several community sporting leagues, and had a mindset which could be described as "zero sum." In other words, there are winners and losers in interactions and relationships. At the same time, teamwork was a concept he appreciated and was an advantage in helping him conceptualize the effort in which he and Louise were engaged. And I was aware that any language suggesting weakness was going to push Glen away. So, I walked a tight line between language that would include Louise and Glen, alienating neither one of them. Using a language Glen understood – sports and teamwork – provided a bridge to analogize what is needed in a healthy marriage.

In an age when international travel for fertility treatment is more common, understanding the native language of your patient and contemporary attitudes to childbearing is critical. For example, if Glen had relocated from a Latin American country to the United States (US) in his teens he would have been steeped in language and customs with a different slant on family creation and images of masculinity that it presents – machismo. Contrary to popularly held beliefs, male college students in a large urban university setting in Mexico were less likely to want children than their counterparts in either the US or Nordic countries [4]. This knowledge would be essential for the fertility counselor to connect well with him and engage him in the process.

Men and Women May Experience Infertility Differently

The literature on infertility is replete with descriptions of how differently men and women view impaired reproduction [5]. For example, masculinity defined, in part, by fertility appears to be a worldwide belief. Greek men tend to suppress feelings of anxiety and experience more psychosomatic illness than their infertile wives. Some African cultures see infertility as exclusively a female problem, leading to male-factor infertility receiving an elevated level of denial from all participants in the process, including caregivers. The belief that male ego requires protection is the norm.

Nowhere could this be truer than in the world of donor insemination. In 1884, the first recorded successful human donor insemination was carried out with the inseminated wife never being told that donor sperm was used [6]. Some have speculated that secrecy would allow the child to better bond with the father who raised her. However, it appears more likely that secrecy was employed to protect the father from the perceived shame of male infertility.

In this case, Glen talked about his sense of being an "incomplete man" due to his infertility. His socialized sense of masculinity was linked with his heavy involvement in sports, and a decreased interest in the emotional aspects of his friends' lives. He did not understand how his wife could become so "emotional," breaking into tears when they talked about their family creation challenges. He was more than reluctant to talk about how he felt. Privately, he told me that talking about feelings was emasculating. It appeared to me that feeling vulnerable was anathema to him. I had to help him see that strength involves being vulnerable at times with the one you love and who loves you.

Fertility counselors are advised to pay attention to these masculine/feminine differences. To do otherwise jeopardizes a useful experience for patients. Given the understandable stressful nature of infertility treatments, anything that will reduce stress is beneficial. For heteronormative couples, normalizing these differences improves the ability to engage the male partner and help the female partner see him in at least a neutral, if not positive light. The same would be true for working with men whose partners are the primary focus of the fertility challenge. My challenge was to help Glen understand Louise's experience and how he could best support her in service of their team effort. We talked about the idea that it would be unusual for them to "be in the same place psychologically at the same time," and that having a different response style wasn't a rejection of the other, "just different."

All of this reflected the differences in how men and women engage in the counseling process. Popular representations of counseling tend to emphasize the verbal expression of emotion. Glen was not in that space! But he had probably seen too many TV programs or movies that depicted counseling as a process with tears, sadness and feeling bad in the forefront. For some fertility counselors who have their own fertility challenges, this is a point when consideration of self-disclosure is at the forefront. Because I was without a personal example to utilize, I told Glen "Many men in your situation have feelings of guilt, regret, etc. Have you experienced any of them?" It helped open the door a crack, and that was sufficient to get Glen talking.

Often, a man whose partner is experiencing a female factor will feel that he must be the protector, staying strong for her. As a result, he may fail to acknowledge how he feels about their situation, sometimes giving her the impression that he does not care, when nothing could be further from the truth. While Glen and Louise did not provide this situation, likely because it was a shared factor case, it would have added another challenge to the therapy.

Social Issues to Consider

Glen worked in a technical field, running a team of computer technology support staff for a large firm. As I expected, he was under constant pressure to produce at work. Quarterly reviews and the price of the company's stock were how he measured success. Numbers were essential to his self-image. I had to take this into account when discussing his semen analysis with him, as I knew that some healthcare professionals were less than adept at discussing these results, often using male-centric terminology that was hurtful such as "you're shooting blanks" [7]. Fortunately, this wasn't the case with Glen. However, performance was an issue for him, and he felt awful about his "performance" with regard to impregnating his wife. We had to find other measures of competence at home to reduce the shame and stigma he felt from this "failure." To that end, we discussed the "wins" he had at becoming a better partner, by understanding Louise's emotions and desire to have a child no matter whose gametes they eventually used.

Another critical variable in this case was improving the way Glen and Louise related to one another. All too often the focus had become on what was wrong between them. We instituted a program to increase positives by focusing on small acts of caring. Each of them was to provide the other with a list of things they could do or say that demonstrated caring in the ways they wanted to be cared for. Upon observing one of their requests take place, they were to provide a small token of recognition, a small piece of paper in this case, that they were aware the request had been fulfilled. Greater detail about the technique, referred to as the Caring Days technique, can be found in Richard Stuart's book [2]. The advantage of this technique for Glen was its game-like quality and the ability to count events, playing into his competitive nature. Providing them with positives in their relationship when they experienced so much loss was important to helping them move forward.

Finally, I had to be aware of Glen's family of origin. He had two brothers, both of whom were married and had children of their own. He came from a family with strong roots to a religion that valued family. There were multiple events each year that drew them together for celebratory meals where he and Louise would see his siblings' children. They both found this difficult, Glen more so because it was his siblings to which he was comparing himself. While his father knew something about their situation, his brothers did not. "It was just too painful," he told me. "Get over it," would not be a helpful response, so we developed a list of things he could say if he was questioned about their plans for a family or if he was too uncomfortable to attend a family gathering.

Personal Implications for the Man

By Glen's account, he had no support network outside of Louise. The one time he had told a friend had been excruciating for him. The loneliness he felt about it was palpable, but reaching out was too difficult. We decided that an online discussion board for men might be the best support option for him. There were no men-only support groups where he lived, and he told me it was hard enough for him to come to counseling. Sitting in a group of men with a similar problem was a nonstarter, even if there had been one available. Fortunately, many men find the discussion boards their best option. They have the advantage of anonymity if they wish and they never have to leave home to participate [8]. Glen's employment in technology and his comfort with the medium were a real advantage and he took to the board easily. I was relieved because he was likely to drop out of counseling with me, especially after the couple moved. There was no male therapist with the necessary skill set where the couple relocated, a frequent problem given the limited number of men in the field.

Mental health in general was a difficult topic for Glen, as it is for many men. Some of the reason for this has to do with popular portrayals of users of mental health services as noted above. Another factor is who a man can identify in his social network that has disclosed their own utilization of mental health services and reported a positive experience with them [9]. Not surprisingly, Glen was at a loss to name a friend or colleague who had a positive experience with therapy. In fact, when he was a pre-teen, he had been in family therapy because his brother was having difficulty and his parents made him participate. It had been an unpleasant experience. With that knowledge I realized what a reach it had been for him to enter my office. I consciously set out to let Glen know I appreciated his willingness and courage to engage in therapy and made sure that Louise understood what an effort this likely had been for her husband.

Glen never reported sexual problems during his time in counseling, even when directly asked. However, it would not have been unusual if they had developed. Erectile dysfunction, rapid ejaculation and delayed ejaculation have all been reported in the literature [10]. Given Glen's personality and performance orientation, a similar problem could have as easily developed between him and Louise, further adding to their difficulties. In fact, their lack of sexual difficulties would be noted as a positive and strength in their relationship.

Using a Donor

There was no question that Glen would be using a donor. He was azoospermic. And there was parity between them because Louise now needed a donor as well. Together they were forced to deal with the bilateral loss of a genetic connection to their child. On the other hand, we had discussed robust observations that children tend to think of the people who raise them as parents and donors as just that . . . if they are brought up with that idea from early on. Fortunately, we had worked on this in several couple sessions. Both Glen and Louise talked about the loss they felt, although Glen was less expressive than Louise was. When he had returned and discussed the "leap of faith" they had taken, I asked about it. He told me they realized that there were no winners or losers in their situation. They would both be "making a sacrifice" to create the family they desired. Glen told me that he had come around to the point of view that their decision was

a sign of strength between them, that they truly were on the same team.

Summary

This case presented many common problems associated with male factor infertility that a fertility counselor must keep in mind. The most important of them being that a man confronted with his own infertility can be at a loss for expressing his shame, guilt, and stigmatization, while at the same time being encouraged by his female partner to understand and talk about his feelings. Understanding that the male experience is not well-reported in popular press, that the typical language of counselors may be a deterrent for the man actively participating, and that support may be best achieved in online forums rather than face-to-face, are all important considerations. For more information on resources for men coping with infertility, please see Addendum 15.1.

References

1. Pedro J, Brandão T, Schmidt L, et al. What do people know about fertility? A systematic review on fertility awareness and its associated factors. *Ups J Med Sci* 2018;**123**:71–81.

2. Stuart RB. *Helping Couples Change: A Social Learning Approach to Marital Therapy*. New York, NY: Guilford Press, 1980.

3. Gottman JM. *The Marriage Clinic*. New York, NY: W.W. Norton, 1999.

4. Place JM, Peterson BD, Horton B, et al. Fertility awareness and parenting intentions among Mexican undergraduate and graduate university students. *Hum Fertil* 2020;**2020**:1–10. https://doi.org/10.1080/14647273.2020.1817577

5. Petok WD. Infertility counseling (or the lack thereof) of the forgotten male partner. *Fertil Steril* 2015;**104**:260–266.

6. Lombardo LX, Polonko KA. Non-governmental organisations and the UN convention on the rights of the child. *Int J Child Rights* 2015;**23**:133–153.

7. Hanna E, Gough B. Experiencing male infertility: a review of the qualitative research literature. *SAGE Open* **2015**;2015:5. https://doi.org/10.1177/2158244015610319

8. Hanna E, Gough B. Emoting infertility online: a qualitative analysis of men's forum posts. *Heal (United Kingdom)* 2016;**20**:363–382.

9. Vogel DL, Wester SR, Hammer JH, et al. Referring men to seek help: the influence of gender role conflict and stigma. *Psychol Men Masculinity* 2014;**15**:60–67.

10. Wischmann T. "Your count is zero": Counselling the infertile man. *Hum Fertil* 2013;**16**:35–39.

Counseling Lesbian, Gay, Bisexual and Queer Fertility Patients

Sarah Holley and Lauri Pasch

Introduction

We are colleagues who provide fertility counseling services at the University of California, San Francisco Center for Reproductive Health (CRH). We provide a range of counseling, psychoeducational and assessment services to CRH patients, including consultations with the population that is the focus of this chapter: lesbian, gay, bisexual and queer (LGBQ)[1] individuals and couples who are navigating the family-building process.

Sarah Holley: I am a Health Sciences Assistant Professor in the Department of Psychiatry and Behavioral Sciences at the University of California, San Francisco, as well as a Professor in the Psychology Department at San Francisco State University. I have provided psychological services at the CRH since 2017, as well as clinical training to students at both universities. My research focuses on the connections between intimate relationship processes, emotional functioning, and mental and physical health.

Lauri Pasch: I am a Professor in the Department of Psychiatry and Behavioral Sciences at the University of California, San Francisco and have directed psychological services for the CRH for 19 years. In addition to being a practicing psychologist, I am also a scientist and educator with expertise in the psychological aspects of women's reproductive health and the use of assisted reproduction.

As noted above, we are both practicing psychologists who are also active in research. Together, we have completed a set of studies examining psychological consequences of infertility treatment for heterosexual couples, with results underscoring the high levels of depression and anxiety that are common in this population. More recently, we conducted a study examining the experiences of female couples who utilized fertility treatment, in order to identify the primary stressors they found to be associated with family building and ways to provide better support. This research informs the approach we describe here.

---

[1] We are using "lesbian, gay, bisexual and queer" and the acronym "LGBQ" as umbrella terms for all sexual minority individuals. We are also using the term "female couple" for all same-sex female couples, and "male couple" as a term for all same-sex male couples. We recognize the diversity of sexual orientation identities and gender identities that can be represented within these dyads, and that identity can change over time.

The case explored in this chapter was drawn from the experiences couples shared with us in our research and highlights some of the major considerations for a counselor when providing support to LGBQ prospective parents during their family-building process. Note that the work we do at the CRH is consultative in nature, that is, we do not provide ongoing psychotherapy. Therefore, this chapter examines fertility counseling with a female couple conducted in a consultative model.

Case Overview

Abby (age 40) and Maddy (age 35) are a married couple in a major metropolitan city. Both are cisgender and identify as lesbian. In terms of family building, they originally planned to do reciprocal IVF (i.e., one partner provides the eggs and the other partner carries the pregnancy). Abby was very connected to her family and had a strong desire to pass on her genes, so they planned to use her eggs. Maddy had always wanted to experience pregnancy and could not imagine having a child she did not give birth to, so she was going to carry. They visited a fertility center for an initial evaluation. At the follow-up appointment, before Abby had even arrived, the doctor informed Maddy that Abby's eggs were not going to be a viable option and suggested they just switch over and use Maddy's eggs instead. Both the news itself, and the way it was delivered, was very upsetting to both of them.

As a result of this experience, they decided to go to a different clinic. They completed their initial visit with the new reproductive endocrinologist. Because they both still wanted to be involved in the pregnancy, they planned to move forward using Maddy's eggs and with Abby as the one to carry the pregnancy. They had already decided they wanted to use anonymous donor sperm and had selected a donor from a sperm bank. The clinic had a policy that anyone using donor gametes must meet with a therapist before proceeding with fertility treatment, so they were scheduled to meet with the clinic fertility counselor.

Counseling Approach

Our approach will depend on where the couple is in the decision-making process, as well as what their reproductive options are. As with the case of Abby and Maddy, counselors are most likely to get involved once the decision to pursue parenthood has been made but before fertility treatments have begun. Couples may or may not have done independent research on the conception process, have friends who can provide advice, or have supportive family. All of these factors can have a major impact on where they are in terms of comfort, knowledge and preparation. Thus, our role is to help the couple navigate whatever issues are relevant to their specific situation and provide psychoeducation and support as needed. Below is an overview of suggested areas to cover in a psychoeducational counseling session.

Set the Stage

We begin by providing an orientation to the purpose of the meeting, which is to discuss the major decisions and concerns that same-sex couples may have when pursuing parenthood. Specific stated goals may involve: (a) helping the couple think through their reproductive options; (b) considering the implications of their decisions; (c) answering questions they may have about the treatment process; and (d) providing guidance to supportive/informational resources. Because LGBQ patients may have already encountered (or be apprehensive of) biased attitudes or discriminatory practices, we try to be aware of and directly address any ambivalent or negative feelings that couples may bring to the meeting.

In particular, for some couples, this meeting may have been a mandatory part of their treatment process. As such, there may be resentment about having to attend the session, or concerns that the meeting is a screening for parental fitness.

Abby: We are here because we were told we had to see a psychologist to move forward with treatment. We are checking a box.

We make it clear that the purpose of this meeting is to provide guidance and support, specify that it is not an evaluation, and provide a defensible rational for why the meeting is mandated. Empathy and validation of negative feelings about the counseling requirement may be important to help foster a therapeutic alliance with the couple. Of note, even if the patients have reservations about the session requirement, they may not express these to the therapist directly. This could be due to the common desire to be a "good patient," or because they still hold the worry that full disclosure of any actual concerns or negative feelings may preclude treatment from proceeding [1].

Collect Background Information and Identify Needs

It is often helpful to start the dialogue with an open-ended question, such as, *"Tell me about how you got to where you are today."* This will help the counselor assess what issues need to be addressed during the session. Some couples may be at the very start of their treatment process, whereas others may have tried various methods (e.g., home insemination). We gather as much information as possible about what decisions still need to be made, and how comfortable each of the partners are with the elements that have been decided already. This is also a chance to see how well-oriented the couple is (or is not) with any upcoming fertility treatment procedures. We work to fill in the gaps as needed with psychoeducation around any relevant medical or emotional demands of their treatment plan.

In the case of Abby and Maddy, they had already selected their sperm donor and knew the treatment plan, so they did not need help with decision-making in these areas. They were, however, still processing the abrupt shift away from their original family-building plan.

Maddy: "I walked into the meeting with the doctor at the other clinic to be told, like, genetics aren't that important and what you want isn't going to be possible and you just need to put that aside and pursue a different path. I think they go to problem-solving, they are trying to be helpful. There just wasn't really a consideration of the emotional attachment that might go with genetics or that might go with carrying."

Abby: "I think because they're used to straight couples where, if the woman has a fertility issue it's like, that's it. I think they view the lesbian couples as, well, you've got back up!

Maddy: "We know we are lucky, we do have this viable 'Plan B.' I mean even though logically we know we are very lucky, emotionally it just doesn't feel lucky. Our solution ended up actually being really tough for both of us to swallow."

For same-sex couples, the fact that only one partner can contribute genetic material or carry does not come as a surprise. That said, partners may still have emotions connected to these aspects of conception and pregnancy [2]. For both Abby and Maddy, the elements each cared about most were not going to happen. So even if Abby were to carry a healthy baby from Maddy's eggs, she might still feel the loss characteristic of infertile women because passing on her genes was part of her definition of what it means to become a mother. Similarly, Maddy was losing the experience of being pregnant and giving birth, which was part of her definition of becoming a mother. Each woman had the difficult task of simultaneously dealing with her loss and trying to embrace the new plan, all while working to support her partner. Thus, it was important to create a space for each to talk about their feelings and mourn their respective losses.

Address Minority Stress-Related Challenges

In addition to the general stress of fertility treatment, same-sex couples may also have to contend with stressors related to their sexual minority status. Sexual minority stress is defined as psychosocial stress resulting from stigmatization and marginalization in a heterosexist society [3]. Sexual minority stress can take many forms, including experiences of discrimination and bias, as well as expectations of rejection, efforts to conceal sexual identity and/or internalized homophobia (see the *Clinical Guide* companion Chapter 16). These stressors can make the already difficult process of fertility treatment that much harder. The fertility counselor's sensitivity to minority stress is important, both in terms of allowing LGBQ patients to feel heard and supported, and to make space for corrective, positive interactions with members of the fertility treatment system.

Some couples will have encountered instances of overt discrimination, or have attributed certain experiences to their sexual minority status. For example, Abby and Maddy felt like the first doctor had handled them differently *because* they were in a same-sex couple. From their perspective, they felt their first doctor was dismissive not only of their family-building goals but of their relationship more generally.

Abby: I feel like there's no way the doctor would have started that conversation about my eggs without both people in the room if it had been a straight couple. The fertility issue would be between the couple, and the doctor would see the need to have both of them there . . . and the same is true for us. I really don't believe that would have happened if we were a heterosexual couple.

Quite commonly, same-sex couples experience minority stress due to the fact that fertility treatment services are largely designed with infertile heterosexual couples in mind. Thus, many standard components of the treatment process can feel off-putting or offensive for LGBQ patients. One of the most oft-cited examples of this kind of heteronormative bias relates to clinic forms [4,5].

Maddy: It seems like forms always have spaces for "the father," "the mother," things like that. I really wish the forms were set up in a way that was just more kind to the various permeations of relationships that are out there.

Same-sex couples may also experience other subtle (or not so subtle) minority stressors based on the heteronormative framework, such as a lack of tailored psychoeducational resources, a sense of invisibility for the partner that is not the identified patient or barriers to insurance coverage [4,5]. Therefore, we actively try to use written and verbal communications that are free from heteronormative assumptions and make sure we are including both partners as co-equal participants in family-building discussions [6].

Minority stress may also take the form of anticipatory anxiety, even absent actual discriminatory events [3]. For example, LGBQ patients may be expecting to encounter rejection or biased attitudes from fertility treatment healthcare professionals, and they may carry the associated worry that revealing their sexual identity could negatively impact their care [7].

Abby: We talk about the fact that you have to "come out" all the time. The minute you go in and check in for a health appointment, someone will be like, "Well, where's your husband?" or whatever.
Maddy: Yeah, they want to check me in next because I'm standing there, right? And I'm like, no I'm with her!
Abby: And they're like, oh, it's so good you brought a friend. No . . . this is my wife. We're constantly coming out, and to complete strangers. It's like, I don't even know your name, you don't know mine, and by the way, I'm gay, and here's my wife, and this is what we're trying to do . . . It's been fine, but you never know what you are going to get in response."

To help counter such anticipatory anxiety within the counseling space, we make an effort to provide clear visual signals that LBGQ patients are welcome. This may include images or LGBQ-focused materials on the website, in the waiting room, and within the counselor's office.

We also listen for indications of internalized stigma that need to be addressed. Familiarization with the literature on LGBQ parenting allows us to point to evidence demonstrating that, for example, parental sexual orientation has no deleterious effects on the development, adjustment and well-being of children [8]. For couples in which one or both members are not yet "out" or are in the process of revealing their relationship to others, we provide referrals if patients are interested in additional support related to the coming-out process.

Finally, we often help couples think through any relevant legal considerations. We are diligent in our effort to avoid providing legal advice, but want to make sure that the couple is aware of legal implications of their family-building plans. If indicated, we strongly encourage couples to consult with a family planning attorney and take whatever precautions are needed (e.g., second-parent adoption, pre-birth orders) to protect the rights of the parents to the child. We also address the feelings couples may have about having to consider these legal issues. For example, Abby and Maddy are married, both their names will be on the birth certificate, and both have a claim to parentage by virtue of genetics and gestation. But because she will not give birth, Maddy may still need to complete a confirmatory adoption if she wants to be absolutely certain her rights are protected, particularly when she travels to other states or countries. The fact of having to adopt her own child can feel disheartening, frustrating, or even enraging.

Planning for Future Disclosure Discussions

Lesbian, gay, bisexual and queer parents may have questions about when and how to talk to the child about their donor origins [9]. We help the couple generate strategies for sharing and discussion. It is recommended that parents start the sharing process early, explaining to the child in a way that is appropriate for his or her developmental stage [8]. Early sharing about the involvement of a donor (and carrier, if a surrogate is involved) helps promote a sense of security within the family, and the conception story becomes naturally integrated into the family's narrative. Parents might start the process with a simple "bedtime story" that introduces the idea that they received help from an outside source. Parents can then fill in additional details as the child gets older and is prepared to understand more.

An example of a bedtime story narrative is presented here. After talking to Abby and Maddy about their plans for disclosure and providing our recommendations, this kind of story can be shared with them. We encourage them to adapt it to make it their own.

"A long time ago, Mommy and Mama wanted to have a family of our own. To make a baby, you need two things: seeds from a woman, and seeds from a man. We knew we were going to use Mommy's seeds, but we didn't have any seeds from a man. So, we went to a special place where

helpers who had more seeds than they needed had given their seeds to share with other families who didn't have any. So, we got some of the helper's seeds, and we got Mommy's seeds, and a doctor mixed them all together and put them in Mama's tummy so that we could have a baby. My tummy got bigger and bigger, and one day the baby came out. It was you! And aren't we so lucky, and we love you so much!"

Mental Health Support

Same-sex couples are not necessarily facing fertility problems, therefore their entry into treatment may be associated with excitement or optimism as they begin the process of family formation [9]. However, psychological distress can be present as a result of minority stress-related factors. Further, for some couples, initial enthusiasm may quickly start to mirror the distress of infertile heterosexual couples as they confront the general stresses associated with fertility treatment: doctor's visits, failed attempts, large bills, waiting periods, and so on. When needed, couples may benefit from ongoing psychological support services (either from a fertility counselor or another LGBQ-friendly therapist) aimed at managing anxiety or depression (see the *Clinical Guide*, Chapter 7), or coping with any communication difficulties or relationship problems that may arise (see the *Clinical Guide*, Chapter 4).

Maddy: I'm starting to now understand why we've found this process so exhausting. There has been a lot we've had to go through ... I'm wiped and the kid is not even here!

Social Support and Access to Resources

If, for example, family members have not demonstrated support (or were outright rejecting) of a LGBQ individual due to her or his sexual orientation, that family is likely not expected to be a reliable source of support during the conception or childrearing process. In this situation, helping the couple connect to sources of peer support will be particularly important. Conversely, if it is the LGBQ peer community that is less than supportive, couples may seek tighter connections with family supports.

In the case of Abby and Maddy, they had the benefit of support from both their families and a robust network of friends. However, the majority of people in their support system were heterosexual. Therefore, though everyone was supportive and they had many friends they could talk to about pregnancy or parenting, they felt relatively isolated with regard to navigating the family-building process as they experienced it:

> Abby: I think being in a lesbian group where people have gone through this process to sort of commiserate on like, oh yeah! I had to fill out those forms, wasn't that stupid. Or whatever. We've had this experience by ourselves in that sense.

Prospective parents value insight into the experiences of others who have already gone through a similar process [1]. For same-sex couples, it can feel particularly helpful to be able to connect with other members of the LGBQ community who have had to deal with similar decisions and stressors [6,7]. Thus, it is important to us to help direct the couple to sources of social support and LGBQ-focused resources (e.g., literature, support groups, community organizations; see Table 16.1 for further information).

Table 16.1 Sample resources for LGBQ patients

Websites
- Connecting Rainbows (https://connectingrainbows.org/)
- Family Equality (www.familyequality.org)
- Gay Parents to Be (www.gayparentstobe.com)
- Our Family Coalition (https://ourfamily.org/)
- Rainbow Families (https://rainbowfamilies.org/)

Legal and Policy Guides
- GLAD Legal Advocates & Defenders (www.glad.org)
- Human Rights Campaign (www.hrc.org)
- Lambda Legal (www.lambdalegal.org)
- Movement Advancement Project (www.lgbtmap.org/lgbtq-families)
- National Center for Lesbian Rights (www.nclrights.org)

Books for Intended Parents
- *Your Future Family: The Essential Guide to Assisted Reproduction* (Bergman, 2019)
- *If These Ovaries Could Talk: The Things We've Learned About Making an LGBTQ Family* (Kelton & Hopkins, 2020)
- *The Ultimate Guide for Gay Dads: Everything You Need to Know About LGBTQ Parenting But Are (Mostly) Afraid to Ask* (Rosswood, 2017)

Books for Children
- *It Takes Love (and Some Other Stuff) to Make a Baby* (Bird, 2014)
- *Zak's Safari: A Story About Donor-Conceived Kids of Two-Mom Families* (Tyner, 2014)
- *The Pea That Was Me: A Two Dads/Egg Donation and Surrogacy Story* (Kluger-Bell, 2014)
- *Daddy, Papa, and Me* (Newman & Thompson, 2008)
- *What Makes a Baby* (Silverberg, 2013)

Note: Fertility counselors should be able to direct LGBQ patients to these types of resources, as well as to other local sources of support

Reflections

Providing supportive, culturally competent care to same-sex couples is a priority for us. As a result of this strong commitment, our particular countertransference reactions may sometimes be characterized by too much of a "righting reflex." That is, we are both so focused on demonstrating our support and lack of heteronormative bias that we run the risk of aligning with the couple so much that we may miss unhelpful beliefs or patterns. Dr. Holley has further noticed that, as a fertility healthcare professional who herself utilized fertility treatment services with her same-sex partner, there is a stronger than usual urge to be directive when supporting LGBQ patients. In such cases, it is particularly important for her to stay grounded in providing nonprescriptive information to empower each couple to make the family-building decisions most in line with their own goals and values [10].

One of the major questions we have grappled with pertains to whether fertility counseling sessions should be mandated. In line with the guidance put forward by organizations like the American Society for Reproductive Medicine (ASRM), some clinics require *all* patients using donor gametes (for whatever reason) to have a counseling session prior to treatment. While in theory that makes sense, in practice (and when viewed through the minority stress framework) we have found it can have unintended and highly negative consequences. We learned from talking to patients like Abby and Maddy that the counseling meant to provide support and guidance sometimes made couples feel they were being screened or judged, which in turn could lead to feelings of defensiveness, resentment or hurt [1]. This was hard for us to hear – we want to be helpful, and it was painful to learn that we sometimes failed at this. Through much consideration about how best to support our patients, we decided to make counseling sessions in our clinic strongly recommended rather than mandatory for female couples using anonymous donor sperm,[2] with the rationale for the benefits of the session clearly articulated. We realize this may lead some couples to miss the benefits of the counseling session if they opt out, but we felt it outweighed the potential harm the mandate was causing. This is not necessarily the "right answer," but the question of how best to approach counseling for same-sex couples in a way that does not add to

---

[2] We note that our clinic does still require a counseling session for any individual or couple using a known donor or gestational surrogate as these tend to be more complex processes.

their minority stress burden is one that warrants careful consideration.

In sum, fertility counseling with same-sex couples will in many ways parallel that done with heterosexual couples, but in other ways it is quite unique.

> Abby: "I think that has probably been the theme of trying to get pregnant overall, and maybe for gay people in general. Things that straight people just take for granted, are just very hard, very hard, and this is one of those things that, along the way, every milestone has been hard."

We as fertility counselors are there to assist same-sex couples with their decision-making, provide psychoeducation and help them to process feelings related to their family-building plans. In addition, we must also be attuned to the ways in which minority stress-related factors can impact couples. As such, we have the opportunity to provide guidance and support, as well as play a pivotal role in helping to facilitate a positive family-building experience for our LGBQ patients.

References

1. Schrijvers AM, van Rooij FB, Overbeek G, et al. Psychosocial counselling for intended parents who opt for donor sperm treatment: which topics do they find relevant? *J Reprod Infant Psychol* 2020;**38**(5):474–484.

2. Goldberg AE, Scheib JE. Why donor insemination and not adoption? Narratives of female-partnered and single mothers. *Fam Relat* 2015;**64**(5):726–742.

3. Meyer IH. Prejudice, social stress, and mental health in lesbian, gay, and bisexual populations: conceptual issues and research evidence. *Psychol Bull* 2003;**129**(5):674–697.

4. Kirubarajan A, Patel P, Leung S, Park B, Sierra S. Cultural competence in fertility care for lesbian, gay, bisexual, transgender, and queer people: a systematic review of patient and provider perspectives. *Fertil Steril* 2021;**115**(5):1294–1301.

5. Gregg I. The health care experiences of lesbian women becoming mothers. *Nurs Womens Health* 2018;**22**(1):40–50.

6. Ross LE, Tarasoff LA, Anderson S, et al. Sexual and gender minority peoples' recommendations for assisted human reproduction services. *J Obstet Gynaecol Can* 2014;**36**(2):146–153.

7. Rausch MA, Wikoff HD. Addressing concerns with lesbian couples experiencing fertility treatment: using Relational Cultural Theory. *J LGBT Issues Couns* 2017;**11**(3):142–155.

8. Golombok S. *We Are Family: The Modern Transformation of Parents and Children*. New York, NY: PublicAffairs, 2020.

9. Ehrensaft D. Just Molly and me, and donor makes three: lesbian motherhood in the age of assisted reproductive technology. *J Lesbian Stud* 2008;**12**(2–3):161–178.

10. Shreffler KM, Greil AL, McQuillan J. Responding to infertility: lessons from a growing body of research and suggested guidelines for practice. *Fam Relat* 2017;**66**(4):644–658.

Transgender Assisted Reproductive Technology

Karen Wasserstein

Introduction

We all go through life sketching our dreams and the paths we think we will take, but sometimes end up in a different drawing. This can happen because time passes too quickly, because we do not meet the person we think we will, or because science slowly catches up with who we are.

When I started my career, I knew I wanted to focus on clients who were dealing with medical issues. No matter how much you plan, no matter how you live your life, dealing with our physical bodies can be so difficult. We can control so much, but not how our bodies behave, respond or line up with our plans and our desires.

I am a clinical psychologist specializing in working with those with fertility journeys. I work with those who come in for consultations for third-party reproduction and with individuals and couples in therapy. My training was eclectic, but all of it centered on seeing the client first, and tailoring my skills to their individual stories and needs. I tend to focus on self-identity and recurring themes that emerge in a person's life. This chapter focuses on the transgender patient and assisted reproductive technology (ART). In some ways it was very difficult to write, as there is no "transgender patient," rather there are people coming to see me who are transgender and who are patients. Nevertheless, there are some specific issues that may be helpful to a clinician to be aware of, and this presentation is a way to highlight some of those issues.

Transgender individuals who want to become parents have several avenues. Some are able to use their own gametes, either because their gametes remain in their primary state, they cease hormone treatments temporarily, or they underwent fertility preservation prior to hormonal or surgical intervention. These clients do not routinely meet with a fertility counselor prior to family building, nor are they usually counseled on their fertility options prior to medical transition. However, many transgender patients do utilize third-party reproduction and these are the individuals that we see in our practices.

While I have seen several transgender clients, they have been only a small percentage of my patients. Therefore, I am even more conscious of what I know and what I do not know, of my questions and of my assumptions. It is my responsibility to examine these interactions to make sure that they are in the best interest of the clients.

The paradox is that when I try not to make assumptions, I am often left with more questions. The "I wonder" lens is helpful when you are trying to help a client explore their deeper issues. However, it is our obligation to "wonder" only for the client's sake and not for our own curiosity or education.

What is different about a recipient consultation with a transgender individual or couple? Should anything be different?

The cases that follow are compilations of my clients and colleagues' clients to represent these stories. Being transgender is hardly the whole story; each patient comes as an individual with their personal story including race, religion, culture, family history, health and mental health history. The same is true regarding the personal story of the fertility counselor (FC). Each aspect is important; the following case studies focus solely on the transgender part of the story in order to help illuminate this variable.

Clients: Sarah and Andrew

FC: Rosemary

Rosemary is a 58-year-old cisgender clinician who has specialized as a fertility counselor for 28 years. She has been seeing more transgender couples than usual and has been thinking about that a lot. She attends continuing education seminars on a regular basis and does her best to stay up-to-date with the literature. However, she knows that when she went to school there were no courses on transgender issues. She wants to be sensitive, but does not want to overcorrect her behavior or her language.

Rosemary has a consultation with Sarah and Andrew prior to their using unknown (de-identified) donor sperm. She walks into the waiting room and immediately notices that they are on time, appear well put together, and are ready for the consultation. She notices that Sarah is a petite woman, 5'5 in height and dressed in jeans and a t-shirt. Andrews is 5'3, also short, and dressed in blue

The addenda referred to in this chapter are available for download at www.cambridge.org/covington-case-studies

Acknowledgement: The author would like to thank Trystan Reese for his invaluable assistance in the review of this case study chapter.

jeans and a button-down shirt. While Andrew has a male name, and is dressed in "male clothing," Rosemary notices "something" in her consciousness about his gender presentation, but berates herself for being conscious of it.

They enter her office and Rosemary, as usual, immediately tries to put the couple at ease. She describes the purpose of the session, reviews the consent forms and asks for questions. She notices that if she closes her eyes, Andrew's voice seems a bit higher than most male voices she has heard. Again, she notices it, but then feels badly that she noticed.

Rosemary begins as usual: "Tell me about your journey and what brings you to be using donor sperm." Sarah jumps in, "Well, considering my husband was born female, we have none!" Sarah and Andrew seem comfortable sharing their story in detail.

Sarah, 30, and Andrew, 31, have been married for 2 years, and have known that they would need to use donor conception. Andrew is a transgender man, which means he was assigned female at birth, and transitioned 4 years ago. He reports that he has never wanted to use his own eggs or carry children.

Sarah and Andrew met about 13 years ago in high school. While many or even most transgender individuals choose not to share their birth name, sometimes referred to as their "dead name," Andrew felt comfortable sharing his former name in the therapeutic setting. At the time, Andrew was growing up with the name Megan and did not share his inner world of turmoil. Megan and Sarah were part of a larger social circle which remained intact through the years. The two were not particularly close, but engaged with one another as part of the group. Megan seemed to disappear about 5 years ago from their social circle.

Sarah, a recently divorced mother to 1-year-old James, soon noticed Megan's absence. Aware of how her own life had recently turned in unexpected ways, Sarah worried about someone who had gone off the radar and deliberately reached out to Megan to see if she was ok. She learned that Megan now identified as Andrew. They provided each other with the perfect ear at the perfect time, and their friendship grew into something more. Andrew began hormone replacement therapy and felt like this was the most important move he could make in his life. The process felt slow but Andrew felt supported, especially by his mother and Sarah. He had known for years that he was in pain and that he had discordant feelings between his personal definition of himself and his body. Andrew had been working with a therapist along with his medical team, and felt very secure in his process. Sarah and Andrew decided to wait to marry until he felt he was at a place of physical and identity stability. Andrew and Sarah live with Sarah's son, James, and want to add two more children to their family.

Rosemary takes in their story and has several thoughts. She is trying to understand gender and sexual identity and this adds to her questions: Is Sarah attracted to men, women, or both? Was she interested in Andrew when Andrew presented as Megan? Or did something change when Andrew presented as male? Or was it just two people who developed a deeper bond through spending more time and more experiences together? It sounds to her that Sarah was in a heterosexual marriage originally, but is that ok to ask? If she was, is James's father involved? What is the role of Andrew to James? Will James be raised with one dad or two? What will it be like for Andrew to raise three nongenetically related children, but to have only been a part of creating two?

Rosemary's thoughts continue: If Sarah was in a same-sex relationship before and used donor sperm, does she want to use the same donor and have her children be full genetic siblings, and how does that play out with the dynamics of her divorce? How does her ex feel about this current relationship?

As Andrew is a transgender man, does he need to pursue second parent adoption to the children born through sperm donation or will he be considered the legal father, as is the case in a heterosexual relationship using donor sperm? Does Andrew plan to be open about being transgender and how does that impact the discussion about disclosure of donor conception with the future children born of donor sperm?

Rosemary's mind is spinning. She begins to filter. What questions are relevant to *this* consultation. What questions will help *these clients*. She decides that who is attracted to whom is not relevant to this conversation, but that the issues of how to parent children with different parents (an ex, and a new spouse) are relevant to explore. She also decides that issues of disclosure about Andrew's journey and identity (and having been born without sperm) and the issues of disclosure of donor conception are intricately linked and therefore should also be explored respectfully. In addition, she helps the couple explore feelings regarding Andrew and Sarah's families, other areas of support and stress in their lives, and issues regarding the creation of their family.

Sarah and Andrew had come into the session knowing that their situation would probably be unusual to Rosemary and were prepared to discuss it. They noticed that Rosemary was thoughtful, tried hard but still made some missteps in her speech, specifically having trouble with using the correct pronouns for Andrew when referring to his past and to his present. They understand, but they wish it would be easier. However, they also noticed that Rosemary brought up some important things for them to consider as they embark on their journey. They thank Rosemary and ask her for additional resources for transgender parents. Rosemary pauses once again. She admits that she does not have any, but promises to ask around and to get back to them as soon as she can. They thank her and the session is completed.

Clients: Scott and Lisa

FC: Denise

Scott and Lisa are prepared for their required consultation prior to ART. They have been prepared forever, as it took weeks to get an appointment. They feel the requirement to meet with a fertility counselor patronizing. Millions of people conceive children without having to see a psychologist. Bad parents even have children without approval, and yet their clinic will not treat them without this appointment. They are frustrated and annoyed to waste their time and money. Scott is 2 years out of college, and is paying off student loans. They have lived together for 1 year at Lisa's mother's home. If they could get pregnant naturally, they could get pregnant cheaply. But they cannot; Scott was assigned female at birth. He has been taking hormone treatments for 2 years and is awaiting surgery.

When Denise calls them to schedule, Scott lays it all out. "We know we are required to do this, but is there any chance we can skip it? After all, heterosexual people do not have to pay for this and what gives you the right to tell us if we can be parents? Just because I transitioned does not mean that you can tell me if I can have children." Denise replies calmly that she understands his point and tries to reassure him that this is a required consultation for anyone who uses any third-party reproduction, regardless of sexual identity, relationship status or any other variable. It is a psychoeducational consultation to help them navigate their way. Scott replies, "What if we don't want 'help' navigating our way?" Denise focuses on the concrete task of scheduling the appointment and presents her availability. They schedule and she says she will send them some forms to complete prior to the session.

Denise pauses and before sending the forms, she reads each one thoroughly for any language that might be heteronormative or nonaffirming to a patient who may be sensitive to these issues. She finds several phrases that are not inclusive and spends hours methodically revising her forms. She feels slightly embarrassed that she has never looked at her forms with this lens before. She recognizes that Scott's resistance led her to use a more critical eye and that other clients could have benefitted from having these revised forms. She is glad she is listening and learning.

Scott and Lisa arrive 10 minutes late to the session. Due to COVID-19, it is a telehealth session. They tell her they would like to do the appointment only with audio and not with video, but Denise stays within her boundaries and explains that she will not do the session unless she is able to see them and they are able to see her. They sit outside where there is background noise and it appears to be difficult to focus, but Denise does not push the issue any further. She begins by explaining the purpose of the session and asking the routine questions.

Scott no longer has a relationship with his parents. He reports that he is preparing to undergo surgery. The couple live with Lisa's mother, who is paying for Scott's surgery. Lisa has always wanted to be a mother but has not had a timeline. Her mother reminds Lisa often that she wants to be a grandmother and that she is not getting any younger. Denise has the sense that Scott and Lisa are dependent on Lisa's mother and that there is pressure to have children. Scott will be undergoing surgery in 3 months. The couple hope that Lisa can get pregnant through IUI at the same time. Scott has a history of depression and anxiety and has been on medication for several years. He had two suicidal attempts when he was younger. It has been mandatory for him to work weekly with a therapist as he prepares for surgery and he reports, "Yeah, I kind of like him. He at least knows about things that are important to transgender people." He reports that his depression has been better since he has committed to surgery and since working with the therapist. His antidepressant medication was changed last week by his psychiatrist as he had plateaued and was not "where he thinks I should be."

Denise really struggles. Her mind filters every question and comment she makes before she says it. Is it offensive? Is there a better way I can say this? What are my assumptions? Am I warm and inviting? Will I ever be able to develop a warm positive regard with this client? How can I help them?

Scott's mental health history concerns Denise. She has seen many people with histories of depression; however, she is not able to get a feel for Scott and his mental health journey. Additionally, Scott has reported two suicide attempts. Scott has been defensive throughout the process and she feels that she has not been able to form a relationship with this client. She is concerned about the couple undergoing treatment to achieve a pregnancy at the same time as Scott's transition surgery. She is also concerned about the influence of Lisa's mother and cannot get a good read on the whole situation.

Denise continues methodically and carefully through the session, but her mind keeps turning. Can I recommend that this couple continue with treatment at this time? What supports would they need to move forward in their plan? She reports to the clinic that the couple has undergone the psychoeducational consultation, but that there are factors, such as upcoming surgery, that will be significant stressors on them currently, as well as mental health issues that are being addressed in treatment right now. She advises that the fertility doctor consult with Scott's mental health team to hear their recommendations as to whether Scott and Lisa pursue fertility treatment at this time.

Denise is both relieved that she had a solution and disappointed in herself that she was not able to make the couple feel comfortable. She feels both a sense of frustration and futility; she had put in so much work to update her consent forms, to be warm and inviting and nonjudgmental, but the couple remained guarded and unhappy. In the end, she knows that they felt judged by her. She also knows that by not saying "I recommend they continue with treatment," she did, in a way, judge them due to their unfamiliar story. While that was never her intention, she knows Scott and Lisa did not feel seen or heard. Overall, she feels like she failed.

Clients: Jacob and Vanessa

FC: Stephanie

Jacob and Vanessa have been together for 6 years. They met at an LGBTQ support group and felt they "just understood each other" in a way that nobody else did.

Stephanie is a 42-year-old cisgender social worker. She has seen many LGBTQ clients in her career. She tries to make everyone comfortable, and feels her way around in every case. She has struggled to discern whether she should ask everyone for their pronouns and has decided not to on a regular basis. However, she is aware that it is a question to ask if she gets any inklings that it would be appreciated. She also knows that she has made mistakes before, and so she is acutely aware that can happen again.

Upon arrival, Jacob and Vanessa immediately tell Stephanie that they have a question to discuss. Stephanie welcomes this and says, "I'll do the best I can – ask away!" Jacob begins, "My family no longer talks to me. I have very few ties to my earlier life. Once I transitioned, I laid down new roots and no one knows that I am transgender. I want to be a father, and to have children with Vanessa. She feels we need to disclose the use of donor sperm. I do not want to. If I love these children, why do they need to know? I am also afraid that my whole story would come to the surface."

Stephanie draws a deep breath. Jacob is asking the right question, but she feels they are jumping into the deep end before she has a chance to learn their background information or develop rapport. She is concerned that if they begin by discussing this question, where each partner has a specific opinion, she might come across as siding with one of them over the other, and she may never have a chance to build trust with both of them. In short, she concludes she needs to slow this down.

This type of "self-talk" is often helpful. When a therapist feels caught up in a wave, they have a choice to make – ride the wave or get out and stand on the beach.

Stephanie decides she wants to stand on the beach. She is honest with the couple, "These are very important issues and questions. I want to address them together and this is exactly the sort of thing to discuss in this session. But first, let me get some background information from both of you so I can know you better as we discuss this. Do you have any other thoughts or questions you want to share at this point to create an agenda that we can get back to later in the session?"

She takes her time, gathers information about their relationship, their stressors, their coping mechanisms and their supports. She asks them medical and mental health histories, asks about their family of origin and their current relationships with them, and about their religion and cultural communities so that she has a better understanding of their journey.

Then they dive in deeper. "Tell me more ... tell me about your thoughts about not disclosing your personal history to any children and how you came to that decision." They explore that area, with Stephanie recognizing and telling the clients that she is not an expert on transgender clients. They have a robust conversation about the interplay between the issues of disclosure regarding Scott's personal story and the use of unknown donor sperm. They discuss the difference between secrecy and privacy, as well as the potential ramifications on children when they discover "secrets" later on.

Stephanie feels she has done all she can. She believes that she has not sided with one partner over the other, but also knows that she discussed the idea of "secrets" and "transparency" which favors Vanessa's position more.

Stephanie ends the session by reminding the couple that the goal of this session was to lay out the land of third-party reproduction and that they do not need every answer right now, but that they want to be comfortable with the questions that will arise. She also recommends that they work with a therapist who specializes in couple's issues with transgender clients. She offers to help find an appropriate referral for them. They suggest that they might prefer to come back to see her in the future.

Overall, the clients seem to feel that the session was helpful and each seem to have understood some of the nuance of their partner's original position. Stephanie feels they have built a solid foundation on which they could potentially hold future conversations about these issues.

Clients: Michelle and Claire

FC: Marcy

Michelle and Claire are relieved to come to their recipient consultation. They were married before Michelle transitioned and it has been a long road. Claire is concerned about the age of her eggs and is excited to be starting a family-building journey. She knows that fertility treatments can be time consuming and are not always easy or successful. The couple has been through so much; donor conception is just their next chapter. They plan to use unknown donor sperm as Michelle does not want to go off hormone therapy and use her sperm. She just wants to be "one of the moms."

Marcy, their FC, notes that there is a solidity to this couple. It is clear that they are very supportive of one another.

Marcy realizes that the past several years has focused on Michelle and her transition. It has included a lot of appointments, the administration of medications and hormones, and a lot of emotional energy expended by both Michelle and Claire. Michelle has been working with a therapist throughout her transition and Claire has been involved in her therapy as needed.

As they discuss this, Marcy talks to the couple about what this might be like as Claire becomes the focus as the identified patient, with a new set of appointments for ART, the administration of medications and hormones, and the physical transition of pregnancy that will take several months. The couple had not thought about this upcoming pregnancy in those terms, but recognize that it will be a significant role reversal.

Michelle and Claire feel heard and seen by Marcy, and they share that they appreciate her insight. They are still excited for their journey but decide to continue in their counseling relationships to help support their marriage during this process. Marcy feels glad that she was able to adapt her style to fit a couple where they are in life. She has not seen many transgender clients, but by listening closely to their unique situation she was able to support them in their story.

Summary

As clinicians, we work hard to try to see each person and couple as individuals. We also listen and learn about groups of people, hoping to be aware of issues that can come up so that we can be on alert to help our clients navigate. Issues of transformation, changing bodies, identification with parental roles, family support, navigating disclosure regarding third-party reproduction as well as assigned sex at birth are all issues to explore with transgender clients. In addition, having resources specific to transgender intended parenting is important and the reader is directed to Addendum 17.1 for further information.

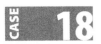

A Racially and Culturally Sensitive Approach to Fertility Counseling

Kimberly Grocher

Introduction

As a licensed clinical social worker, I have worked with women and couples across the lifespan in various contexts for almost two decades. Over the course of my career, I noticed the issues women face around their reproductive health and the impact this has on their mental health (and vice versa). As a Black woman, I was also personally, as well as professionally, aware of the issues and barriers Black women face when accessing reproductive and mental health services. I sought specialized training in fertility counseling and maternal mental health to be able to address the nuanced challenges many of my clients face when fertility challenges are part of the mosaic of struggles they face in life, especially my Black Indigenous and People of Color (BIPOC) clients. In addition to providing psychotherapy, I am a yoga and meditation teacher and often incorporate yoga and mindfulness meditation into my work with clients experiencing fertility and/or maternal mental health issues.

The following case is fictitious and inspired by several clients I have worked with over the years. The names in the case study are also fictitious.

The Case of Ashley and Dr. Yancy

"I'm just feeling so alone and isolated from the people I thought would support me throughout all of this, the people who I have gone out of my way to support whenever they needed me," Ashley frustratedly exclaimed while peering into the screen of her iPhone making what she thought was eye contact with her therapist. Ashley Brown is a 40-year-old bi-racial woman who identifies as Black living in Brooklyn, NY with her long-time partner, Wayne, a Southeast Asian man, and his 8-year-old daughter, Sienna.

Ashley's struggle with fertility has taken over her life and highlighted other areas that need a "renovation" as she describes. Chief among them is her current position as an attorney at one of the top law-firms in Manhattan, where she is the only Black woman in her division. She has been struggling with managing the work demands that include being available until the early morning hours, multiple clients, and several organizational meetings a day. Now there is the added responsibility of being "selected" for the firm's diversity, equity and inclusion (DEI) committee, which ultimately adds another lengthy meeting to her calendar each week, taking time away from billable hours, with the minimum billable hours seeming to rise despite being in the midst of a global pandemic.

Ashley was referred to counseling by her acupuncturist. Ashley has a close relationship with her acupuncturist and would often confide in her about the struggles she was facing on the fertility journey and how it impacted the other areas of her life. She would occasionally consider seeking therapy but was reluctant, since none of her close friends or family members had been in counseling and so she wasn't sure what to expect. She didn't want to find herself in another professional relationship where she had to play a role. Her acupuncturist recommended one of her colleagues, Dr. Lynelle Yancey, a licensed clinical social worker, who was also a woman of color. The following week, after another unsuccessful egg retrieval, Ashley reached out to Dr. Yancey for an appointment.

During the initial phone consultation, Dr. Yancey conducts with all potential new clients, she engaged Ashley in a conversation about her current concerns and how they were impacting her life. Feeling comfortable with the conversational style of this consultation, Ashley also opened up about her concerns with seeking counseling and what her loved ones would think if they knew she was seeking therapy, especially for her fertility challenges. She expressed that her mother and friends would often ask how the process was going and then casually offer other options, like adoption, for Ashley to consider. She was frustrated and hurt and knew that she needed a space where she could share her feelings without fear of judgment or unsolicited advice. She also expressed relief that Dr. Yancey was another Black woman and that she hoped to be able to address the racial issues that were also apart of some her challenges.

In the *pre-engagement phase*, Dr. Yancey was intentional about engaging Ashley in a conversation during the initial phone call about her concerns and encouraging Ashley to take the lead by sharing her story, as well as any questions that she might have about the process. Dr. Yancey did have a few pointed questions, such as had Ashley ever been in counseling before (no) and if she felt that things were so overwhelming that she had considered harming herself (no). These questions were asked during the initial conversation and after Dr. Yancey invited Ashley to ask any questions that she may have about the process or Dr. Yancey's way of working. Dr. Yancey and Ashley ended the consultation call by agreeing to meet virtually the following week due to COVID-19 restrictions. Dr. Yancey's role in the engagement phase did not end with the conversation. Dr. Yancey also identified as a Black woman and began conceptualizing what she knew about Ashley so far from this initial conversation. She considered what she would like to learn more about from Ashley in the intake session. She also thought about herself in relationship to Ashley and what she would need to be aware of as they built rapport. First and foremost was being careful not to assume that she and Ashley had similar life experiences or shared the same political, social or spiritual views.

Dr. Lynelle Yancey decided to specialize in fertility counseling after her own struggles with carrying a pregnancy in her late thirties, while working toward her Ph.D. in social work. Dr. Yancey and her partner, Simon, knew that they wanted to have children when they met during their doctoral studies. After dating for several months, Lynelle learned that she was pregnant. Admittedly unplanned, both Simon and Lynelle were elated about the surprise pregnancy. Unfortunately, their elation turned to devastation when Lynelle miscarried late in her first trimester. Simon, who was in his early forties, consoled Lynelle, but ultimately became distant and eventually ended the relationship, stating that having a family was a priority for him and that he worried about Lynelle's ability to have children at her "advanced age."

Heartbroken and struggling with the losses, Lynelle sought her own counseling. Though she had been working as a hospital social worker for several years, she had been reluctant to engage in her own therapy. The first therapist she met with was a White male psychologist who came highly recommended by one of her classmates. The initial session started well enough but took a turn when she began to open up about the miscarriage and the psychologist remarked, "I'm sorry for your loss .... I didn't think most Black women struggled with fertility. It's not something you often hear about." She didn't return for a second session but began to search for a therapist of color who specialized in working with pregnancy losses. She eventually found Clara Perez, a licensed mental health counselor, who identified as Latina. Her work with Ms. Perez helped her with processing her grief while also inspiring her to transition into clinical social work and working with women

experiencing fertility challenges. She knew how she struggled to find a fertility healthcare professional that could help her navigate the nuances of her experiences with fertility as a Black woman and wanted to provide that support for other Black women. When she felt she had reached a point in her own treatment where she could begin to hold space for the grief and pain of others, she began seeking training in fertility counseling. Since that time, Dr. Yancey's family life has grown to include her twin sons, conceived with donor eggs, who she is raising with her wife, Sabrina.

When Ashley and Dr. Yancey met for the initial session, Dr. Yancey invited Ashley to start with any questions that she might have and then asked Ashley if she'd like to share her story of what had led up to this moment. In the initial intake questionnaire Dr. Yancey asks all her clients to complete prior to the first session, the client is invited to share their race, ethnicity, gender, sexual orientation and spirituality/religion. The queries are open-ended questions that empower the client to use their own words to describe how they identify in each area. During the *teaching and learning phase*, Dr. Yancey asked Ashley how her identities have an impact on her current struggles. Ashley thought for a moment and then admitted that they did in ways that she had not intentionally considered before.

Throughout the *participatory evaluation phase*, Ashley and Dr. Yancey explored what would make this process meaningful and effective for Ashley and how she would know that for herself. Ashley shared that she wanted to be able to cope with the ups and downs of her fertility treatment. As of now, she felt that she vacillated between going numb and feeling as if she was drowning in her emotions. She stated that she would know she was coping better when, "I feel like I'm on a life raft, I can feel the motions and I am aware of what's happening, but I'm hanging on, I'm floating, I'm just riding the wave." Ashely and Dr. Yancey agreed to check in every few sessions to see how the process was going with regard to Ashley's goals and expected outcomes.

Over the course of the fertility counseling process, Ashley began to open up about her struggles on her fertility journey and how it related to other themes she struggled with in her life, especially when it came to her well-being. Ashley spoke openly about her struggles with being a bi-racial Black woman at work and in the healthcare system. At work she felt that she was often overlooked for opportunities to grow in the firm but was often tasked with work deemed too challenging for some of her colleagues or paired with other associates who needed additional guidance. The firm was making an effort to address race and diversity issues within the business by creating committees and sponsoring groups through their Employee Assistance Program (EAP) for BIPOC employees. This program provided a space to reflect on the current and ongoing racial tensions being felt across the United States (US) in the wake of the multiple murders of Black men and women by law enforcement throughout the country. While Ashley and her other BIPOC colleagues appreciated the gestures, they all agreed it wasn't enough, as the day-to-day microaggressions and stereotypes continued in the workplace.

Ashley was raised primarily by her African American mother, a college professor, after her parents divorced when she was a toddler. Her Caucasian father, also an attorney, relocated to California shortly after the divorce and married her stepmother, a Mexican American woman with three children from a previous marriage. She spent random holidays and a few weeks each summer with her father and his family. Growing up in Brooklyn, NY she was aware of the racial differences in her family and what that meant in the larger world, but for her personal world she felt loved and accepted by both sides of her family. There were the occasional warnings about being in the sun too long due to her darker skin tone from her stepmother and stepsister when they were basking in the sun on beautiful Californian beaches, but she never thought to let the comments bother her.

Ashley became more aware of the complexities of her identity in college, law school, and when she entered the workforce. She noticed the slights of being overlooked in her Ivy League classrooms – being singled out for comment when issues of race, social issues or anything associated with "otherness" came up; and the look of surprise on the faces of her White friends and colleagues when she brought them to her mother's beautiful historic brownstone for dinner. There were, also, the occasional assumptions that she was a scholarship recipient for diversity reasons and not because of her excellent grades. She experienced these issues as an observer as they almost felt surreal, like she couldn't quite claim them as an issue because she didn't always feel in touch with her "Blackness" as an adult. She didn't always feel accepted by her Black peers. She claimed her Black identity because of how close Ashley felt to her mother and her desire to identify with her mother as a child, wanting to feel that she belonged to her mother even though her features resembled her father far more.

Race and gender certainly impacted her fertility journey. She often wondered how it was possible for the medical system in the US to be so archaic when it came to women's reproductive health in the twenty-first century. In her counseling sessions, she recounted her experiences of being talked over and looked over during invasive procedures in the most intimate places on her body. There was one specific incident that stood out clearly in her mind that occurred when her physician, Dr. Paul, was away and was being covered by someone else in the practice that Ashley did not know very well. Since the timing of the procedure was critical, she agreed to let the covering physician complete the procedure. What she did not know is that medical students would be observing the process. As the students filed into the small room and took their places at the foot of the exam table where she had been placed in stirrups by the nurse only minutes ago, her voice caught in her throat. She wanted to let the physician know that she was not ok with having this procedure viewed by medical students, but something in her held back. The doctor was methodical as he described what he was doing to everyone in the room, though she knew it was more for the student's benefits than her own. At one point, the procedure became unusually uncomfortable to the point of pain. She told the doctor that she was experiencing pain to which he replied, "If you could please try to relax, you won't be in as much pain." She felt humiliated and unable to speak and attempted to use the breathing exercises that were part of her yoga practice to no avail. Her body's response to the pain only frustrated the doctor and he asked several of the medical students to assist Ashley with holding her body still and "legs open."

Ashley left the appointment feeling ashamed and violated. While she was very angry with the covering doctor for the way he disregarded her pain and discomfort during the procedure and didn't inform her beforehand that medical students would be viewing the procedure, she was angrier with herself. Why hadn't she said anything? She was an attorney who was skilled at speaking up and advocating for others. What had caused her to go mute when it came to her own body? Her anger only increased later when she explained the incident to Dr. Paul. To his credit, he empathized with her experience and asked if she had requested anesthesia. Ashley hadn't known that she could ask for anesthesia nor had anyone talked to her about requesting it if in pain. Instead, she assumed that it would be administered if needed, especially since she had expressed that she was in pain. Ashley vaguely recalled a conversation with a close friend, Nina, also a Black woman, about something Nina read where Black women were perceived as having a higher tolerance for pain. At the time, Ashley thought the notion was ridiculous and hadn't given much thought to it until Nina's words came floating back to her in Dr. Yancey's office while she was discussing the event.

Through the course of fertility counseling, Ashley became more aware of how her social identity as a Black woman also played into the process. Dr. Yancey provided a safe space for Ashley to explore these complexities as they arose in the context of Ashley's fertility journey, without imposing her own ideas of what Ashley's experience might be as another Black woman. She had done the research on the state of reproductive health for Black women in the US and knew, also, from her own personal struggles with fertility. Through supervision and knowing how countertransference may impact the therapeutic process, Dr. Yancy allowed herself to be curious about Ashley's experiences and the meaning they held for Ashley, while using her knowledge to validate and empathize with Ashley's feelings. She also realized that even if she didn't possess this knowledge, her role was to validate and not to question Ashley about whether this was an issue related to her race. She realized that race and cultural issues are subjective and based on objective cultural and power dynamics in a given society. This seemed to be particularly helpful to Ashley when she found herself questioning her own reactions, whether this could indeed be attributed to race.

The fertility counseling process helped Ashley to notice themes of being the observer in her life, being hesitant to speak up for herself because she wasn't sure if her perceptions or experience were valid. She found herself in situations where she thought she would have power, but often felt the opposite, completely powerless. The fertility journey was a culmination of these themes. She often found herself shouldering her issues alone, as the people in her life assumed she had it all together and could take care of herself.

These issues spanned into her relationship with Wayne. While Wayne was eager to have a child with her, he also had a daughter, and Ashley often felt the fertility process wasn't as urgent for him as it was for her. She often went to her fertility treatment appointments alone, not wanting to disrupt his or Sienna's schedule, even when she could have used the emotional and physical support after pulling all-nighters for work. It was difficult for her to acknowledge that beneath her "I have it handled" appearance was deep grief, anger, and a sense of inferiority that she was unable to give Wayne a child.

Ashley and Wayne, a Southeast Asian man born and raised in New York City, already faced challenges as an interracial couple, and this added to the complexities. Ashley didn't feel particularly embraced by Wayne's family and her challenges getting pregnant seemed to only widen the divide. At a recent gathering she overheard his uncle tell him "... it's not as if you're married yet. Maybe you might have an easier go of it with one of your own. You and Sarika had no problems conceiving Sienna. Maybe that's a sign." Through the work she did in fertility counseling with Dr. Yancey, Ashley began to voice these concerns in her relationship. She and Wayne decided to go to couples counseling to help them navigate the fertility treatment process and their different backgrounds so they could learn how to support one another on this journey.

After working together weekly for 8 months, Ashley brought up ending fertility counseling, bringing them to the *termination phase*. Dr. Yancey and Ashley had been checking in regularly about her desired outcomes in the counseling process and how they were (or at times, weren't) progressing in those areas. Ashley valued the process and felt that she had reached the place where she found her raft, she was able to be present with her emotions, feel them, and manage them in a way that allowed them to be present in the rest of her life. She was also feeling more supported in her relationship with Wayne and had recently joined a yoga fertility group with other women who were at various stages of their fertility journey. Further, she was able to set healthier boundaries at work and with her family and friends. While she was still grieving the fact that up until this point her fertility treatments had not been successful in the way she hoped, Ashley was not ready to give up and felt that the work she had done in therapy helped her cultivate the resilience to continue.

Conclusion

Dr. Yancey respected and supported Ashley's decision to end therapy at this time. She noted in the *action and accompaniment phase* of working together, shifts in Ashley's ability to manage her emotions and apply the coping skills they explored in their sessions to her fertility journey as well as her workplace stressors and her relationship. Ashley was no longer pushing past her emotions – she was aware of them, engaged them and most importantly showed herself compassion for having them and gave herself permission to ride "the raft" she metaphorically constructed when her emotions threatened to overwhelm her. She and her partner were actively engaged in the couple therapy process and were making significant changes in their relationship which included Wayne being more available to accompany her to appointments and both empathizing with the other's perspective on their fertility challenges. They were also engaging in challenging conversations related to their cultural differences and the impact this has on their relationship and the future family they are committed to creating together. While Ashley had not yet been able to conceive, she demonstrated acceptance for where she was currently on her fertility journey.

Dr. Yancey also recognized that psychotherapy could have continued to be a support to Ashley during this time and respectfully offered ways that psychotherapy might be beneficial to her in the near future. Ashley agreed with Dr. Yancey and expressed gratitude for knowing that she could return to therapy if needed, but ultimately decided that she wanted to terminate the process right now. Dr. Yancey suspected that Ashley was still uncomfortable with the concept of "being in therapy" while also understanding and experiencing how beneficial it can be. Ashley admitted during one session, "sometimes coming here is a reminder that I am broken, my body is broken, my mind is broken, my emotions are broken ... and I need all these treatments to put me together again although I'm not always convinced they can ...."

In her clinical supervision, Dr. Yancey was able to reflect on challenges with managing her emotions during sessions where Ashley's experience triggered memories of her own fertility journey. She also examined the places where she needed to remain curious about Ashley, not assuming that their lived experience, or that the meaning attributed to similar experiences, were alike. At the same time, she needed to lean in when Ashley reached for connection around their similarities of being Black women in America. Early on, Dr. Yancy shared with Ashley that she was interested in this work due to her own experiences, and while that seemed to relax Ashley in the moment, there was no further inquiry from Ashley about her experience. Knowing that there was this connection seemed to be enough. Dr. Yancy also needed to come to terms with her definition of "success" for Ashley in therapy and how it differed from Ashley's definition of "success" for herself. By being able to recognize and manage her own triggers, experiences, expectations and their potential implications on the therapeutic process, Dr. Yancy was able to provide Ashley with the support she needed in a way that Ashley benefitted from and in a frame that was meaningful for Ashley's fertility journey.

Resilience in Reproductive Loss

Irving Leon

Introduction

I am a clinical psychologist who has been in practice for 40 years and an Adjunct Associate Professor at University of Michigan Medical Center for 20 years. While my training was in traditional psychodynamic therapy, my current approach is more eclectic and Rogerian in its emphasis on empathic engagement with the client as the primary vehicle of change. My initial interest in reproductive loss was based on having a number of child cases in which perinatal sibling loss was an important unrecognized dynamic. But my lifelong dedication to this area was decided after my wife had several ectopic pregnancies followed by infertility and the adoption of our son.

What follows is a detailed case summary with italicized commentary. For didactic and confidentiality reasons some material was altered and composite characters drawn.

Unexplained Infertility

Susan is a 34-year-old woman with unexplained infertility who has been trying to become pregnant for 5 years, having had five IVF rounds resulting in two miscarriages, the last one 3 months ago. She was so visibly distraught in our first session, her husband, Paul, did much of the talking (he also arranged the consultation). I didn't call attention to her silence and distress to allow the interaction to unfold. Eventually she joined in, remaining on the verge of tears, expressing her deep frustration and embarrassment over how out of control she felt her life was, including her emotions. She can't stand how she starts crying when she talks about her medical treatment and so sometimes, prefers to be silent.

It is not unusual to have this extreme distress upon initial presentation, often mistaken for greater disturbance than is the case. It felt paramount to demonstrate and ally with her having some control in her life. This violates the almost instinctive therapeutic strategy of facilitating her grief, which might only have intensified her feeling out of control in this case. This is an example of tailoring the interaction to meet the needs of the client. Importantly, she distinguished her life not being literally out of control, but it feeling that way.

I asked her if there were any areas in her life where she felt effective and in control. Brightening a bit, she still enjoyed and felt she did well at her job of doing applied research in the medical school. I told her that was great, both in and of itself, as well as providing a welcome distraction from the infertility and its treatments, with which she agreed.

She clearly resonated with having an arena of competent functioning, preserved by compartmentalization, suggesting some areas where her self-worth still flourished. I also endorsed her using repressive coping [1] as a valuable defensive tool to avoid unpleasant thoughts and feelings. The cumulative trauma of multiple losses and invasive treatments due to infertility is often recalled by clients as just as devastating, if not more so, as single reproductive losses, evidenced in this case by it initially leaving her speechless.

She has been much more private in sharing her feelings with family and friends than her gregarious husband. Infertility doesn't appear to affect him the way it tears her apart, but she feels he is compassionate when she needs his support. He will at least listen to her. She can't tolerate being with mothers with young babies, because they have what she so much wants. Due to time constraints, she has cut back her aerobic exercising from four to five times a week to only once or twice a week, a major deprivation for her. At the end of the first session, I normalized her intense feelings of frustration at the beginning of the session, and strongly encouraged her to find the time to resume her exercise regimen, as it would help her to feel better and begin to get back some of her prior life. I also validated her wanting to avoid seeing infants right now, something that virtually all women in her situation feel.

Without labeling her earlier feelings of embarrassment when she cried at the outset (which could serve to only shame her more), I normalized her intense distress and avoidance of seeing other babies. In categorizing her reactions as typical of women struggling with fertility issues and the treatments they endure, it is important that one conveys genuine empathy for those feelings, lest it be experienced by her as dismissing her pain and it not warranting any help. Encouraging her to resume her earlier exercise frequency was intended to improve her depressed affect and, just as importantly, covertly demonstrate that more is in her control than she actively asserts (though I am aware that telling her what to do may not be the optimal way of helping her to recover some sense of control). I chose not to highlight her primary issue (at least up to now) of loss of control, as I wanted more material on that, expecting it would re-emerge in a later session because it often is such a major issue for high-achieving couples [2]. I also suppressed the urge to introduce the potency of societal stigma of infertility [3] instigating feelings of embarrassment, fearing that would lead to her feeling more isolated and rejected rather than providing a normalized explanation which might reduce her shame.

We scheduled individual sessions to enable me to get a better sense of how each of them was handling the fertility issues. Paul minimized its impact on him, stressing he was coming in for her. He found relief in talking to others and playing golf. He could not offer any specific goals for himself in therapy. He believed it was especially important to reduce his wife's stress, fearing that was another factor interfering with her becoming or maintaining a pregnancy. While I acknowledged that was possible, I was concerned that emphasizing that to his wife might only serve to increase her sense of responsibility and self-blame, thereby increasing her stress.

As is true of many, though far from all, men in this situation, his motivation was to help his wife get pregnant but not to meaningfully participate in the therapy. Similar to most men, his distress was significantly less than that of his wife, as the woman is culturally saddled with responsibility for fertility issues even when causality is unknown or there is male factor. He did maintain his support for his wife throughout the therapy, but felt no need for himself to come in. While pressure could have been exerted for him to participate directly, their being neither estranged nor negatively entangled in their marriage led me to leave it up to him (and her) to decide who should come in, which he chose not to do. It would also provide a more concentrated focus on her distress and difficulties.

In my first individual session with Susan, she was much less tearful, especially when discussing her life apart from the infertility. She felt it helped to hear what I had to say, thinking of sharing more of what she has been through and increasing the frequency of her exercise. She bitterly complained about how hard it was not to know the cause of the infertility and how much IVF was disrupting her life. She was always able to accomplish what she set out to do, was a good student, followed all the rules, and now she can't even plan vacations. She had

less intercourse with Paul and had to deal with her work schedule in turmoil due to the unpredictability of the IVF process. While she still believed in God, she felt estranged from Him, believing she didn't deserve this. "It's unfair that everyone from all over the world can do this," while knowing more than 15% of the US population struggled with fertility issues at some point in their lives. She felt her life had been like a race she had always won or finished well, while, now, everyone was passing her and she was frozen in place. Her usual upbeat approach to life and self-confidence now seemed a thing of the past. She felt alienated from couples becoming families. While it usually helped when her family empathized with her pain, sometimes it bothered her when friends made too big a deal of it, which only validated how awful this was. I told her it made sense that the fertility issues had been so difficult because it challenged some of her fundamental ways of viewing the world as safe and fair, that if you worked hard and played by the rules, good things would come to you. It's as if someone had pulled the rug out from under her and everything before that felt manageable now felt out of her control. Not having the successes that helped make her feel good about herself now left her feeling like a failure. Pausing a moment, I went on to say with conviction that these challenging circumstances needn't determine her future. Her long-standing faith in herself, her sense of efficacy in achieving her goals, and her positive attitude would guide her back to her former happy life. I said I thought we might try and tackle her feelings of things being out of control, noting how she already was able to assert more control by increasing the frequency of her exercising. Perhaps there were other aspects of her situation where she could exert more control, while paradoxically relinquishing the expectation of almost total control that was both impossible as well as a burden to try to realize.

Susan was able to tell us in vivid detail that the central issues for her appear to be a profound loss of control in her life, which includes a loss of meaning and blaming herself for not producing a child. I tried to empathize with what her infertility meant to her, cognizant of her not mentioning the most intense deprivation it causes for most couples with infertility, denying them the experience of parenting their own child. This, of course, does not mean that loss is not significant, but importantly it is not cited as her most pressing difficulty, and, as such should not guide our treatment plan and interventions. Her personal strengths are cited as crucial supports for returning to a more solid sense of well-being. In fact, those effective attributes correspond to many of the elements of resilience that she possesses but bypass her now. Her potent sense of loss of control and reduced efficacy speak to the current diminishing of her usual mode of active coping [4] in challenging adverse circumstances, perhaps the most important element of resilience. Contextualizing her distress in the loss of meaningful expectations of reward for good work helps her to make sense of her current spiritual confusion, a beginning to making meaning of her acute distress, another important ingredient of resilience [5]. More work in this area will need to be done in paring down the expectation of total control, alluded to at the end of my last remarks. Finally, while masked by her current hopelessness, her history of positive emotions (another source of resilience) [6] speaks well to her likely momentum in improved functioning once she hits her stride. I did not overtly respond to her dissonant reaction to a friend's empathy, but dialed down my empathic resonance with her, instead supporting her capacity to weather the rough waters ahead.

There was significant, immediate, emotional relief when the couple, under Susan's direction, decided to take a couple of months off from trying the next IVF cycle. I supported her sharing the situation and the distress it brought with several close colleagues at work, enabling her not to feel so alone. She did not feel ready to check out the recommended self-help group for infertility, RESOLVE. It was an important revelation to observe that she could feel connected to a good friend who had just given birth, due to this woman's consideration in not discussing her baby much with Susan.

Susan deciding to take a vacation from IVF not only enabled her to feel more in control of her life and treatment, but also implicitly challenged the expectation (and reality) that IVF is now a regular part of life, rather than a decision to postpone or even stop. Sharing the infertility with close colleagues enlarged her support network, and it was especially valuable to include several trusted co-workers who could provide consolation if she received bad news at work. They could also run interference for her by sharing (or not) the situation with other colleagues, if Susan wished, rather than her being put on the spot answering unwanted questions. Sharing also helped to undercut the stigma and associated shame which is magnified by feeling this condition must be kept secret. Although attending RESOLVE meetings can be liberating and can facilitate feeling not so different from others by seeing oneself as part of a larger group, for some it can feel a violation of privacy by "coming out" to strangers, and relinquishing the sense of control – so important to Susan – in deciding who and when others are told. Susan appreciated her friend's form of empathy that did not involve resonating with her feelings, but having the sensitivity to be aware of how hurtful it would be to Susan for her friend to be gushing over her baby.

In subsequent sessions, Susan's distress and sadness considerably lessened, with greater ability to talk about the fertility issues in and outside of therapy without crying. Feeling she could decide when treatments would be, as well as recognizing the unrealistic nature of believing she could control the outcome, helped mitigate the earlier profound sense of losing control of her life. She could now see how much of her life was under her control, including the pace of treatments, whether and with whom to share her feelings, her schedule, her exercising, etc. She was also increasingly realizing she could not tolerate doing IVF indefinitely with these results, and was considering she would do only one more cycle. She would be very sad if it didn't work out but she would get over it. We reframed this not as "giving up" or losing the race, but as a realistic understanding of other options, including adoption or being childfree. While Susan reported that Paul was sad to hear she was moving away from ART if the next attempt didn't work, he didn't pressure Susan to stick with it. He didn't feel he could adopt and raise "someone else's" child. But he found his life more than satisfying, was delighted to see Susan showing more of her old self, so not having children held some appeal.

By talking through many of the feelings of infertility, Susan could tolerate her distress more and cried less. Even though we welcome crying as a natural expression of grieving, many clients feel gratified when they can get through a session without tears, as a sign of mastery and active coping (sometimes unfortunately called "being strong"). By accepting more and more that she couldn't control the outcome of IVF, Susan could feel more in control of her daily life. Nor did IVF not working make her a failure or a loser, even if it was disappointing. In the process of making her schema of having to be in control less absolute and rigid, she could make sense of her predicament by incorporating a more tragic view of life, where we don't always get what we want, as deserving as we may be. Identifying the final IVF may be helpful in controlling its usage, if not the outcome, anticipating processing the many conflicting feelings of grief, relief, sadness, and freedom that follow.

One session was marked by a return to tears and sadness as she approached her thirty-fifth birthday without the family she hoped and expected she would have by then. Her grief was normalized and supported, with my encouraging her to go out with her friends, even if she was determined it not be a celebration. Ultimately, she felt gratitude for the family and friends who did care about her.

It was important for Susan to see that she could grieve for something worth grieving – a cherished dream of having a family by 35 years old, a lifelong narrative that was not to be and might never happen [7]. Some clients fear this sadness will set them back to square one when instead it is a reminder that grieving infertility is slowly, sadly and meaningfully relinquishing all the wishes along the way projected onto our planned future. There is the next session, without tears, as life goes on.

With her dramatically diminished distress we began meeting less frequently. She was much calmer as she was preparing for what she expected would be her final IVF attempt. We reviewed how much she felt she had her life back, being able to decide when and if to make any IVF attempts. Her tension and stress lessened considerably with her resuming her more frequent exercise regimen, as well as planning to distract herself when anxious during a cycle by socializing more. She observed she was less of a "control freak." She reported feeling gratitude for not having an even worse situation, such as a friend preparing to parent a disabled baby. It felt good to be able to reach out to others who had losses so they wouldn't have to silently suffer. She took deep pleasure in mentoring new researchers at work.

Not only did Susan resiliently retain many of the aspects of her old self, she demonstrated nice examples of posttraumatic (or postloss) growth [8], gains resulting from the adversity she faced. Instead of focusing on what she had lost, she appreciated the goodness in her life, especially not taking her friends for granted, and trusting them to be caring confidants when needed. While still counting on herself to get what she seeks and works hard for (it did get her far), she recognized she can't determine all outcomes and gave up some of her need to be in total control. Finally, even though it did not appear her loss of parenting was the central issue it is with most women dealing with infertility, apparent postloss gains are evident in sublimations of those wishes witnessed by her pleasure from increased nurturance in both reaching out to those suffering losses and mentoring younger colleagues.

After meeting for 4.5 months, we tentatively planned for her to get back to me sometime during or after her upcoming final IVF cycle, but I never heard back from her, even after trying to contact her about a month later to follow-up.

It is not possible to know exactly the reason for her choosing not to follow-through with our plan to touch base. If the IVF procedure was unsuccessful, she perhaps didn't want to risk sharing a painful though understandable return to past, present, and future reproductive losses, which a session would likely have triggered. If the procedure was successful, there might have been a similar motivation despite the different circumstances, wanting not to be reminded of her struggles with infertility and trying to now put it behind her. A nonending ending such as this does not disqualify the many gains she made during her therapy. But it may leave her therapist frustrated and disappointed that as a participating listener to her narrative, he is left hanging, perhaps a fitting conclusion to losses that leave traces of open-endedness that may never be completely resolved.

References

1. Bonanno GA. Loss, trauma and human resilience: have we underestimated the human capacity to thrive after extremely aversive events? *Psych Trauma: Theory, Res, Pract, Policy* 2008;**8**:101–113.

2. Leon IG. Understanding and treating infertility: psychoanalytic considerations. *J Am Acad Psa Dyn Psychiatr* 2010;**38**:47–76.

3. Whiteford LM, Gonzalez L. Stigma: the hidden burden of infertility. *Soc Sci Med* 1995;**40**:27–36.

4. Stroebe M, Schut H. The dual process model of coping with bereavement: a decade on. *Omega* 2010;**61**:273–289.

5. Neimeyer R. Searching for the meaning of meaning: grief therapy and the process of reconstruction. *Death Studies* 2000;**24**:541–558.

6. Rutten BP, Hammels C, Geschwind N, et al. Resilience in mental health: linking psychological and neurobiological perspectives. *Acta Psychiatr Scand* 2013;**128**:3–20.

7. Jaffe J, Diamond MO. *Reproductive Trauma: Psychotherapy with Infertility and Pregnancy Loss Clients*. Washington, DC: American Psychological Association, 2011.

8. Tedeschi RG, Calhoun LG. Beyond the concept of recovery: growth and the experience of loss. *Death Studies* 2007;**32**:27–39.

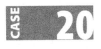

Reproductive Trauma and PTSD: On the Battlefield of Fertility Counseling

Janet Jaffe

Introduction

As a clinician in private practice for over 25 years, it has been my privilege to work with hundreds of men and women on their reproductive journeys. I became a psychologist after surviving my own fertility issues. There was so little support and understanding at that time; I felt like I could make a difference and help others through their trauma. So, back to school I went!

My training was in psychodynamic psychotherapy, but as will become evident in reading this chapter, I combine dynamic work with an eclectic mix of narrative therapy, cognitive therapy and grief work. I am always aware that patients initially arrive in a traumatized state: nowhere in their hopes and dreams for a family did they expect that fertility issues and reproductive losses would take such a toll.

The case I present in this chapter is about Evelyn, who has just turned 33 years old.[*] A professional actor, she splits her time performing in the community and teaching children in a theater school. A creative and talented person, she began therapy feeling depressed, traumatized, and full of self-doubt. She and her husband, Jayden, who is an ethnic studies professor, started trying to conceive about 2 years ago, first "on their own," followed by a series of IUIs. Recently on a "break" from treatment, Evelyn did conceive naturally, but had an early miscarriage.

This chapter serves as an illustration to concepts discussed in the accompanying *Clinical Guide* volume, focusing on the trauma of infertility and pregnancy loss. As noted there, reproductive trauma is usually not a single event, but very often chronic in nature. So many of our patients struggle with the seemingly never-ending time they are in fertility treatment, and sadly may also deal with pregnancy losses as well. In the case I present here, we will listen to Evelyn's reproductive story, how she thought things would go, and how she has coped with being on the battlefield. Whether you are new to this specialty or are a "seasoned" fertility counselor, I hope that this will offer new ways to conceptualize reproductive trauma. I have attempted to provide

[*] This case is entirely fictitious; any resemblance to someone, living or deceased, is purely coincidental. It has been compiled from several sources to illustrate issues that typify reproductive trauma and loss.

reflections of my process as well, from both a theoretical and emotional viewpoint.

Evelyn's Reproductive Story: The Beginning of the Battle

The early sessions with Evelyn focused on the course of her fertility journey: her story started with excitement and joy about creating a family. She and Jayden finally felt ready, but were shocked by how difficult it was for them to conceive. She was grieving, her self-esteem was at an all-time low, and the expectations she had about her life were fracturing.

"I never thought it would be this hard," she began. "I thought I would just stop birth control, you know, and boom. A baby. I'm just so exhausted. And after all that, to *finally* get pregnant on our own and then have a miscarriage – it's just too much! I don't understand why this has happened to us. What did we do to deserve this? And now we are really confused about what to do next. Should we try again on our own? The fertility clinic suggested we do IVF. Should we bite the bullet? It's so ridiculously expensive. I mean, it's just so unfair!"

Evelyn gave insight into some of her deeply held core beliefs and assumptions [1]: (1) getting pregnant would be easy; (2) they must have done something wrong to deserve this; and (3) life is fair. Interwoven into her current trauma, I listened to her worries about what was going to come next. In taking her history, I also learned that her mother struggled with alcohol abuse, her father died when she was an adolescent, and she felt responsible for taking care of her younger sibling; more events in her life that were traumatic and unfair. We discussed how she coped with the early trauma in her life.

"I don't think I ever really did cope with it . . . I'm still dealing with it now, to be honest. Back then . . ." she sighed. "I just sucked it up. I had to, for my little brother. My mother was barely functional." She paused and again tried not to cry. "It was such a shock; my father collapsed at work. I stepped in and took over: made sure bills got paid, made sure dinner was on the table. I guess I was the strong one – at least on the outside." It was clear that this was difficult for her to talk about. "When I think back on it now, that was when I got involved in theater. Playing different characters allowed me to escape into another world – at least for some of the time. Don't get me wrong, I cried a lot too, only I did it when no one was around."

"Sounds like you had to play a role at home as well as in your theater classes. You had to act the part of being strong and invincible," I said.

"Totally," Evelyn replied. "I've really never thought about it that way, but you are spot on." After a pause she added, "It's really awful when a kid can't be a kid. I don't want my child to have to take care of me. Ever." We spoke about the beginnings of her reproductive story [2] (see Chapter 20 in the *Clinical Guide*) and its development throughout her life. I gained insight into how she coped with adversity, and I appreciated her need to be in control. Her early narrative and the need to cope with the death of her father and an alcoholic mother was formative in the foundations of her adult self. She developed a strong outer façade, while internally shouldering intense feelings. Having a child of her own would not only give her the opportunity to parent in a different way than she was brought up, but also to re-parent herself.

"Do you feel the need to be strong and invincible now?" I queried, bringing her back to the present.

"Well, I do feel the need to be strong, but guess what?" she half-chuckled, "I am falling apart! I guess that's why I'm here."

Challenging Assumptions and Grief Work: The Battle Goes On and On

As our weekly sessions continued, a pattern unfolded: we focused on family of origin dynamics; the pain of her current trauma of infertility and pregnancy loss; her feelings of guilt and self-blame; and her anxieties about the future. We discussed using the reproductive story as a way of coping with her relentless fertility battle. Knowing she was presently in the middle of this narrative was helpful in many ways. First, it was important for her to tell her story in as many intricate details as necessary – not just about her fertility issues but also about her life and relationships. Telling her story in depth was essential to her growth in coping with trauma and loss. I encouraged her not to shy away from details: her internal fears, ambivalence and shame.

Secondly, knowing that she kept things bottled up informed me that I needed to gently probe and challenge her faulty assumptions about herself and her life. These assumptions (discussed at length in the accompanying *Clinical Guide* chapter), about how the world is and how the world should be were blocking her from moving forward. She was beating herself up for her fertility struggles; it was important to challenge her negative thinking and cognitive distortions.

Lastly, the reproductive story provided Evelyn with a sense of control. She realized that there would be an end to this battle, even though we couldn't be sure what that would look like at this point. Knowing that she still had some ability to edit and rewrite her story allowed us to explore her future.

The following are excerpts of our work together.

Grief and Loss: The Miscarriage

"I had a dream last night that hundreds of bugs were trying to get through the screen window. They kept banging their heads against the screen, such an awful sound, and then they started to die. It was so frightening and I couldn't do anything to save them."

She recognized the symbolism of the dream: how difficult conception had been, and the guilt of not being able to protect her unborn child. I encouraged her to talk more about the details of the miscarriage. While it can be uncomfortable for the therapist to hear, the need to tell one's story in depth is part of the healing process. She spoke about her ride to Urgent Care, how she was treated there, the sterile room where she had an ultrasound, the look on the clinician's face. These are the kinds of images that are often replayed over and over in our patient's minds; being able to speak them out loud and share them with me took some of the punch away and made them less unbearable. Even so, her self-blame was profound. "Even before my baby was born, I can think of so many things I did wrong," she cried. "At the theater I moved some of the set pieces out of the way. They weren't that heavy, but . . . and I also had a glass of wine before I knew, not thinking I could possibly be pregnant."

Self-blame, guilt and anxiety are so common in fertility patients. My own reaction to hearing her emotional distress was like a knee-jerk reflex: I wanted to take the pain away and assure her she did nothing wrong. Her assumption – if something went wrong it must be her fault – was flawed, and I knew if I challenged it too soon, I would stop her from unloading her feelings. Instead, I encouraged her to tell me more.

"I know it's not rational but I keep wondering why my body is not working right. Is there something wrong with me? Sometimes I feel like I'm not supposed to have a baby – like there's something or someone out there deciding who should have children or not. I know that sounds ridiculous, but sometimes I really believe it."

"Your feelings are not ridiculous"; at this point I needed to reassure her. "When people have been traumatized, they often ask *why me*? We want to understand why – and we blame ourselves, even if it's not rational." It was important to normalize the self-blame; I purposely used *we* to convey that she was not alone in her thoughts and feelings. "In many ways it feels better to blame oneself instead of having no reason at all. It gives us a sense of control – if we believe we know what caused the problem, we can avoid repeating it."

"The night before my dad passed away, he yelled at me for having the music on too loud. I did that typical teenager eye roll thing; I was so annoyed. But I've never been able to play that music again." I nodded. Her ability to make the connection between feeling responsible, grieving both the past and the present, and trying to let go of the guilt was significant.

Self-Blame and Stress

At another session, her focus turned to her mother. While her current relationship with her mother is better, Evelyn still feels the need to take care of her, and finds it necessary to hide her fertility struggles from her. "She tries to be a support, but her attempts just fall flat. Actually, she gives advice, not support, like *you're just too stressed*. She told me she heard from one of her friends about this herbal cream that supposedly enhances fertility. My first thought was snake oil! But I mean if I don't try everything does that mean I don't really want this to happen? I feel like I'm a bad mother if I don't do it all."

At this juncture, it was important for us to disentangle some of these feelings. Using a blend of cognitive techniques, we discussed how faulty assumptions could lead to self-distortions and self-blame. Our patients often feel as if they need to continue their battle with infertility, just to prove they've done everything, even if their attempts defy logic. As discussed in the *Clinical Guide*, Chapter 20, the core belief that *I can achieve what I set out to do if I just work hard enough* was at play. Evelyn needed to regain trust in herself and her decisions. It was also essential for her to decouple stress from her fertility problems. "I don't know anyone who isn't stressed and distressed when they're struggling with reproductive problems," I said, trying to normalize her feelings.

Feeling Stuck

Many of our patients feel trapped by fertility issues. Because Evelyn felt that she couldn't leave the battlefield, other decisions about her life were on hold.

"There's a play coming up that I'd love to be part of . . . the director actually has me in mind for a great part," she began. "But what if we do go forward with IVF? There are so many appointments . . . what if they interfere with rehearsals? And what if I get pregnant? I suppose we could try to plan it all around the show schedule, but that would mean pushing IVF out. And what if I get pregnant before then?" She was clearly becoming distraught.

We discussed what it would feel like to say "no" to this opportunity. "Just awful," she said. "It would feel like another loss. But I'm worried – I don't want to let anyone down."

Over the years of doing this work, I have heard many patients struggle with these kinds of decisions: putting off vacations; delaying the purchase of a home; waiting to change jobs. Having grappled through some of the same kinds of decisions in my own fertility battle, my inclination was to jump in and advise Evelyn to take the part in the upcoming show. This, however, was part of *her* process; it was another area where *she* had to take control and feel good about it. What was of value was her analysis of her own feelings: what there was to gain, and what there was to lose. Being mired in so many losses she felt it was inevitable things would go south, no matter what her decision. Here was yet another assumption we could focus on, and in doing so, not only did she have to believe in herself, but I, too, had to trust that her choice would be right for her.

Left Out and Left Behind

"Tell me more about the teaching you do. How old are the kids you generally work with?" I asked.

"I work with kindergarten kids. They're so sweet and creative, full of beans! But it's also challenging."

I urged her to say more. "The hardest part is not about the kids, truth be told; actually, it's interacting with their moms that's the issue. Many of them are having their second or even third kid. They come with little ones in tow. There's a stroller brigade outside the classroom. Some of the moms are even younger than I am; makes me feel like an old crone. It should be me."

Once again, I needed to normalize and label these negative feelings. "How could you not feel jealous?" I asked. "It must seem like everyone can get pregnant, when and how they choose. I don't think most of us are aware of how much we believe this. It's so ingrained in us, that we don't even realize it until we hit a brick wall. Problems having children happen to other people, not us." Here, I was echoing notions of her reproductive story.

"Yup. I am feeling exactly that way with friends too. There's a group of us – they're all either pregnant or have babies. I'm the last one standing – so to speak. I feel like such a bad friend. Social events are more and more difficult – I just want to stay home, which is not like me. Sure, I'm happy for them on the outside, but inside I just want to crawl into a hole."

She was reporting another layer of grief and trauma: feeling left out and left behind. The battle she was fighting was creating a chasm between her and her peers. The expectation that she would be able to fit in and be part of the parenting "club" was deep within her reproductive story. It was also reminiscent of how she coped with her father's death: for all intents and purposes appearing strong outwardly, but in reality and privately, in intense pain.

This insight led us to explore other ways she might be able to cope: if family and friends understood, would they be more supportive? She decided to try talking about her reproductive battles more openly, where it felt safe to do so. In essence she was willing to try teaching others about infertility and pregnancy loss: how deeply traumatized she felt by the experience. She thought this would help raise her self-esteem: letting others know what to say and what wasn't appropriate would allow her to feel in charge. We also discussed the possibility of finding a support group where she didn't have to explain herself over and over.

Leaving the Battlefield: How Does the Story End?

The idea of the reproductive narrative having an end point was continually woven into our sessions, as Evelyn was not only grappling to make sense of the past and the present, but also of her future. Even though she had conceived without medical intervention, her clinic recommended IVF as the next step to increase the odds of a live birth. She and Jayden were clearly faced with a major decision. Should they try again on their own or should they move forward with the medical plan laid out by the clinic?

"These decisions are part of the trauma I'm experiencing, aren't they? Most people don't have to consider this at all. This is part of my assumption that 'life is fair.' I'm getting it! This whole thing has been out of my control!"

"Well, yes, to a great degree," I replied. "But you and Jayden get to make the decision – albeit a very difficult one – about what to do next; you get to consciously write

the next chapter of your story. This part is in your control and you do have options."

We considered the possibilities, one of which was to remain childfree. As she adamantly rejected that, we discussed the plusses and minuses of trying on their own versus using IVF. I suggested that she and Jayden separately write down their feelings about each, why one would be a better or worse option in each of their estimations. My own opinions needed to stay in check. I have grown to recognize that these moments are difficult for me; I can get overly invested in wanting my patients to have a baby. My countertransference is something I have learned to acknowledge and use; it is undoubtedly related to my own reproductive story of trauma and loss. While my story has since been resolved, it still creeps in, as I want to cheer others on to a happy ending. When the feelings surge in me and I get the urge to "do more," I reach out to colleagues. Supervision is essential in our line of work!

I also know that many fertility counselors have not resolved their story and may find themselves in a similar "middle" as their clients (see Chapter 24 in the *Clinical Guide*). Having a shared experience with clients can both enhance treatment but can also muddy the waters. It can be difficult to keep clear boundary lines. That impulse to "do more" may be even more intense; there may also be feelings of jealousy and competition with the client, especially if they become pregnant during the course of therapy, but the fertility counselor does not. Another situation, which can trigger strong countertransference, occurs if the patient has had a pregnancy loss, while the counselor is pregnant. It can be overwhelming to be feeling vulnerable oneself, and have a patient who is in the midst of a crisis. Compassion fatigue and vicarious trauma (see Table 20.1 in the accompanying chapter in the *Clinical Guide*) are areas of concern for therapists, especially if they are feeling emotionally at risk. Here again, seeking supervision is critical.

Ultimately, Evelyn and Jayden decided to take their doctor's advice and try a round of IVF. The strongest negative for them was the cost of the procedure; the strongest reason to move forward with it was the potential to produce several embryos and have them tested while Evelyn's eggs were still relatively young.

"I know we're not out of the woods yet – there may be many more traumatic moments – but it feels so good to finally make a decision about this," she said. She recognized that part of the trauma was being so unsettled about this decision. Making a choice about her treatment allowed her a reprieve from the battle, even if only for a short time. "The pieces are starting to land in place. I know I'm going to be anxious, but at least I know which foot to put in front of the other." Evelyn was excited but also realistic about the possible losses ahead.

Summary

For the fertility counselor, using the premise of the reproductive story can help organize how we address client issues. So many assumptions about pregnancy and parenting go awry when the reproductive story takes a detour from the desired course: the losses that amass, the feelings about the self that can be so destructive, the anxiety and depression, guilt and self-blame that occur – all this amounts to trauma in the truest sense of the word.

Listening to the narrative our patients present allows us the opportunity to find the meaning behind their core beliefs, and likewise helps them understand their internal conflicts to a greater degree. Helping them leave the battlefield intact, whether they are able to have a family or not, is the goal.

References

1. Cann A, Calhoun LG, Tedeschi RG, et al. The Core Beliefs Inventory: a brief measure of disruption in the assumptive world. *Anxiety, Stress Coping* 2010;**23**(1):19–34.

2. Jaffe J, Diamond MO. *Reproductive Trauma: Psychotherapy with Infertility and Pregnancy Loss Clients*. Washington, DC: American Psychological Association, 2011.

Introduction

I am a clinical psychologist who has been in practice for 40 years and an Adjunct Associate Professor at University of Michigan Medical Center for 20 years. While my training was in traditional psychodynamic therapy, my current approach is more eclectic and Rogerian in its emphasis on empathic engagement with the client as the primary vehicle of change. My initial interest in reproductive loss was based on having a number of child cases in which perinatal sibling loss was an important, unrecognized dynamic. But my lifelong dedication to this area was decided after my wife had several ectopic pregnancies followed by infertility and the adoption of our son.

For didactic and confidentiality reasons, some of the case material to follow was altered and composite characters drawn. The first study provides a case summary with italicized commentary. The second case draws upon dialogue to illustrate clinical interaction of especially important segments.

A Perinatal Loss with Infertility

I usually start the first session by asking, "Where should we begin?" Even though this client is coming in due to the recent loss of a twin which I know by her first phone call, her story may start earlier, alerting us to prior issues, resolved or not. This beginning question also invites her to be the author of her narrative, empowering her to organize her personal experience rather than being the passive patient with the medical records being the dominant vocabulary. Finally, she may choose to talk about something lighter or marginally related to the loss, wanting to test the emotional waters first to see if it is safe to trust this therapist who initially is a stranger with credentials. I give her the time and space to go at her own pace.

"So where should we begin?" Alice, a tall woman in her early forties, began the session almost cheerfully, "I remember how happy I was when I learned almost a year ago that I was pregnant with twins." *[The fact that she can retain those feelings of being thrilled by the pregnancy and put such a positive spin and affect in introducing herself are early signs of her being resilient.]* She then described in much detail the long journey of trying to become pregnant over the prior 10 years. This included many unsuccessful attempts at IVF (without any explanation for her

infertility), tensions with her husband over her unwillingness to consider adoption yet, when he was ready to give up medical treatments, and finally becoming pregnant with donor egg. *[She can describe the disappointments and stresses of her infertility, helping us to appreciate she can grapple with major challenges, and not avoid those feelings or slap a happy meme on depressive circumstances.]* She beamed with pleasure, proudly announcing how she hit the jackpot. It was two for the price of one. *[Paradoxically, she prides herself achieving this, while chalking it up to luck in winning the jackpot. Maybe the financial metaphor is a playful swipe at the often high cost of assisted reproductive technology (ART).]* Wistfully, she momentarily recalled her high school days as a star athlete, but was sidelined due to injuries. *[Her taking credit for the pregnancy may be an attempt to compensate for her body injuries leading her to leave sports with regrets.]*

She gave birth abruptly at 30 weeks. She goes into much detail in describing her birth – how unexpected and frightening it was to happen so suddenly; how small and helpless her babies appeared; how much she ached to hold them but couldn't due to medical interventions; how much she blamed herself for not holding onto her babies longer so they could be fully nurtured by her body; and her fears for their not having normal development due to their prematurity. *[This is perhaps the most crucial part of the session, when she gets to tell her story. It enables her to begin to process a sudden, traumatic birth, which by organizing her experience in some coherent fashion reduces her sense of helplessness and being overwhelmed. She is already beginning to grieve the loss of early contact with her babies. Most importantly for her therapeutic relationship, she enables the therapist to vicariously participate in and empathize with her traumatic birth, forging a strong bond between them. I have been let in to her private experience and am no longer a stranger.]* Her daughter, thankfully, was fine. *[As by now a regular illustration of her resilience, good news takes precedence over bad.]*

Pushing back tears, she said how her son Jim had a rampaging sepsis which he succumbed to within a day. While this occurred over 3 months ago, she still can't believe it happened, starting to cry more openly. *[She clearly was overwhelmed by the loss, still struggling with the reality of an event that often gets experienced, simultaneously, as having happened just yesterday or years ago. Her not believing it happened may be understood as the last stand of a defense against fully feeling the impact of her loss, allowing her to cry more openly, a sign of recognizing her baby is gone].* She pulled back again from crying, voicing her fear that her daughter, Jill, would pick up on her sadness, preventing her daughter from having a happy life. She was also afraid this would blot out how thrilled she felt over being a Mom. She paused long enough for me to comment. *[Her pause lets me know she is ready for me to speak. Up to now, more than midway through the session, I had verbally said very little, save for the occasional empathic comment to let her know I was taking in what she was saying. This was her story to tell and she didn't need (nor ask for) any help structuring it or questions about it. In psychotherapy lingo, she was on a roll. But I was far from absent during my verbal silence. I made quiet uh-huhs and nods in synchrony with her affective states, resonating in sadness with her grief while shifting into smiling enjoyment during the happier parts.]*

I told her I could see (more accurately feel) how painful it was to so unexpectedly lose Jim. "What a shock it must have been. Perhaps you are just coming out of it now. The emotional gestation was much longer than 30 weeks. It was more like the 10 additional years of trying to have a baby. I could also see how great it was not only to be pregnant, but pregnant with twins. It brought back those great high school athletic days when you felt your body was strong and capable of doing anything." *[My task here is to demonstrate my empathic understanding of just how shocking and devastating this loss is, weaving in her prior infertility as part of the gestation of this pregnancy. I also connect the bodily achievement of making twins with her pleasure of her own high school athletic achievements. These observations are not interpretations of unconscious content she is unaware of, but part of the strategy to deepen her understanding (and being understood by me) of why her reactions make total sense, providing meaning and normality to her experience. Translating the chaotic swirl of conflicting feelings into words helps process her traumatic grief.]* She smiled appreciatively. "You bet," she said, "no more losing and failing for me." *[She lets me know my empathic understanding was accurate as well as the impact of her adolescent bodily injuries and possibly unsuccessful infertility treatments.]*

Perhaps that was why, I went on, it was so important that she created these babies from scratch rather than their being adopted. She looked dismayed, *[she quickly lets me know I am off target]* saying that making the babies seemed less important than her being able to nurture them during pregnancy. After all, they were not her

eggs and that felt OK to her. I told her I could see the distinction she was making and appreciated her correcting my misunderstanding. *[Inevitably empathic failures or misunderstandings occur. I didn't recognize the much greater significance for her of being the gestational, nurturing mother rather than the genetic, blood mother. The former is defined by what her body did in sports and pregnancy which mattered a great deal, while the latter signaled a much less important part of her maternal identity. Empathic failures often, though not inevitably, occur when we project our own issues into the therapy. My being an adoptive father who is sensitized to the stigma adoption carries when blood kinship takes precedence over psychological ties caused, I believe, my erroneously assuming she would feel the same because of her earlier statement of not wanting to pursue adoption. Similarly, I brought up adoption out of the blue, without it being meaningfully connected to what she was discussing. When we find ourselves as therapists inserting tangential explanations or allusions, we may want to check our own thoughts and associations to what might be provoked in us. Such empathic failures are inevitable, especially working in a field where it is common for therapists to have their own reproductive losses never fully put to rest and ready to be activated. Rather than problems, they may more accurately be understood as therapeutic opportunities if honestly acknowledged by the therapist and discussed in the therapy as necessary, not burdening our clients with sharing our understanding of our error but rather the impact of the misunderstanding on her. Integrating the expectation that such failures will occur from time to time can deepen the collaboration between therapist and client; empower the client to not only write but edit her narrative; undercut the usual placement of the therapist at the top of the hierarchy with the client in a one-down, less able and more passive position; and offer a more realistic though generally softer portrayal of the harsher world where such empathic failures occur with greater insensitivity.]*

Over the course of the session, she reported a happy childhood, no prior history of depression or other emotional problems, and a very supportive husband, many friends and a caring family. *[If there is sufficient time it is useful to obtain a brief history, to be expanded upon in a later session. That way we don't run the danger of defining her solely by her current situation and crisis, doing an injustice both to her and our understanding of her. Her benign history, with no major psychological problems, excellent coping and managing intense feelings with internal and social supports, make it more likely that she will have an adaptive, shortened recovery from her loss [1].]*

No matter how deeply she grieved, I told her I was very impressed with how smoothly she balanced her different feelings over the course of the session, when to allow the tears to flow for Jim and when to nurture Jill. She said, "Yep. It's hard to read books about parenting during the day and then read about grieving at night." I completely agreed with how difficult that can be. But I strongly believed she would not be in this position a year from now and would not have to be doing nightly or even necessarily weekly readings on grief. *[Rather than conceptualizing the process of grieving as a sequence of stages, a more balanced model developed by Stroebe and Schut [2] describes how grieving and restorative coping oscillate between two poles. This envisions grieving, unlike depression, not as a constant, unchanging state – though right after the loss it may feel that way – but an intermittent emotion, often likened to waves crashing the shore and then receding. This dual process model of bereavement also explains why one's energy is not consumed entirely in grieving, but devoted to doing the many tasks mourning dictates, such as informing others, planning a funeral or memorial service, performing religious rituals, etc. For Alice, her coping would be embodied in parenting her surviving twin. Over time, as grieving subsides, there is more energy available for returning to work and getting back to a new normal life. Because of the fears of this acute grief never lessening, whenever feasible and realistic (based on the benign clinical picture I mentioned), I try to more accurately normalize how much the intensity of her grief will diminish over the next 6 months to 1 year, without suggesting that she will ever completely "move on" and leave her grief behind. As sad as the loss was and will be, she could be comforted by knowing that emotionally and spiritually that baby would be a part of her as it initially was physically. Typically, I give feedback in the form of a summary at the end of the first session, ideally helping her to feel understood by me, with something she can take away from the session. Then I would advise finishing the consultation by gathering a more in-depth picture of her past and current functioning, in biopsychosocial terms, before presenting a tentative outline of some of the issues we might explore over the following 3 or 4 months. This turns out to be her continued anxiety of Jill being negatively affected by her grief, her lowered self-esteem due to the infertility and her perinatal loss, the special circumstances of losing a twin, and the toll the loss took on her relationships, expanding topics all introduced in the first session.]*

The next session a week later, she said our first meeting helped a lot. Being able to talk about the whole experience lifted a load off her shoulders. "It helped me to see things could get better and I might not always feel

this way." *[I try to begin the second session by asking about her/their thoughts and feelings after our first meeting. It gives some sense of how helpful it was, but also encourages feedback to the therapist as an important part of developing a collaborative relationship and common goals for the therapy. The load lifted off of Alice's shoulders could be traced to feeling understood by the therapist's words, not feeling so alone and burdened, due to his emotionally sharing her loss and providing a realistic basis for a happier future once her grief had subsided.]*

We met for about a month weekly, reducing at her request to every other week for another month and then once a month for the final 3 months. *[While many clients prefer the last sessions scheduled less often to "test out" how they will tolerate not meeting, I usually favor meeting at the same pace to the end in order to maintain the momentum of therapy. I usually agree with their wishes of how to end this relationship, perhaps aiding healing of the prior loss of which they had no control.]*

A Pregnancy Termination Due to Fetal Anomaly

The following case preceded the US Supreme Court overturning of Roe v Wade and thus the increased illegality of all pregnancy termination in many states is not a factor here. However, the current experience of pregnancy termination in the US will likely be more logistically and psychologically problematic in ways that cannot yet be fully appreciated.

(Wfe) is wife, (Hd) is husband and (Th) is therapist.

Learning of the Anomaly

At 20 weeks, the couple had recently been told by the OB of their baby having a potentially very severe case of spina bifida (a neuro-tube defect where the spine doesn't close) associated with paralysis, bowel and bladder problems, and potentially major disabilities in neurocognitive development, mobility, etc. The actual severity of the disability will not be known until after birth.

(Th) I know this can be terribly painful, but please tell me your first reaction to learning about the medical condition so I can better understand what it was like for you both?

[I try to provide some warning of the potential traumatic impact of revisiting this event, explaining I am asking so as to vicariously experience what they were going through, preparing to absorb some of that pain.]

(Hd) We looked at each other and thought this can't be right. They must have made a mistake. (Wfe) I thought these things happen so rarely it couldn't happen to us. We even picked out a date in a couple of weeks to celebrate learning the sex of the baby. *[It is common to have profound disbelief because the news is so shockingly unexpected and many women go into prenatal testing viewing it as a formality rather than something that could go wrong [3]. Most women vastly underestimate the incidence of pregnancy loss, believing, for example miscarriage occurs in 5% of pregnancies when it is three to four times that number [4].]*

(Th) I can see this was something that you couldn't even imagine happening, let alone having to make any decisions about regarding the pregnancy.

[The therapist aims to empathize with the enormity of this situation, anticipating how difficult it will be to think of deciding about the continuation of the pregnancy.]

(Hd) Yes, I thought there must be something they can do to make the baby better. But they told us nothing could be done, that he might be like a vegetable. (Wfe) I couldn't bear his talking about our baby that way. We wanted him so much (she begins to cry) and it's so hard to let him go (cries harder).

[While not intending to be cruel, the health care professional (HCP) callously overlooked how much love went into this baby and how tremendously disorienting and disappointing this news is. There is an important distinction to make between the formerly healthy baby, who was claimed as their baby and was wanted so much but is no more, and the actual disabled fetus/baby whose personhood by the parents has not yet been established. She is already beginning to grieve the healthy baby to whom she was so attached but now must give up [5].]

(Th) Yes, I can see how understandably indignant you felt over his not talking about your baby with the respect he deserved (with a flash of anger). I also hear your devastating disappointment and grief that the baby you loved so much is gone (with much sadness).

[I empathize with her feeling outraged by the HCP calling her baby a vegetable, legitimating her reactions as normal. By resonating with the client's sorrow, my identifying the feelings of disappointment and grief are not gratuitous and don't ring hollow. My words help integrate the power of her feelings with their verbal meanings, enabling a deeper processing of both trauma and grief.]

Defining the Loss

(Th) Some couples can find it useful to talk over what the loss literally means to them. Is this a baby or is this something else, not quite a baby? [6]

[This designation often becomes clear over the course of the conversation. But, if not, it can be helpful to know as it has implications for making the decision to terminate the pregnancy.]

(Wfe) I know this must sound weird, but I don't know what to call "it." I know I got furious at the OB for calling it a vegetable but aren't I doing the same thing by denying his being human? Because if I make him human, I feel such guilt, like I murdered him. But if I make him not a baby, not the baby I dreamed of having, then I haven't even let him come into being a person who existed. (Hd) I don't know if we can do this. It feels like we're playing God.

[This articulates the dilemma parents face, whether acknowledged and discussed or not, between viewing the loss as a child they killed or something less than human whose existence is denied. While the prohibition of playing God often emerges in making the decision between life and death in continuing or ending the pregnancy, it can appear earlier in the husband questioning whether he is entitled to decide what is human or not.]

(Th) Most parents can't tolerate being in this situation *[empathizing with the husband's wish to extricate himself]*. But only the two of you and no one else can decide if this is an "it" or a person or something in between. *[Intended to validate their perception as what matters, and not the Pro-life versus Pro-choice abortion wars. But, perhaps sensing the husband's tuning out, I realize I may be felt as too pushy.]* But you know you're not obligated to make this designation now and permanently. Some couples do have their sense of what the loss is change over time. *[I appropriately back off.]*

(Wfe) Well, I carried it for over 5 months. I have been feeling it kick for weeks now. If that ain't a baby, I don't know what is. I just can't think of it as anything else right now. (Hd) I am not there yet. My relationship with it was less personal and more mental. I didn't feel him kick me or anything like that. But I know I am going to miss him if we don't go ahead with the pregnancy *[cries softly]*.

[When couples disagree over how the loss is experienced it is more common, though not inevitable, for the woman to feel an earlier and more powerful attachment, even though she had just expressed indecision, perhaps the difference between a reasoned and gut response. Even when one designation is favored, each goes back and forth between "it" versus a baby. As is often the case, especially with men, the disavowal of personhood along with an incipient attachment is uttered in the same breath.]

Deciding to Terminate the Pregnancy

(Wfe) Trying to decide what to do is driving us crazy. We keep going back and forth between continue or terminate. It's like we're all over the place. (Hd) And we always seem to be taking the opposite side of the other, not getting into fights about it, but making us question what is the right answer because whatever we choose makes us feel terrible (said with some desperation by both). And then time is running out to decide and we really don't have enough solid information as to what the outcome will be (heightened desperation). What would you do if you were in our situation?

(Th) I think what you're feeling and going through is normal, not crazy. You have not faced such a decision like this (after that was established earlier on) which is so life-changing, so time pressured, where so much is based on not knowing what the actual outcome will be. You're not crazy, yet being in this situation can feel that way. I think you're trying out different choices and going back and forth makes perfectly good sense as a way of trying out and feeling your way into deciding what is best for you both and what each decision feels like. And best does not mean you will feel good about what you decide to do. The best may be doing what is less intolerable. When I see your suffering with not feeling you can decide, I do wish I could give you the right answer, but I don't believe there is one and if there was, I doubt I could confidently tell you what that was. I can say I will work on this with you as long as you feel it is helpful and I will support whichever choice you decide.

[Because there are similarities between couples on the tasks of deciding whether to terminate a pregnancy with fetal anomaly, what I say for one may resemble how I respond to another. But the wording of what I say and my attention to their affect hews, as much as possible, to what they bring in without, of course, parroting their words. So, I normalize their reactions and help them appreciate how taking different perspectives is a wise way of evaluating the alternatives. I resonate with their desperate wish to be told what to do so that when I inevitably decline to do that, they hopefully do not feel personally rejected, reinforced by my pledge to see them through this process. The necessary neutrality in taking a position on the decision-making contrasts with compassionate understanding of what they are going through emotionally over deciding what to do. When they are at virtually an utter loss of how to problem-solve or strategize the decision-making process (which is not the case with this couple), I might offer McCoyd's [7] model of balancing all they know about the medical condition –

needs, demands, deficits and positives – with the family's strengths, challenges, resources, emotional limitations and financial situation, in order to come up with if not a decision, a better and more realistic understanding of the parameters which can help making a decision. For a more detailed distinction of the many additional tasks couples need to navigate who are dealing with the decision to continue or terminate a pregnancy where there is a fetal anomaly, see Table 21.2 in Chapter 21 in the Clinical Guide.]

The Next Session

(Wf) I think we have come to a decision to terminate the pregnancy because we just don't want him to suffer the disabilities he is likely to have. We wish we could consult with him about that but, of course, we can't and have to respond on his behalf. (Hd) But we feel guilty knowing this would be best for our family, knowing the burdens and stressors we already have. We just can't take on a child with this many needs. Do you think we are bad people for doing this? That we are taking the easy way out?

[While the most commonly given rationale for doing the termination is concerns about the child living a miserable life with such disabilities, almost all couples state with some guilt and shame that the burdens on taking care of such a child would be too much to handle [8]. Viewing themselves as saving a child from suffering may help alleviate their earlier guilt of feeling like they murdered their child, that it was done out of mercy rather than selfishness. But the husband still has doubts.]

(Th) Considering what you went through in making this decision would hardly lead me to think you took the easy way out. Far from it. You made this decision as seriously and carefully as anyone could. And when you look back on this, I hope you can give yourself credit for considering everyone's needs were at stake.

[The husband's guilt is closely aligned it appears with being judged by others, most notably the therapist. The therapist shouldn't try to play God himself and give absolution. But if the therapist has it in his heart to be moved by the husband's moral dilemma, he can and does provide a more compassionate and humane perspective.]

Some Concluding Thoughts

Reproductive loss can be the emptiest grief. When grief is embedded in people who are known, there are the memories of them which are initially a source of deep yearning but may eventually become a solace borne of remembering. But for those suffering reproductive loss there are initially no memories to turn to, which is why constructing those memories through rituals, mementoes and other links to the loss may eventually construct an identity of who this baby might have become. Reproductive loss is losing a creation or creative potential. Healing involves creating a loss that may be wholly grieved when before there was none.

Whatever treatment model is used, empathy needs to be one core ingredient. It is important that the bereaved parent feels understood, combining the emotional realm with verbal cognition. Empathy is robust. In this pandemic era when remote psychotherapy is becoming a norm, much to my surprise, I learned that even with grainy images, distorted sound, and eyes not making contact, a human therapeutic bond can usually be forged and sustained. This is not intended as an endorsement of technology that sometimes constrains interaction by putting a digital wall of notetaking between client and therapist. It is a reminder that when the foundation of all relationships, that of parent and child, is ended before it was able to begin, another intimate, this time therapeutic, relationship must be created to fathom the depth of this loss.

References

1. Lasker JN, Toedter LJ. Predicting outcomes after pregnancy loss: results from studies using the Perinatal Grief Scale. *Illness, Crisis Loss* 2000;**8**:350–372.

2. Stroebe M, Schut H. The dual process model of coping with bereavement: a decade on. *Omega* 2010;**61**:273–289.

3. Sandelowski M, Barraso J. The travesty of choosing after positive prenatal diagnosis. *J Obstet Gyn Neon Nurs* 2005;**34**:307–318.

4. Bardos J, Hercz D, Friedenthal J, et al. A national study on public perceptions of miscarriage. *Obstet Gyn* 2015;**125**:1313–1320.

5. Solnit A, Stark M. Mourning and the birth of the defective child. In Eissler RS, Freud A, Greenacre P, et al. Eds. *The Psychoanalytic Study of the Child* (vol. 16). New York, NY: International Universities Press, 1961, pp. 523–537.

6. McCoyd JL. Women in no man's land: the abortion debate in the USA and women terminating desired pregnancies due to foetal anomaly. *Br J Soc Wrk* 2010;**40**:133–153.

7. McCoyd JL. "I'm not a saint": burden assessment as an unrecognized factor in prenatal decision making. *Qual Hlth Res* 2008;**18**:489–500.

8. Koronromp MJ, Page-Christiaens G, van Den Bout J, et al. Maternal decision to terminate pregnancy after a diagnosis of Down Syndrome. *Am J Obstet Gyn* 2007;**196**:149.e1–149.e11.

"A Little Bit Pregnant": Counseling for Recurrent Pregnancy Loss

Mia Joelsson

Introduction

My own fertility struggles brought me to this field as I learned myself how isolating and traumatic infertility and pregnancy loss can be. Being able to support others going through this journey has been so important for me personally and has helped me grow professionally in ways I never imagined. I have a Bachelor's Degree in Psychology from the Pennsylvania State University (Penn State) and a Master's Degree in Social Work from The University of Pennsylvania (UPenn). I worked for family service nonprofits for over a decade doing outpatient mental health work, clinical supervision, program management, and outcomes development and tracking. Later I went into private practice, where I have now been specializing in reproductive health since 2008.

I would describe my clinical work as integrative, but leaning toward cognitive-behavioral therapy (CBT), solution-focused, humanistic/existential and strength-based interventions. I have also incorporated significant trauma and grief training into my work and find that I learn and adapt what I do to every unique client's needs. I am forever grateful to my colleagues for their support and much needed humor at times, and to the clients I have worked with over the years for the trust they place in me at a very vulnerable time in their lives. I have been changed personally by these experiences and could not imagine doing any other kind of work.

Recurrent Pregnancy Loss: The Case of Susan

Recurrent pregnancy loss (RPL) is defined as a "spontaneous loss of two or more pregnancies" [1] and it affects approximately 1–2% of couples or individuals, although it's hard to determine the exact prevalence [2]. For those who experience RPL, it is incredibly distressing, especially since an underlying cause is found in fewer than 50% of such couples or individuals [3,4], leaving them without any answers for why this has happened and whether it might happen again. RPL involves grieving several losses at once, as an individual or couple

The addenda referred to in this chapter are available for download at www.cambridge.org/covington-case-studies

must grieve the loss of the pregnancy itself, the lost child, the loss of a dream of parenting that child [3,4], as well as a lost "reproductive story" that may have been a narrative they began constructing many years earlier [5]. As a result, many individuals or couples experiencing RPL find their normal coping tools and self-care strategies lacking when it comes to managing the experience of suffering more than one pregnancy loss. Reaching out for therapy takes courage and the hope that having professional support will help to reduce isolation and manage the experience.

My goal in this chapter is to capture the experience of counseling RPL clients and share my own feelings and techniques I often use when I'm working with a client who has suffered multiple pregnancy losses. The case presented in this chapter is made up from a compilation of clients and represents common themes in counseling RPL clients. While the client in this chapter is a cisgender female in a heterosexual relationship, the struggles presented are universal for a pregnant person whether they are single or partnered.

The Beginning: Lost in a Storm at Sea

Susan (38) called me to start therapy after her second pregnancy loss. She told me that she and her husband Tim (40) had their first miscarriage at 6 weeks gestation while trying to conceive on their own. Their pregnancy had been confirmed by Susan's Ob/Gyn but before they were due for their first pregnancy ultrasound, Susan miscarried at home. She described the miscarriage as "scary, painful, and lonely."

Susan stated they tried to conceive on their own for another 6 months without success and then sought help from a fertility specialist. Susan described the initial testing as "invasive" and said that she had a growing fear that "something was wrong with me" and "my body was broken" which was only intensified by all of the fertility testing. She was relieved to hear that all of the testing came back "normal" except that her egg quality was diminished, which her doctor said was normal at her age. They continued to try to conceive but were monitored this time by the fertility practice and given some medication to try to enhance the odds of success. Their second cycle resulted in a pregnancy and they were thrilled. Susan had increased anxiety about this early pregnancy but began to relax when she saw the baby's heartbeat at their first ultrasound. She started allowing herself to envision her life in the future with a baby and she even told a few close family members and friends about the pregnancy. Susan had the usual early pregnancy fatigue and nausea and felt reassured that those symptoms indicated a healthy pregnancy. She returned to the fertility doctor for a second ultrasound and was devastated to learn that the baby had stopped developing around 6–7 weeks and there was no longer a heartbeat. Not long afterward, Susan had a surgical procedure (D&C). She called me to begin counseling the following week.

Susan asked me in that initial phone call if I had ever had a miscarriage or experienced infertility and we had a productive conversation about this that resulted in me deciding to disclose to her that I had experienced infertility and pregnancy loss myself, while keeping my disclosure brief and vague. She stated she felt she could only work with a therapist who personally understood what she was experiencing.

Susan arrived for the first therapy session and she began crying as soon as she sat down on the couch in my therapy office. She was embarrassed about crying and we processed how emotionally raw she felt. I was able to normalize that her feelings were incredibly common for people going through multiple pregnancy losses. She nodded and took a deep breath to compose herself. We spent the majority of that first session talking about her reproductive story and how it had not gone the way she planned.

My goal in the early part of therapy with pregnancy loss clients is to build a strong therapeutic relationship as quickly as possible and help them gain some tools for grieving and coping with their losses. Part of my job is to hold some of the grief and fear for them so they can face the uncertainty of continuing to try to build their family. As much as I often want to rush to the skill-building part of therapy, I know I also need to slow down and sit in their pain with them. My ability to provide empathy and warmth are just as important as any coping skill they could learn in our sessions. I focus less on history taking and more on hopefully providing some connection and relief in that first session. I do often assign homework in the first session to bring a list of strengths to the next session and we then talk about those strengths and how we can use them to build resilience to work on grieving their losses and continuing to try to build their family.

When clients ask about my personal history of pregnancy loss or infertility or if I have children,

I always have to pause and catch my breath. This question is uncomfortable for me despite my years of training and experience with this client population. I stop to think, "what does she really want to know?" Usually, clients want to know that I understand, beyond training and clinical experience, what it feels like to lose a wanted pregnancy and to fear that they may never be parents. Sometimes it's enough to talk about those feelings from their point of view and normalize the feelings. Other times, they really do need to connect to me by knowing I've been through this journey personally. And I have. As a result, I do disclose that fact to them at times, but only in very general terms, and I pay close attention to how they are reacting to my disclosure. The reaction is usually relief, as they want to know that I "get it."

Many clients have told me that they had a therapist they enjoyed working with but that the therapist didn't understand their journey with pregnancy loss or that their prior therapist said some things that were ignorant or hurtful about their RPL journey. Thus, they deliberately set out to find someone with personal and professional experience with pregnancy loss and/or infertility. What I find most uncomfortable in these moments is that I know my infertility and pregnancy loss journey ended happily with two wonderful children (this part I almost never share with clients unless they ask directly and seem to really need to know this information), and I know that I can't guarantee them the same outcome. Processing this in peer supervision or with a trusted colleague helps tremendously to remember where my boundaries should be, both for my client and for myself.

Over the course of our first few sessions, Susan shared how "broken" she felt. Family members and friends checked in with her to see how she was doing but this only added to Susan's shame that "everyone knows I'm a failure." She was able to state her deepest fears: "I'll never be a mom," "It's my fault this keeps happening," and "I'm being punished for something." She struggled with shame and uncertainty, longing for a much-loved child, and blaming herself for not being able to make it happen. She shared that she felt like she was lost at sea, in the massive ocean without a life raft and no sense of direction or safety. This became a metaphor that we used throughout our work together.

Susan stated she felt like she was failing at everything, even grief itself, because her husband had been able to "go back to normal, as if this never even happened" while she felt unable to concentrate or think about anything other than the pregnancy losses and her own sense of brokenness. We talked about different styles of grieving. She was comforted to hear that everyone grieves differently and that her husband was still grieving, even though his expression of grief was different from hers.

In those first few weeks after the second pregnancy loss, Susan was unable to resume fertility treatment cycles even though getting pregnant again was something she desperately wanted to achieve. She had to wait for her hormone levels to return to baseline before she could start another cycle and the uncertainty of how long this would take was only adding to her grief and anxiety. We talked about trying a "worry period" where she would intentionally delay her worries to one 30-minute block of time after dinner. At her "worry time," she could let herself worry for an entire 30 minutes and then she would immediately find a relaxing activity to distract herself from the worries for the rest of the evening. This strategy appealed to Susan and it became a very successful way to manage her need to worry about the process but not have it take over her day. She would keep a notebook with her and jot down worries that popped in her head so she would know to worry about them later at her "worry period." We also worked on learning about the difference between productive and unproductive worry and she would often use her worry period to see what worries she could categorize as productive and work to solve them versus which worries were unproductive and needed a different strategy. Another tool we used was the Positive Reappraisal Coping Intervention (PRCI) which she kept in her purse on an index card and used when her anxiety spiked in any type of waiting situation.

Talking about how everyone grieves differently and educating clients about Intuitive versus Instrumental grief has been very helpful in my RPL cases. So many of my clients, like Susan, demonstrate predominantly Intuitive Grief symptoms and process their loss emotionally, while their partners often exhibit more Instrumental Grief expressions like returning to work, building savings for their future family, researching treatment options, etc. [7]. It can feel like a big disconnect to grieve so differently and, thus, normalizing this is often helpful. It's easy for me, even as the therapist, to forget that the instrumentally grieving partners are still grieving; it just looks different. It's easy to assume that the partner is in denial about their grief or just not that affected by the loss, but I've found that if I listen closely and invite the partner in for a session, I learn that they are grieving in their own way. I also want to give the partner an opportunity to share their own experience with the pregnancy losses, as partners can often feel left out in the RPL experience. Understanding the way their partner is grieving often helps my clients feel less alone in their own grief and more able to share it with their partner.

Table 22.1 Recurrent pregnancy loss coping toolbox

- Worry period
- Productive versus unproductive worry
- Mindfulness
- Breaking down goals into smaller chunks
- Identifying and challenging negative thoughts
- Building social support
- Positive Appraisal Coping Intervention (PRCI)
- Setting boundaries with others
- Assertive communication techniques
- Grounding techniques (example: 54321)
- Daily self-care
- Physical activity

Helping clients to identify and cope with the shame and catastrophic fears they are experiencing can help them move through this phase of grief. We work on building a toolbox of coping skills that they can access for different situations and feelings. Concrete tools that they can practice and use in different situations can give them a sense of control over the roller coaster of emotions they are experiencing. The PRCI is an example of a readily accessible intervention for managing worry in the moment and has shown benefit in research studies with RPL [3,4]. Two other worry management tools that I often use are mindfully delaying worrying until a specific "worry period" each day [8], and educating clients about productive versus unproductive worry [9]. Table 22.1 explores some coping tools for RPL that I often use with clients in this phase of treatment. Addendum 22.1 provides more information on intuitive versus instrumental grieving as well as some of the Coping Toolbox techniques including the worry period, productive versus unproductive worry, the PRCI and grounding techniques.

The Middle: In the Life Raft

Once Susan was able to process her grief, gain some new coping skills, and feel more stable emotionally, we began to talk more about trying to conceive again. She told me that she was starting to feel like she was in a life raft paddling to shore but trying to conceive again felt as though her life raft would disappear.

As she approached the time to try another cycle, we spent time creating a plan for how to communicate her needs with her fertility treatment team, including that she wanted her nurse to email her with test results instead of calling so that she could process the information on her own terms and not have to remember all the details to tell her husband. We visualized the treatment cycle from beginning to end and practiced coping with different outcomes. Two more cycles of medicated IUI ended without a pregnancy and these losses continued to feel challenging. We used her new coping tools to manage the disappointment and continued fears during these cycles.

On the third cycle, she was pregnant again. She was more guarded and detached from the pregnancy this time and we were able to talk about how normal this is. Her anxiety was high and she was hypervigilant about what she ate, her activity level, and the stressors she faced. We were able to talk about what she could control in this process and what was out of her control. Her lifeboat was in choppy seas sometimes, but she could see the shoreline ahead. We practiced breathing techniques and other grounding tools, like the 5–4–3–2–1 exercise, to help her stay in the present moment when she felt anxious.

Control is often a big theme with my RPL counseling clients. Their bodies, pregnancies, feelings, and future all feel out of their control and this creates anxiety. In the therapy room, I often feel powerless to help them in their moments of intense anxiety, trauma and grief because I can't control the outcome either. I must remember that my job is to provide a safe place to process their journey but not to "fix it" for them. They frequently need support between sessions and we formulate a check-in plan so that they can contact me as needed to help them cope between our meetings. I identify with their helplessness and anxiety, and feel like I can support them by holding their feelings during and in between our sessions.

The detachment that RPL clients experience from their subsequent pregnancies is common. They are using a phenomenon called *emotional cushioning* to brace themselves for the possibility of experiencing another pregnancy loss (see Chapter 22 in the *Clinical Guide* for review.). I sometimes find myself practicing my own version of *emotional cushioning* while I wait to get updates from them in between sessions. I hold my breath along with them as they go through treatment cycles. I brace myself for their updates and prepare for the support they may need from me.

I use the same tools I teach my clients to ground myself to stay present and not become triggered by the level of despair that RPL clients often feel. My own commitment to self-care and healthy lifestyle practices are essential for this to work. The 5–4–3–

2–1 exercise is one grounding tool that I use quite often in session with RPL clients and also for myself (see Addendum 22.1). Table 22.2 highlights my goals for counseling RPL clients. I don't always use all of these with all clients; rather I choose what seems to fit each client as each client, situation, and pregnancy loss are unique.

The End: Reaching the Shore

Susan continued to attend regular therapy with me throughout her pregnancy. We continued to process her grief and work toward finding some meaning in her losses. Her anxiety decreased considerably by the twentieth week of pregnancy and she enjoyed the rest of her pregnancy. We spent the second half of her pregnancy talking about the meaning of her pregnancy losses and how to integrate them into her reproductive and family story. She stated that before she started therapy, she felt that RPL would be the title of the story of her life and now it felt more like a chapter in the story of her life that might turn out to have a happy ending after all. We processed how much great work she had done to successfully integrate the pregnancy losses into her reproductive narrative.

She continued to use her coping toolbox (see Table 22.1) and found that these tools worked for other worries or difficult waiting periods as well. She gave birth to a full-term baby boy and we met for one final session a few weeks after he was born. She stated her coping tools and self-care routines were holding strong and helping her through some occasional postpartum anxiety. We were able to reflect on her journey and our work together and she shared that she felt therapy had been her life raft, keeping her afloat during this scary and uncertain time. Our last session ended with a short breathing exercise focused on her transformation to motherhood.

Table 22.2 Counseling goals for recurrent pregnancy loss clients

- Process trauma and grief
- Reduce mood and anxiety symptoms
- Reduce shame
- Build coping toolbox (see Table 22.1)
- Identify and use strengths to promote resilience
- Prepare for another pregnancy
- Improve self-esteem
- Evaluate what they can control versus what they cannot control
- Identify and modify negative thought patterns
- Find meaning in the losses

It is a gift to be able to work with RPL clients through their grief and fears, their ups and downs, their vulnerable and raw emotions. I feel honored to be entrusted to hold their grief and fear in the hard times and celebrate their joy and success in the good times. The trauma and grief of RPL are intense and personal. Helping clients to explore ways to find meaning in their losses can be crucial in continuing to integrate their grief [6]. I often use existential and spiritual themes in this phase of therapy with RPL clients to help them create a meaningful way to integrate their losses and honor the babies they won't get to meet. We work on finding a "new normal" where they know they have been changed by the losses but are able to be invested in their life as it currently is and feel the full range of human emotion again.

I always like to invite RPL clients back for a free postpartum session to talk about their birth and postpartum experiences and to meet their baby. That final session is also a good time for me to remind them of their strengths and coping tools to use with future stressors and difficult life experiences. It also provides a good check-in for postpartum adjustment. Having a safe therapeutic space to process their feelings and gain skills to cope can be a true life raft to navigating the treacherous seas of RPL. I've since used this analogy with other clients and found it resonates with many of them. The life raft you create for your clients may look different than mine, but I hope this chapter was useful in providing a possible framework for working with RPL clients.

References

1. American Society for Reproductive Medicine. Definitions of infertility and recurrent pregnancy loss: a committee opinion. *Fertil Steril* 2020;**113**:533–535.

2. European Society of Human Reproduction and Embryology. ESHRE guideline: recurrent pregnancy loss. *Hum Reprod Open* 2018;**2**:1–13.

3. Ockhuijsen HDL, Boivin J, van den Hoogan A, et al. Coping after recurrent miscarriage: uncertainty and bracing for the worst. *J Fam Plan Reprod Health Care* 2013;**39**(4): 1–7.

4. Bailey, Bailey C, Boivin J, et al. A feasibility study for a randomized control trial for the Positive Reappraisal Coping Inventory, a novel support technique for recurrent miscarriage. *BMJ Open* 2015;**5**:e007322. https://doi.org/10.1136/bmjopen-2014-007322

5. Jaffe J. Reproductive trauma: psychotherapy for pregnancy loss and infertility clients from a reproductive story perspective. *Psychotherapy* 2017;**54**:380–385. https://doi.org/10.1037/pst0000125

6. Wenzel A. *Coping with Infertility, Miscarriage, and Neonatal Loss: Finding Perspective and Creating Meaning.* Washington, DC: American Psychological Association, 2014.

7. Doka KJ, Martin TL. *Grieving Beyond Gender: Understanding the Ways Men and Women Mourn.* New York, NY: Routledge, 2010.

8. Borkovec TD, Sharples B. Generalized anxiety disorder: bringing cognitive-behavioral therapy into the valued present. In: Hayes SC, Follette VM, Linehan MM, Eds. *Mindfulness and Acceptance: Expanding the Cognitive-Behavioral Tradition.* New York, NY: Guilford Press, 2004, 209–242.

9. Leahy RL. *The Worry Cure: Seven Steps to Stop Worry from Stopping You.* New York, NY: Crown Publishing Group, 2005.

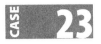

CASE 23 Pregnancy and Postpartum Adjustment in Fertility Counseling

Laura Winters

Introduction

As a fertility counselor also trained in perinatal mental health, I have enjoyed working with clients during their fertility journeys and seeing them through the postpartum period. I began my career working with children and families before changing my focus to perinatal mental health. Becoming a mother for me was both life- and career-changing, as I appreciated first-hand the struggles that come with the postpartum period. I found a new passion in working with pregnant and postpartum clients. As I gained more experience with perinatal individuals, I began to hear more stories of infertility treatment. This peaked my interest and so I pursued training and mentoring in fertility counseling.

I have been in practice for 19 years now, with the last 13 years being in private practice. I take an eclectic approach to therapy, drawing on cognitive-behavioral therapy, psychodynamic therapy, and attachment theory.

The cases I have presented here are intended to illustrate concepts identified in the *Clinical Volume*, Chapter 23. These cases are fictitious and do not represent any one person. They are based on various themes I have seen in working with fertility clients through their pregnancy and postpartum journeys. It is my hope that these cases offer the reader a clearer picture of the various ways that perinatal mood and anxiety disorders (PMADs) may present, as well as identify some of the special considerations for working with fertility clients in the perinatal period.

Pregnancy and Postpartum Anxiety: Megan

While undergoing fertility treatment, Megan and her husband had suffered a miscarriage and had to terminate another pregnancy due to medical reasons. While she had grieved the miscarriage, her grief over the second loss was complicated by the burden of having to make the heart-breaking decision to end the pregnancy. The couple moved forward with treatment and, after two more IVF cycles, she was pregnant again. This news caused Megan's anxiety to spike. Despite feeling happy about another

The addenda referred to in this chapter are available for download at www.cambridge.org/covington-case-studies

pregnancy, she could not help but fear that she would receive devastating news again at some point in this pregnancy. Her anxiety level remained fairly high as the pregnancy progressed and increased around significant dates or scheduled tests. I had Megan complete the Edinburgh Postnatal Depression Scale (EPDS) in order to provide another measure of her symptoms so that we could track and refer back to, as well as administer again in the future.

To assist Megan in coping with the anxiety, we utilized cognitive-behavioral therapy (CBT). First, we worked on relaxation techniques, focusing on breathing to calm her nervous system. Megan found relief in square breathing or simply placing her hands over her heart while breathing deeply. Once she had a way of lowering her anxiety level, we were able to examine her thoughts and identify the cognitive distortions she was experiencing. Megan found herself falling into the trap of many "should" statements and "fortune-telling." She would often say, *"I should be feeling happy that I'm pregnant again"; "I should be thinking about the babies that I lost more"; or "I should be more connected to this baby."* Examples of fortune-telling thoughts included, *"There will be something wrong with this pregnancy and I won't be able to handle it"* or *"Something terrible will happen to my husband."* After identifying the cognitive distortions, we evaluated the validity of these notions and created a more balanced thought. One example of a balanced thought we used was, *"What is true today is that I am pregnant. My baby is healthy. My doctor confirmed that at my last appointment."*

Megan struggled with feeling detached from the pregnancy. The idea of losing another pregnancy was too painful, and so she felt safer maintaining some distance and not letting herself think too far into the future about the pregnancy or the birth. She felt extremely guilty that she was scared of attaching to this baby.

Detachment during pregnancy is a common theme I see in working with fertility clients. Their anxiety and grief from prior loss prevents them from being able to fully embrace this pregnancy. There is a sense of holding their breath until the next milestone is achieved. For some, this will bring only slight relief, while other people may experience more. Common significant milestones include passing the time in which the other pregnancy was lost, the completion of each trimester, and each ultrasound or other diagnostic test. Regardless of how much their anxiety may have decreased before, most clients report not being able to completely exhale until the baby is born and they get to hold their child.

This can be challenging work supporting clients through pregnancy after loss and fertility treatment. Countertransference issues can arise. There may be an inclination to comfort and reassure, or to encourage them to find the joy in this pregnancy and work on attaching to the baby. I certainly have found myself reflecting on these issues in my work. With Megan, at times I would question whether I should be challenging her detachment from the pregnancy and helping her to find ways to connect to the baby. I recognized that this was my own discomfort or desire for my client, rather than what was beneficial to her. What she needed was to be validated that her reaction was typical after the losses and trauma she had experienced. Sitting with those feelings and being validated, Megan could gain a new perspective on her behavior and start to release her guilt.

What I have found to be true is that grief is ongoing. It does not follow a series of steps and then reach an endpoint. Pregnancy, and even a new baby, does not cure it. It can be quiet for a while and then reappear, overwhelming our clients with emotion or fear. Grief theories recognize the importance of processing the pain following a loss. This emotional pain can be too much to bear for many people in our clients' lives. Friends and family tend to offer reassurance in attempt to fix the hurt. But reassurance is not what helps people to heal. What helps is validating their emotions and holding space for however messy that may look from one session to another.

The rest of the pregnancy was uneventful medically. Megan's anxiety continued to rise and fall. She experienced periods of intense grief, particularly as her due date approached. Megan was struggling with maintaining a connection to the baby she had lost, Luke, while welcoming this new baby. She feared that she would somehow forget Luke or that he would become less important to her. Megan is a spiritual person and found comfort in wearing a memorial necklace as well as speaking to Luke and asking him to watch over this baby. The necklace helped her to feel more connected to him on a daily basis and asking for Luke's protection proved to be a meaningful way of keeping him a central part of the family.

The postpartum period presented more challenges for Megan. Breast-feeding was very difficult and became a source of anxiety, insecurity, and frustration. She struggled with the decision to stop nursing, as this made her feel guilty and ashamed that her body was "failing" her once again in motherhood. To address her all-or-nothing thinking, *"I'm a failure if I can't breastfeed my child,"* we challenged this idea with questions. *"What are some examples of mothers who are failures and those who are successes? Who will know the difference between breast-fed and formula-fed children when they all are in kindergarten together?"* Megan realized that she was judging herself much harsher than she would other moms. She acknowledged that a successful mom is one who loves her child and a failure would be abandoning your child. This was in sharp contrast from the meaning she was assigning to herself. She appreciated the ridiculous thought of trying to discern who, in a room full of kindergarteners, had been breast-fed. To help Megan problem-solve, we included her husband in session and weighed the pros and cons together of continuing or discontinuing breast-feeding. Ultimately, she decided to switch to formula-feeding, as this would allow her husband to assist more with feedings and give her the opportunity to get more sleep.

We processed this loss of what breast-feeding meant to her. For Megan, breast-feeding represented being able to do something that comes naturally as a mother. After being an infertility patient for years, she viewed her body as broken. She had hoped that breast-feeding would restore some of her faith in her body and its capabilities. I held space for this loss and validated Megan's feelings first. Then I gently challenged her "all-or-nothing" thinking. *"What would you say to a friend who had been through what you had? Would you think her body was broken? Is breast-feeding the only way your body can nurture your child?"* I also normalized how common breast-feeding issues are, regardless of a prior history of fertility issues.

Sleep was another source of anxiety for Megan. She was anxious about SIDS and often would stare at the baby on the monitor or would get up to check on her. Megan could not rest or sleep for very long while her daughter was asleep. Recognizing that this was further exacerbating her anxiety, Megan decided to consider medication. She met with a reproductive psychiatrist for a psychotropic consultation and began the medication that was recommended and prescribed.

Grief reared its head again after the birth. Megan struggled with reconciling how to maintain a connection to Luke, while still enjoying the life she had with her daughter and husband. She was afraid that she was forgetting Luke, as she was not thinking or talking about him as often as she had. She also would feel badly when she mistakenly referred to her daughter as Luke. She cared very much about keeping Luke's memory alive in their family and was grappling with what that looked like at this time. We reframed mistakenly calling her daughter Luke as an indication of her love for him and her intention to keep him an important part of the family. I normalized how common it is for parents to refer to one child by their other child's name, sometimes even the family pet's name, for that matter. I explained that she had mistakenly called her daughter Luke because he was a part of their family even though he was not physically here on this earth with them. Megan appreciated this notion and found relief in this idea.

Pregnancy and Postpartum Obsessive Compulsive Disorder with Intrusive Thoughts: Kelsey

Research shows that 88% of fathers and 91% of mothers experience intrusive thoughts of harm coming to their baby, partner or themselves [1]. These types of scary intrusive thoughts are extremely common, and I find it helpful to share this statistic with clients in order to normalize their experience. Some parents are able to have these thoughts without them interfering much in their day. They simply notice the thought and may have some mild anxiety in the moment, but are able to continue on with whatever they were doing. Other parents may experience these thoughts quite frequently and become extremely distressed by them. The latter are the parents who are experiencing an anxiety disorder, most likely obsessive compulsive disorder (OCD). It is important to note that intrusive thoughts are also present in postpartum psychosis (see the *Clinical Guide,* Chapter 23 for a more in-depth discussion on the differences between OCD and postpartum psychosis).

Kelsey sought treatment 2 months postpartum due to anxiety and intrusive thoughts. Kelsey and her husband Jake had been through several rounds of unsuccessful IVF cycles and one miscarriage. She had been experiencing intrusive thoughts during the pregnancy but did not seek treatment because she was ashamed, convinced she was off to a terrible start in motherhood. Well-intentioned family members had suggested that she was just stressed about the pregnancy and she would feel better once the baby arrived.

Cultural and societal views play a major role in how one experiences parenthood. There are messages, some obvious and some less so, that get conveyed and reinforced in the media, in social interactions, and among families. These ideas have the potential to either assist individuals in their transition to parenthood or to hinder their development. In this way, they can also influence how safe the parent feels in seeking support for themselves.

During pregnancy, the thoughts were primarily focused on harm coming to the baby. Kelsey worried about contaminants in the environment affecting the pregnancy, or getting into a car accident and losing the baby. During the postpartum period, the thoughts centered on harm coming to herself and the baby. She was fearful of dropping the baby in the bathtub and had vivid images of her injured baby floating in the tub. Knives were also distressing to her as she had intrusive thoughts and images of stabbing herself and the baby. She could not walk past knives or use them without her anxiety spiking. Kelsey avoided them as much as possible.

After meeting with Kelsey for the initial appointment, we met one more time to administer the Yale-Brown Obsessive Compulsive Scale (Y-BOCS). The Y-BOCS is a helpful tool in identifying all of the obsessions and compulsions experienced, as well as their severity. The information gained from the Y-BOCS is used to create a fear hierarchy, which serves as a guide in implementing exposures. After this session, we met with her husband in order to involve him in her treatment plan. It is important for the partners to have an understanding of what their loved one is experiencing. You can take the time during those sessions to clear up any myths about postpartum mental health and explain what the mother is experiencing and what the treatment plan involves. The partner plays an essential role in helping mom to feel better. It is crucial that partners are given correct information on diagnosis and how to support mom. They are an integral part of the client's support system and treatment plan.

Jake was relieved to have the knowledge about what Kelsey was going through and to know that there was a plan in place. He wanted to be a supportive partner and assist her in overcoming this anxiety. After Jake had an understanding of symptoms, we explored ways he could best assist Kelsey, paying particular attention to anything he may have been doing unintentionally to reinforce the intrusive thoughts. We discovered that Kelsey would often turn to him for reassurance around her scary thoughts. While it is a natural tendency to comfort someone in distress by reassuring them, this response actually serves to reinforce the anxiety. With this information, we were able to develop alternative ways Jake could respond to Kelsey's anxiety and also monitor how often he may still be offering some reassurance. Jake agreed that when Kelsey sought reassurance, he would point this out and remind her of coping strategies she could utilize instead, such as getting a hug or going for a walk. We also made the distinction between offering reassurance around the fear versus being Kelsey's cheerleader and reminding her that she can tolerate the anxiety. The latter was a helpful way Jake could provide comfort, whereas the former would reinforce the obsessive thoughts.

Once a plan was in place for how Jake could best support his wife, Kelsey and I were able to begin addressing her intrusive thoughts with Exposure and Response Prevention (ERP). Reviewing our fear hierarchy, we agreed upon which exposure we would start with. In vivo exposures were conducted together in session and Kelsey was given exposures to practice on her own in between sessions. We started with the bathtub fear, as this was lower on her fear hierarchy. The initial exposure involved sitting on the bathroom floor next to the tub. As anxiety was fairly tolerable after sitting for several minutes, we attempted to increase her level of distress by stating out loud, *"I could drop my baby in the tub."* As intended, Kelsey's anxiety intensified, and she allowed herself to tolerate the uncertainty of what could happen without engaging in reassurance-seeking. Future exposures for this fear involved variables such as filling the tub with water and imagining bathing her child. Kelsey responded well to ERP and made great progress. The intrusive thoughts decreased significantly in frequency. She was able to bathe her baby alone and was able to look at and, with similar ERP work, use knives without experiencing intense anxiety.

Pregnancy Anxiety and Surrogacy: Carrie

There are many myths surrounding pregnancy and childbirth. When it comes to the mental health of parents, it is commonly believed that one can only experience a PMAD if they are the person carrying the pregnancy. As discussed in the *Clinical Guide*, Chapter 23, PMADs affect all parents, regardless of who carried the pregnancy, as there is an adjustment to parenthood.

Carrie and Sam, who had been trying for years to conceive, with multiple miscarriages and several unsuccessful IVF cycles, were recommended by their doctor to use a gestational carrier (GC) and decided to move forward with this. The first transfer with the carrier was a success. Like Megan, Carrie was very anxious during the pregnancy and was holding her breath for each milestone to be reached. Fortunately, the pregnancy proved to be healthy, and Carrie was able to focus on her grief and anxiety in therapy.

A few issues arose during the pregnancy that are unique to using a GC. Carrie continued to grieve not being able to carry a pregnancy. These feelings intensified at times and then softened, only to repeat this cycle over and over, as is the cyclical nature of grief. This recurring pain was very difficult for others to tolerate. Whenever she did share her grief with friends, they often tried to comfort her and point out all the things about pregnancy that were not enjoyable. While these friends were well-meaning, their comments tended to make Carrie feel misunderstood and alone in her grief. Our sessions were a safe place where she could express these emotions and be validated. It was heart-wrenching to see Carrie break down and mourn the loss of carrying a pregnancy to term. Validating her experience and encouraging her to speak freely was helpful in facilitating her grieving.

As her therapist, it was challenging to sit with all of Carrie's grief and hear her deepest fears about the pregnancy and motherhood. I was aware of my countertransference as I wanted her to find some hope to hold on to, rather than feeling so scared and sad. I didn't want this to be her entire experience of the pregnancy. Recognizing this was my reaction and not what was needed, we found that what worked best was sitting with the feelings and processing all of those scary, unpleasant thoughts. After that, we restructured her thoughts so that they were more balanced. For Carrie, this meant focusing on what was true for today. They were still pregnant, that was a fact. Staying present and in the "here and now" helped Carrie to contain her anxiety in between sessions.

Learning about the baby's development was both exciting and sad to experience this second-hand. Carrie felt disconnected from the pregnancy and baby. She had concerns whether the infant would bond with her since she was not the one carrying the baby. Carry envisioned the birth, being handed her newborn and worrying that the baby would reject her. She pictured the baby crying in her arms and then being placed in the carrier's arms and finding comfort. After validating her grief, we explored ways that she and her husband could bond with their baby during pregnancy. We discussed making audio recordings of their voices talking to the baby, reading a story, and a playlist of their favorite music for the GC to play throughout the pregnancy.

Sharing pregnancy news later in the pregnancy also stirred up grief. People sometimes asked intrusive questions about using a GC or made insensitive comments – "Is the baby actually related to you?" or "At least you don't have to worry about the baby weight." To assist Carrie in dealing with similar future exchanges, we discussed ways she could respond to these comments. She decided that when she felt up to having the conversation, she would explain to the person that their comments were, while hopefully well-intentioned, insensitive, and then provide them with resources, to help educate them on the topic. Carrie acknowledged that there were other times when she did not have the energy to engage in these discussions.

Later in the pregnancy, Carrie questioned what type of childbirth classes she would feel most comfortable attending. Going to a traditional childbirth education class with a room full of pregnant individuals created anxiety for her. She did not want to have to explain their circumstances to a room full of strangers and deal with their reactions. She and her husband investigated online and private class options, as this would allow them to focus on the information, rather than explaining their story to strangers.

The birth also created anxiety for Carrie. Because their carrier lived several hours away, she worried about what would happen when labor started. Would they be able to get to the hospital on time? Would both she and her husband be allowed in the delivery room? What if a cesarean section was necessary? She and Sam contemplated who they wanted, if anyone, at the hospital with them. Because they had a GC, nearly every aspect of expecting a child was shared with others. Carrie longed to have some things that were just between her and her husband. With that in mind, we worked on identifying ways they could create moments shared just between the two of them. The birth was one opportunity. Carrie and Sam agreed that they wanted their parents to come to the hospital, but decided they would take time alone with the baby for the first couple of hours following the birth. They also found comfort in preparing the baby's room together.

As the pregnancy progressed, Carrie felt safer discussing the birth and postpartum period. We were able to review typical challenges that arise with a new baby and began to create a postpartum plan. Postpartum plans serve as a safeguard against perinatal mood and anxiety disorders, highlighting risk factors and key areas that need to be addressed in order to protect the mental health of parents. For instance, sleep has a significant impact on mood, and it is particularly difficult to get adequate sleep with a new baby. The postpartum plan can help parents identify some strategies to maximize the amount of sleep they each get and consider if they have support people who can assist with that. For an example of a postpartum plan, please see Addendum 23.2[1].

Postpartum plans also provide fertility clients with a sense of control, which is often lacking in their parenthood journey. Carrie and Sam created their postpartum plan on their own and we reviewed it together in session. Other than experiencing the common struggles of welcoming a new baby, Carrie and Sam coped quite well in the postpartum period.

I always suggest scheduling a follow-up session after the birth, with baby present, and normally do not charge for this meeting. I like to take that opportunity to admire baby and comment on the ways the parents are doing a great job caring for the child. I find this to be incredibly healing with a surrogacy birth. As grief and anxiety have been the prevailing themes prior to the birth, it is a beautiful transition to witness our clients holding their much-anticipated child and feeling joy. This session also serves as a time to assess how the parents are feeling and discuss the birth.

Summary

As fertility counselors, we can help prepare our clients to navigate pregnancy and the postpartum period. We can provide education about PMADs, review risk factors, and identify referrals to therapists trained in perinatal mental health, as well as other support professionals. Unfortunately, expecting parents are often not given information on PMADs until they are suffering and seeking support. By introducing information early on to our clients, we arm them with the knowledge to recognize what they may be experiencing and potentially remove a barrier to reaching out for help.

References

1. Abramowitz JS, Khandker M, Nelson CA, Deacon BJ, Rygwall R. The role of cognitive factors in the pathogenesis of obsessive-compulsive symptoms: a prospective study. *Behav Res Ther* 2006;**44**(9):1361–1374.

Walking the Tightrope: The Pregnant Fertility Counselor

Laura Covington and Janet Jaffe

Introduction

This chapter serves to explore and illustrate the topics addressed in the accompanying *Clinical Guide* volume. While the case chapter is not a how-to guide, we hope it helps to shine light on some of the issues that may arise within us, as therapists, and within our interactions with our fertility patients. We also believe these issues reflect similar struggles in any reproductive medical healthcare professional who is pregnant and working with infertility patients.

Laura Covington (LC)

From an early age, I remember an innate desire to help others. I even walked into my first-grade class and repeated a mantra I had heard about what it takes to be a therapist by asking my teacher, "What does it mean to you? How do you feel about it? Tell me more ..." Of course, this was part of my upbringing. I was raised with an acute awareness around the struggles many had to grow their families. It was a part of our family narrative that my parents had their own pregnancy losses. The apple doesn't fall far from the tree, and while my mother, Sharon Covington, influenced my interest in this work, it was a journey for me to decide to pursue fertility counseling.

A few years after I finished my Masters of Social Work, I returned to obtain a Ph.D. to focus on fertility counseling. While in school, I met a veteran who suggested I do my dissertation on combat-related injuries that cause infertility. I dove into the fertility counseling world, learning the ways this work could make a difference.

My theoretical orientation is blended. While psychodynamically rooted and family systems trained, I use a mixture of cognitive-behavioral therapy, mindfulness, supportive therapy, and grief work. Patients come in with different histories and different needs; it is often the first time they are seeking counseling, as their journey to grow their family takes an unexpected detour.

As this chapter is about the pregnant fertility counselor, I, as the therapist, will be the case study.[1] With self-disclosure, transference and countertransference concerns, I talk through clinical issues that came up at various points in my pregnancy journey, discuss the need for consultation and supervision, and explore the reactions of my patients.[2]

Janet Jaffe (JJ)

My reproductive journey was the impetus for pursuing fertility counseling as a career. When I was in the midst of fertility treatment and losses, many moons ago, there was very little support to be found. I was lost in a sea of despair, shame and grief, and in searching for a lifeboat, decided to go back to school and obtain my Ph.D. in psychology.

It has been a long time since I was in the midst of my own reproductive trauma; since then, I have used my training as well as my personal experience to talk about it, write books and chapters about it, and counsel patients so that they may not feel quite so alone in their quest to have a family. My perspective, with my trauma resolved and the pursuit of pregnancy long past, affords me clarity to supervise and consult with other fertility counselors. Working with Laura on this chapter has been wonderful: her courage to share herself combined with my more distanced and seasoned view will hopefully provide you, the reader, with insights. As you will see in this chapter, my role will be as a peer consultant to the fertility counselor to help her understand and explore what it takes to "walk the tightrope" with our patients.

Entering the Tightrope

As fertility counselors, we hear countless stories about failed conceptions and pregnancies. Because of my own strong desires for a baby and knowledge of how difficult the process could be, I had a lot of anxiety as I began trying to conceive: *What will my journey be like? Is it even possible to have a baby naturally? How will I manage my own anxieties if I struggle to conceive? How do I keep my emotions separate from the therapy space? Will my patients be upset if I get pregnant? What will I tell them?* All this jostling around in my brain before I even started to try to get pregnant!

---

[1] While I will be using parts of myself for this chapter, the case study highlights a combination of various clinicians and readings I have done to illustrate a broader range of issues that can arise during the pregnancy process. This is not entirely a reflection of myself.

[2] All cases have been de-identified, altered and do not represent any one patient.

Maya: When to Tell

Maya came to see me after her previous therapist went on maternity leave. After trying to conceive for 2 years, Maya remembered looking at her therapist's belly and wondering if she was pregnant, but Maya never asked. Weeks later, the therapist finally brought it up, noting her "growing belly in the room." The therapist observed that Maya had not said anything and wondered why. Maya discussed with me the many feelings she had and the pressure she felt from the therapist that she was supposed to bring up the pregnancy. This story weighed on me as I imagined being in the therapist's position, and I knew I would handle it differently.

Maya was in her 2-week wait after a frozen embryo transfer (FET). She discussed "symptom hunting" to determine if she was pregnant. A previous pregnancy had ended in a miscarriage, and she wondered if she had the same symptoms now. I sat there completely distracted by my own thoughts: *Could I be pregnant too?* As Maya ran through the symptoms, I found myself wondering if I was feeling those symptoms also.

Maya's next appointment was extremely painful; she had had a chemical pregnancy. "Why didn't this work? They said it was a 'perfect' embryo, and my uterus looked 'beautiful,'" she lamented. While I was heartbroken for her, I was also incredibly conflicted. I had just found out that I was, in fact, pregnant. My worries started to kick in: *Would mine be a viable pregnancy? Would I miscarry like Maya?* Staying present was challenging, as I held this secret. I knew it would be a while before I would tell her, but it made sharing all the more real, as I contemplated what it would be like for me to disclose and for her to receive this news, especially after her experience with her previous therapist.

I began to wonder: *When should I tell my patients? How are they going to react?* All I knew was that I wanted to bring it up myself, rather than waiting for them to bring it up, like Maya's previous therapist tried to do. One thing lingered for me, *What if someone asked before I was ready to share?* I knew I needed to be honest if I was asked, even if the timing wasn't perfect.

Ideally, I wanted to share after my 20-week ultrasound. I thought I would feel more secure that all was well with my pregnancy after that ultrasound. I was conscious to wear flowy clothes and baggy sweaters to hide my growing belly. I was thinking about sharing with my first patient and who that would be.

Consultation

LC: *I know it's time to address my pregnancy, but I am so anxious about hurting my patients. What if they don't want to continue to see me?*

JJ: *Your sensitivity to their needs is so apparent. I am sure your caring will come across, but you have to remember that each person's reaction will be unique. We may need to think of some referrals if they aren't comfortable seeing you. The key is to allow them to process their feelings with you, and then you and I can process your feelings.*

Amy: Not Ready to Share

Amy and her husband, Drew, had been experiencing both male and female factor infertility. Her husband, although in remission for about 4 years, had a history of cancer and had to have one of his arms amputated. Prior to his cancer treatment, they had frozen his sperm. Amy also had polycystic ovarian syndrome (PCOS). Sadly, about 4 months before Amy began psychotherapy with me, she had a traumatic pregnancy termination for medical reasons due to complications for her and the baby.

One afternoon, as Amy followed me back to my office, she shouted out, "Are you pregnant?" *I was caught.* I had been planning to tell her during the next session, but I wasn't ready today! I repeated to myself: be honest, be direct. I knew more or less what I wanted to say, and so with a deep breath in, I exhaled: "Yes, I am. I was planning to bring this up before you wondered, but I am glad you asked." I went on, "I am due the beginning of May, and I will be taking about 3 months leave. I will have someone covering for me during that time, and I will let you know when I have figured out those details. I want this to be something we can talk about, as I know it may bring up many feelings for you. How do you feel knowing this?"

Amy countered back, "I hadn't wondered until you were walking back, but you were walking differently. How does it feel to be pregnant? Is this your first child? Did you use fertility treatment?" I wasn't sure where to go from here. I was not used to opening up and sharing this piece of myself. *How much do I share? How much do I answer directly or explore her questions?* I responded back, "I know that this may bring up many questions for you, and I am happy to answer the questions if they would be helpful. But before I answer questions, I think it would be important for us to talk about what this is bringing up for you and to understand where your questions are coming from."

Amy discussed finding out recently that her friend was pregnant. "A bunch of us were out to lunch when my friend shared it with the whole group," she recounted. Amy described feeling a pang of sadness and anger run over her as her friend made her announcement. At

8 weeks along, she seemed to have no anxiety, and it felt like she didn't consider Amy at all, even though she knew Amy was having difficulties. Yet, Amy also felt bad that she wasn't feeling happy for her friend. We discussed holding two conflicting feelings at one time, feeling happy for her friend while, also, feeling sad for herself. I eventually responded back, "I wonder how these feelings about your friend relate to knowing about my pregnancy." Amy minimized her feelings about my pregnancy. I reminded her at the end of the session that feelings may come up for her about me, and I wanted to have an open space to explore them.

Consultation

When I finished seeing patients that day, I called Janet to process what it was like. My nerves had been high, and while I felt like overall it went well, I was filled with emotions.

LC: *I used the script I had practiced with Amy, but I gave too many details all at once. It wasn't natural. How much of my own story should I share?*

JJ: *I get the feeling that you needed to fill the space with details about having someone cover for you because of your own anxiety. Seems like you wanted her to know that even though you are pregnant, you still understand what she's going through. In the future, it may be helpful to allow space to process the feelings about the disclosure before talking about your leave. The leave is important for them to know, but not everything needs to be said at once. You did a great job in bringing it back to her and her feelings. But an important question to ask yourself: Who will benefit from the details of your story?*

During this consultation I realized that my desire to share wasn't necessarily for the patients' benefit but my own. I wanted them to still believe I was able to help. This self-knowledge was crucial as I made decisions about how much to share and to which patients. I tuned into my own anxiety as a cue to take a deep breath and encourage patients to express their feelings and concerns. My mantra became: "Is this in my patient's best interest, or is this about me?", knowing that I had my own support system in place to process my feelings.

Amy was a resilient woman, and I anticipated that it would be easier to share with her. At our next session, I asked if she had "any thoughts, feelings, reactions" since our last meeting. Amy then retorted, "Honestly, I thought about cancelling and not coming back to see you. But I thought maybe I should come in for just one more session." I commented on how brave she was for coming back in and asked her to share more with me. My anxiety was creeping in; I didn't want to lose her, but rather than get defensive I let her continue. She said, "I

don't know if I can continue to come, seeing another pregnant belly that's not mine. I have a hard time talking about infertility, and this is the one place I thought would be safe. Now it feels weird to talk about." Validating how difficult this must be, I realized this was the first time Amy really acknowledged her dwindling hope. Amy felt I would no longer understand; she worried she would never get to that point of being pregnant. Amy and I came up with a plan together: we would meet for another four sessions, and decide how to proceed after that. I offered to provide names of other clinicians if she didn't feel comfortable continuing with me, but she said if she stopped seeing me, she probably wouldn't use any of those referrals.

Sadly, this felt like a no-win situation. I felt guilty that I had betrayed Amy, but I also wanted her to believe and know that I did still understand and care about her. I wanted to go out of my way to make sure Amy continued therapy, and I felt even worse that she said she wouldn't see another therapist if she stopped seeing me.

Consultation

JJ: *You offered Amy a great solution: come in for a few more sessions so we can process all of this together. You might gently remind her that being able to work through her anger, feelings of betrayal, and grief with you in therapy will help her be able to deal with these situations with friends and family outside of therapy. You might also remind her that whatever her feelings are towards you, you will understand and be ok.*

Staying on the Tightrope

I was at a point where I could no longer hide my pregnancy. This was around the time several of my patients were going away for the holiday season. After consultation, I decided to wait until they returned, as I didn't want to tell and then there be several weeks before we saw each other again. It was hard not to disclose: I couldn't hide my belly much longer: I wanted to rid myself of my secret and put it out into the therapy room. Wanting to share before the holiday was about my anxiety, not in the patient's best interest, so I decided to wait.

James and Jennifer: No Room for Error

James and Jennifer began therapy with me after experiencing their third miscarriage. James had reached out as he didn't know how to support his wife. She was crying daily. In the beginning weeks of my pregnancy, they too conceived but had a miscarriage before they even knew that I was pregnant. My anxiety was extremely high as

I imagined they would have a lot of difficulty with my pregnancy.

I had made the decision to tell James and Jennifer at our next session. They would be one of my first patients to tell, and I was naturally jittery about it. Jennifer began that session saying, "Well, my sister is pregnant, again! I am happy for her, but no one seems to get that this is hard for me. I am constantly worrying about everyone being pregnant. I thought my friend was pregnant, and she was, but I found out that she had a miscarriage." James commented that he was not having the same concerns, but visiting family had been extremely hard. He wanted to know how to help Jennifer.

As Jennifer and James went on, my mind began drifting: *Was she worrying about me being pregnant? Would her anger transfer to me? How were they going to take this? Is this the "right time" to tell? Is this yet another place where James will feel Jennifer can't be supported?* I knew I had to share, but when? It is such an awkward position to be in, with the focus on me rather than them.

Consultation

JJ: Listening to your inner voice is the key to countertransference. Their feelings of anxiety and helplessness were informing you of your own feelings. There really isn't a "right time" to tell, but putting it off will make you less present for them.

While I didn't want to start the session with my disclosure, I also knew that we would need time to process it. After about 20 minutes into the session, I tried to find a way to bring it up organically. I empathized and normalized, "It is unfair that you aren't pregnant yet, and it must be hard to have anxiety wondering about others." We continued on, and time seemed to be flying by. When there was about 15 minutes left in the session, Jennifer slowed down, and after a natural pause, I spoke up, "There is something I think is important for me to share as I don't want you to wonder about me too. I am expecting and due in May. I know this is probably hard for you to hear, and it is hard for me to share." James followed up, "Congratulations" as he grabbed Jennifer's hand. Jennifer looked up and said, "Thank you for telling me. I had not wondered if you were pregnant, but in some ways it feels like a relief to know. We were supposed to have a baby in June." I knew my face was visibly red, and my voice a little shaky, so I wanted to acknowledge my own feelings. I went on, "You two have had a hard journey, and I have been nervous to share because of this. However,

I do want this to be a place for us to talk about your feelings about my pregnancy, unlike other times in your life, as I know it may bring up a lot for you both. I also understand if you feel like you can't continue to see me." Neither Jennifer nor James had much to say, and the conversation slowed down. I finished off the session noting that there may be feelings that come up, and we could discuss any and all of them.

I wondered what would happen next; would they come back? When they did return, I sighed with relief, and we began by talking about the last session. Jennifer and James seemed to be okay. I was extremely surprised: not only were they willing to talk about their feelings, but it also seemed less impactful for them. Wanting to make sure they weren't minimizing their feelings, I emphasized that lots of feelings could arise, that I would check-in during future sessions, and they were free to talk about my pregnancy when they needed. A few sessions later, Jennifer noted, "I really appreciate that you wear flowy clothes to hide your belly. When you told me, it's not like I thought you would come in with your 'clubbing' clothes on, but I kind of did think that." I thanked her for letting me know. I had been purposeful in the clothing I wore; I had been very conscious about trying to make the pregnancy less present. I was doing my best to be sensitive to my clients' needs.

Ginny and Brad: We Can't See You Anymore

Ginny and Brad, having taken a break from counseling when using their own gametes had not worked, returned because they were considering egg donation. When Ginny called, she stated, "I want to come back to see you so I don't have to go through my whole story again." While I was ready to start immediately, they delayed for 2 months. Had they made an appointment sooner, I would have told them about my pregnancy in person. However, by the time they scheduled, I was showing significantly and I had to let them know over the phone.

"Before we schedule," I began, "I want you to know that I am pregnant. Although I wanted to tell you in person, I didn't want you to be surprised when I came into the waiting room, so I thought it was better to tell you now." Ginny congratulated me as she began to cry. I spent the next 45 minutes on the phone talking to both Brad and Ginny. I struggled to end the call with them; my feelings of guilt were soaring. I wanted so much to help them. I knew how much they wanted a child, and I, too, wanted them to have a baby. I felt like I had hurt and betrayed them by being pregnant. I got an email from Ginny a few days later saying that they did not want to meet with me, after all. I tried to follow up, and let her know that was okay and to help her connect to another clinician. However, Ginny didn't respond to my call or email. I never knew what happened.

Consultation

JJ: *I can only imagine how this made you feel.*

LC: *It was awful. It was exactly what I was trying to avoid.*

JJ: *You might want to reach out to them again in a week or two, sending them a note. As you did with Amy, you can offer them an in-person session to deal with this more thoroughly, and include referrals in case it is too difficult to see you. If they refuse, however, you have to know that you did everything you could.*

Keeping Balance: Entering the Fourth Trimester

As the baby's due date comes closer, anxiety can rise for both the clinician and the patient, not knowing when the baby will arrive. While a stop date with patients is important to establish, a baby can arrive before then. Having a plan between the fertility counselor and patient can help to decrease some of the unknowns and uncertainties.

Charlie: Same Due Date, Different Arrivals

Charlie came to see me as she and her wife were using fertility treatment with a de-identified sperm donor to grow their family. Charlie, a lawyer, also had a history of depression. She reached out to me at her wife's insistence after their sixth intrauterine insemination (IUI) didn't work, and they were planning in vitro fertilization (IVF). After two embryo transfers, Charlie conceived, and our babies were due at the same time. As Charlie was also pregnant, I thought it might be easier to disclose my pregnancy, and in some ways it was. However, there were also challenges.

It was surprising to me that Charlie jumped into panic mode when I shared my parental leave plans with her. She began to worry about her own postpartum. She was clearly anxious about her own maternity leave and the pressure she had as a lawyer. She had observed the difficulties in her practice when other colleagues went on parental leave. I became aware that my leave felt like an inconvenience for her. My countertransference of anger

was boiling up. Intellectually I knew therapy was the place for her to work out her issues, but I started to feel dehumanized, as if my experience and needs didn't matter. My inner thoughts and feelings made it clear that I needed to reach out for consultation.

Consultation

LC: *I am having such a difficult time with Charlie. She is treating my pregnancy as a nuisance and at the same time keeps asking me about my plans. It's as if she wants to do everything that I do, but then dismisses me.*

JJ: *It must be hard to know what to do with the anger you are feeling. I also struggle with this: patients are allowed to be annoyed with us, but we are not "allowed" to show our anger towards them. With Charlie, it might help to think of her as being very frightened. She needs to be in control. The good news is she is connected to you and trusts you. Preparing her for postpartum may help reduce her anxiety and at the same time reduce your anger.*

Because Charlie had a history of depression, it was clear to me that she was worried about postpartum depression, even though she denied it. She was not currently on medication, but I had referred her to a reproductive psychiatrist to consider medication, especially postpartum. In laying out a plan for postpartum her wife came in for a session. It was important for the two of them to discuss a postpartum plan[3] and to watch for signals of distress after birth.

I also referred Charlie to an interim therapist, Amelia, who was covering for me while I was on leave. Charlie signed a release for me to speak to Amelia, and we had planned on having a three-way virtual session together to ease the transition. Unfortunately, this never happened, as I went into labor a month early.

Because of my unexpected labor and delivery, Amelia had to contact my patients for me. I was supposed to see Charlie that very day; there were so many loose ends I felt I had with her. I reached out to Charlie soon after I was back from the hospital. I wanted her to know that the baby and I were doing okay and to discuss the transfer of her care to Amelia while I was gone. In the height of my own trauma and lack of sleep, I expected a quick call with Charlie; instead, I was overwhelmed with her state of panic. Thinking only of herself, she told me all the reasons why she could not deliver early. My countertransference was again piqued. *Did she really believe that I wanted to have my baby a month early?* I sat there mostly quiet, as

---

[3] Please refer to the *Clinical Guide* and *Case Studies* volumes, Chapter 23 on Postpartum Adjustment, for additional information about postpartum planning.

she bellowed out her worries about having her baby early. I tried to reassure her but knew I was not in any state to be helping her. I was finally able to interrupt her and said, "I hear you are feeling anxious about all the uncertainties with your baby's arrival. These sound like important things to talk to Amelia about. Would you like me to have Amelia reach out to you, or would you like to reach out to her?" While reassuring her, it was important to set a boundary with Charlie. I was not available as her therapist at this time.

Consultation

JJ: Her lack of concern for you is telling, but you handled this with therapeutic grace. I know you felt conflicted: you wanted to make sure she was okay, but you also needed to take care of you and your new baby. Lessons learned?

LC: Yes … don't reach out to a patient when you are in your own state of panic!

JJ: I agree. So important to remember that self-care is essential, especially with difficult therapeutic cases. Charlie will be okay, as you set up care for her while you are on leave.

Returning to Work: The Fifth Trimester

Returning to work was something I didn't think about when I was pregnant. I was so worried about sharing my pregnancy with my patients that I didn't think about what it would be like to return postpartum and how I would manage this with them. What a juggling act! I had to figure out childcare and felt guilty when I was away from my daughter. I needed to schedule time to be able to pump or nurse. When I was doing telehealth, I would at times hear her cry and felt awful that I couldn't go help her; I also worried that my patients could hear her and wondered what feelings it would evoke for them. One of the biggest challenges for me clinically was that my patients now knew I had a baby. How much should I discuss my baby with them and bring her into the therapy room?

Charlie . . .

My work with Charlie was more challenging upon return. She was now a mom as well! Even though I was aware of my countertransference, I struggled with how to use it beneficially. I was furious when she commented on how easy breastfeeding was and how her baby was sleeping 8 hours, when I was lucky if I would get 3 hours. Her competition with me was profound.

Consultation

LC: My daughter keeps coming up in Charlie's sessions – I'm not bringing her up, Charlie is. She keeps letting me know what her baby is doing as if this were some sort of contest.

JJ: This is how Charlie sees the world: it is a contest to her. Do you think Charlie might have you on a pedestal and is feeling insecure about her own parenting? Is there a way to move her in that direction? I think this is going to take time, but if Charlie can gain insight into this competitive dynamic, the therapy will likely go to deeper levels.

James and Jennifer . . .

My first session back with James and Jennifer occurred as they were entering into a FET. They wanted to know how I was doing, and asked me if I had a boy or girl, the name, and how the baby was doing. I answered the questions with short answers, "I had a girl. Her name is Margaret, and she is doing well." Unlike my interactions with Charlie, their concerns about my daughter and me felt sincere. Although I knew talking about my baby brought up so much for them – their pregnancy losses and the upcoming FET – we were able to do so in a supportive and productive way. I struggled with how much to share now that they knew I had a baby.

Consultation

LC: This is such a delicate dance. How much do I tell them? My daughter is clearly a part of this therapy, and it feels so daunting.

JJ: Rule of thumb: follow their lead. You can let them know that although you are happy to answer their questions, you wonder how it makes them feel. I actually think you've done a great job doing just that! This is all so new to all of you – perhaps it would help to share that as well.

In one session, doing telemedicine with them, it was clear that they could hear my baby crying in the background. They could probably see from my face how uncomfortable I became. I felt like I was on the hot seat and wasn't sure how to respond. So many thoughts rushed into my head in an instant: *Were they judging my parenting? Did they think no one was taking care of my baby? Was this making them uncomfortable because I had a baby and they didn't?* From consultation, I knew it was important to use my own feelings and face the conflict head on, and so I asked what this was bringing up for them. To my surprise, they both smiled and said it was great to know I was human! It made me realize that I should never assume how a patient may feel.

Summary

For the fertility counselor, becoming pregnant and having a baby can bring up complications and new dynamics for therapy. Being pregnant while working with patients who are trying to become pregnant, have issues with fertility or pregnancy loss, can bring up various transference and countertransference issues. Understanding transference and countertransference dynamics in considering how much to share about trying to conceive, the pregnancy, and the postpartum journey can create roadblocks to the therapeutic alliance but can also deepen the experience for both patient and therapist.

25 Telemental Health in Fertility Counseling

Carrie Eichberg and Lauren Magalnick Berman

Introduction

Lauren Magalnick Berman (LMB): I am a clinical psychologist and the owner of the Fertility Psychology Center of Atlanta, having been in practice since 1989. I am a past-chair of the Mental Health Professional Group of the American Society for Reproductive Medicine and a founding board member of the Jewish Fertility Foundation. While a Rotary Scholar in Israel, I conducted my dissertation research on the impact of stress on the immune system. I have extensive training in posttraumatic stress disorder, having been an EMDR practitioner since 1997. I have been studying and researching telemental health for more than 10 years and am a certified telemental health specialist. I was drawn to work with fertility patients by my deep interest in the mind–body connection, commitment to helping patients heal from trauma, passion for psychotherapy, and my delight in helping patients to build their families.

Carrie Eichberg (CE): I am a licensed psychologist with over 20 years of experience in private practice. I currently live in Boise, Idaho and specialize in reproductive psychology. My work focuses on counseling clients on a variety of reproductive issues including infertility, donor conception, gestational surrogacy, postpartum depression, miscarriage, and grief and loss. I also conduct psychological evaluations of donors and gestational carriers. I became interested in reproductive psychology through my own infertility challenges, ultimately building my family with the aid of a gestational carrier and egg donor. My passion is helping others through their reproductive journey, particularly teaching parents about sharing their conception and birth story with their children.

The following three case studies demonstrate how telehealth has changed our practices. Traditionally, mental health professionals are trained to conduct psychotherapy and assessment in-person. There is something unique about sitting with someone face-to-face

that just can't be replicated via telehealth. However, telehealth has given us the ability to serve clients when the burden of traveling long distances to a healthcare professional's office is cumbersome or when there is no other choice considering circumstances like a global pandemic. However, the decision to provide telehealth should not be done without thought and thorough risk assessment. These cases illustrate how different telehealth is for both clinician and client, including unexpected successes, anxieties, and the clinical and ethical questions that arose for us as fertility psychologists. The following telecounseling and telepsychological assessment case studies are a compilation of cases reflecting salient issues in reproductive counseling via telehealth. All names and identifying information have been altered and changed so as not to reflect any one person.

Case 1 (LMB): Same Gestational Carrier, Same Intended Parents, Different Assessment

When the COVID-19 pandemic hit, many of us avoided gestational surrogacy evaluations. Principally, this was because gestational carrier evaluations carry a great deal of risk for all stakeholders – intended parents (IP), baby, gestational carrier (GC) and her family, as well as legal liability for all professionals involved in the case. Additionally, we had no data as to whether a remote evaluation would be valid, and we had little evidence on the validity of psychological assessment tools administered remotely. Parenthetically, the MMPI-2 and MMPI-2-RF were not yet tooled for remote assessment.

However, when GC candidates, whom I had recently assessed and who underwent a successful surrogacy were referred to me again, I agreed to evaluate them remotely. After careful risk assessment, I viewed these cases as updates of previous evaluations. I had previously met with all of these candidates and their spouses in person, and I had previously administered psychological testing, namely the Personality Assessment Inventory (PAI), in person.

In November 2020, IPs Simon and Greg contacted me to tell me that they had a beautiful 8-month-old son from their surrogacy with Courtney and that they would like to do a second journey with Courtney to have another child. They told me that the experience with Courtney worked out beautifully and that she was interested in doing a second journey but her time frame for this was narrow.

Simon and Greg are a stable, loving, same-sex couple who have been married for 5 years. They met in an exercise studio and have been together for 8 years. Both are healthy and active. Simon is a corporate executive and Greg is a journalist. Simon was raised in a military family and Greg was raised in a divorced family, mostly by his mother.

Courtney is a 31-year-old case manager for a social service agency. She is a veteran, and she has been married to Jonathan, also a veteran, for 8 years. They have a 6-year-old son together and they are raising Courtney's older son from a previous marriage. Courtney and Jonathan own a home and they have their own health insurance policies. Courtney has a serious, intelligent and guarded demeanor. She acknowledges that she is not very sociable, and she likes to spend leisure time alone, reading. She has no medical issues and no reported history of psychological treatment.

When Courtney was assessed in-person in 2019, her PAI validity scales were within the normal range. This presented the high likelihood that the assessment accurately reflected Courtney's underlying psychological dynamics. Her profile was absent of indicators of clinical psychopathology. The findings did suggest that Courtney is likely to be socially aloof, sharp in her verbiage, controlling, pragmatic and potentially demanding. Courtney's profile was not typical of the gestational carrier candidates that I usually screen. Many of the gestational candidate carriers I see are women who seek connection. They might be people pleasers or women who crave attention. Many are direct and dominant, like Courtney, but their presentations are softer and more amiable.

Outside of the concerns about Courtney's social presentation, there were no other concerns about her candidacy. She was educated, intelligent and able to understand complex instructions. She was in a long-term, stable relationship and worked in a responsible position at her job. She had no criminal record or reported psychological or medical problems. There was no suggestion of financial

or emotional coercion. Concerns about her personality style were discussed with the IPs and they believed that the fact that Courtney did not need much social connection suited their busy lifestyle.

My 2020 pandemic year interface with Courtney was quite different. First and foremost, the clinical interview of Courtney and Jonathan was done through a HIPAA-compliant videoconferencing platform. Courtney and Jonathan were seated in their lovely home with their dog coming in and out of the frame. At one point, one of the children requested something and Jonathan left the videoconference to see to the child's needs. Courtney reported no job changes since our previous meeting and no changes in lifestyle. Jonathan was supportive and amiable in our meeting. Both reported that the previous surrogacy had been a positive experience for the family.

I administered the PAI remotely, but Courtney and I remained on the videoconferencing platform throughout the testing. I advised her that I was there as a proctor and to answer clarifying questions. The results of the PAI were surprising to me. I had expected Courtney's validity scales to be similar or even lower than in the first administration. GC candidates and egg and sperm donors tend to produce "fake-good" profiles. "Fake-good" profiles are akin to an old business called Glamour Shots, which would have professionals do a customer's hair and makeup prior to taking photos and then retouch the photos before selling them. The fake-good profile comes out when a candidate is trying too hard to present as psychologically healthy and, instead, presents as too good to be real. Logic would predict that once a candidate had already been cleared and undergone a gamete donation or a surrogacy, the motivation to fake a good presentation would be lower. That was not the case for Courtney. In the telemental health administration of the PAI, Courtney's validity scores were in that fake-good range, indicative of positive distortion.

In the PAI (and the MMPI-2), positive distortion suppresses the clinical profile. For example, if a candidate is truly struggling with obsessive-compulsive disorder, a PAI profile with average validity scores would reveal obsessive-compulsive measure in the clinical range. However, in a fake-good profile, the candidate's score on this measure would not reveal clinical psychopathology. However, the PAI offers a wealth of methods for analyzing positive distortion and getting a clearer picture of what might be underneath the distortion.

The clinical results of Courtney's remotely administered PAI were quite different from the previous results obtained 1.5 years before. Most significantly, the results from the remote administration indicated much higher levels of hypervigilance and social withdrawal. They also suggested concerns about verbal aggression, risk-taking, distrust of others, impaired empathy and rigidity.

Had this been Courtney's first PAI rather than her second, I would have counseled the IPs to find a new gestational carrier. However, in the in-person administration, Courtney presented as open and honest, not guarded and defensive. The results of the remote administration were perplexing, and I conducted an item analysis with Courtney to help understand the reasons why she selected certain responses. The item analysis did not change the results or my understanding of them. What might account for the changes in result?

A possible explanation is that Courtney's remote assessment results were an accurate indicator of her responses to the COVID-19 pandemic itself. During a pandemic, it is likely that many of us became more hypervigilant, more irritable, more rigid, more socially withdrawn and, potentially, more verbally aggressive. This explanation is face valid given what we all experienced during lockdowns, quarantines and teaching our children while working in our jobs.

However, it is also possible that these differences were influenced by telemental health and remote administration of the PAI. Might it be likely that a candidate will respond more defensively when she is being monitored via videoconference? Might a candidate even feel more paranoid to glance up from responding to test items to see the clinician's face on the screen? If so, might it be less threatening for the examiner to turn off her own webcam so that the candidate does not have a face hovering over the test? Or might the knowledge that the examiner is there but not seen be even more intimidating? Finally, are remote assessments as valid as in-person assessments? These are questions that will need to be addressed by future research if we are to continue doing remote assessments when face-to-face contact safely resumes.

The decision about whether to clear this GC was a difficult one. It required weighing experience and clinical judgment against objective testing. My assessment mentor and PAI researcher, Dr. John Kurtz, has told me that objective data is critical. I absolutely agree with this advice. In the end, however, I weighed Courtney's past experience as the most significant variable. She had undergone a positive surrogacy journey with Simon and Greg and she delivered during the beginning of the COVID-19 pandemic. She worked well with them, followed the advice of her physicians, and showed flexibility when curve balls were thrown her way. I discussed my concerns about Courtney's PAI results with Simon and Greg and cautioned them about potential issues. They had an awareness of her limitations and yet worked well with her. They began a second journey together shortly after our meeting.

Case 2 (CE): The Psychotic Sperm Donor

A few years ago, I accepted an offer from a sperm bank to provide their office with donor evaluations. The practice is located in a state where there were no qualified reproductive psychologists. I was licensed there but I didn't live there. It was a dream job. However, the evaluations would need to be done remotely. I had preached in conferences and to my local referrals, face-to-face evaluations are always best. And I still believe that, but I really wanted this job. As this was several years before the pandemic, teleassessment was still in its infancy. Excited about my new opportunity, I researched everything I could find on teleassessment. There wasn't much. I wondered what colleagues would say if they found out I was doing remote assessment. Would they judge me negatively? Would they whisper that I was a hypocrite, that I would be taking on too much risk, and not doing a complete enough evaluation. I wondered that myself. I only told my closest psychologist friends my plans. As someone who is overly neurotic about the possibility of board complaints and malpractice, I reached out to my insurer which offers consultation from psychologists who are also lawyers. Surprisingly, they gave me the green light to proceed, if I did my due diligence with having the right HIPAA compliance [1], the literature to back it up [2–8] and documentation of reasons why I would need to conduct the assessment virtually. They warned me, it wasn't without risk.

I consulted experts in psychological testing who also supported the use of telepsychological assessment. I hired a computer company to help me arrange the logistics. I flew to the sperm bank headquarters, met the team, and left them with a computer full of PAIs for virtual administration. The plan was for the sperm donors to come to the sperm bank where their identity would be validated by the donor team and the PAI could be monitored in the agency office. I was able to control the computer I left at the sperm bank remotely from my office in my home state.

Nobody else I knew was doing this. At all the ethics and malpractice conferences, they tell you the best way to prevent a problem is to make sure that you, as a psychologist, aren't doing things that your colleagues aren't doing. Well, that certainly wasn't the case here. The way I saw it, the train of burgeoning psychological technology was already on the tracks, and I could either get on it, or let it pass me by. It came down to this: as a psychologist who did an internship and fellowship in psychological assessment and had been practicing reproductive psychology for over 10 years, I could provide a really well-done evaluation, but it would need to be conducted remotely. The alternative was for the agency to continuing having their evaluations done by a mental health professional who could see the donor in-person yet who was likely completely untrained, nor familiar with third-party reproduction and assessment. I decided that such an arrangement would not serve anyone well.

Having carefully thought out the risks and benefits of this offer to do telehealth assessment, I graciously accepted. For the first few years, it went swimmingly! I was doing multiple evaluations a month. The sperm bank and associated medical teams were pleased with my work. I was building positive relationships with the staff and donor team. And then, as always seems to happen when things start off so well, I saw dark storm clouds gathering in my direction.

As part of my evaluation, I ask sperm donor candidates to complete consent and detailed intake forms prior to my appointment with them at the agency via videoconference. Occasionally I wouldn't get the forms back before the appointment, which I note. This speaks volumes about a person's organizational skills, motivation, ability to follow directions and follow through on required tasks. At this point enters Sam, a new candidate who did not complete the forms prior to his telehealth appointment. I emailed the donor coordinator about the missing forms, and she agreed to call the applicant, have him arrive early to complete the forms and she would get them back to me before the meeting. This did not happen. Sam arrived late to the appointment and when the coordinator sent me the forms, he had barely filled them out. Everything he wrote was "not applicable." He did not report any history of mental illness for himself or his family members, no medications, nor any substance abuse history.

When we began the video conference, Sam appeared disheveled. His hair was a mess, and his clothing was dirty. He wasn't looking into the camera. He seemed to be mumbling to himself every once in a while. I thought perhaps that the rush to the sperm bank had caused him distress. I began with my typical review of the consent and then dove into the evaluation. I asked Sam what motivated him to be a sperm donor. He had quite an unusual

answer. He said, "I just think I would make perfect children and it's hard to find a job right now." This was the strangest answer I had ever gotten for wanting to be a donor.

The interview progressed and Sam verbally denied a history of any mental health problems. When we began talking about his childhood and family relationships, he became very agitated, complaining bitterly about how his parents treated him. He, then, began to perseverate on this. His speech became illogical, difficult to follow, and his thoughts had loose associations. At first, I wondered if perhaps my difficulty following him was due to our internet connection. He took a longer than usual time to answer questions. He appeared disconnected. Then, while taking the PAI, Sam told me he heard yelling in the next room. He was becoming annoyed and agitated by this, and said the voices were telling him that he is annoying and worthless. Again, I was unsure as to what was happening and thought perhaps he was hearing the voices from the streets or in the waiting room. I started to question my reality (which was important clinical information!) so I needed to check it out.

On my mobile phone, I called the sperm bank coordinator to ask about the noise and to go to the room to check on Sam. She told me she did not hear anything unusual in her office, waiting area, or outside and then went to see him. When the coordinator asked him if he was OK, he told her that the people stopped talking to him because the coordinator must have scared them away. Sam said he felt good about continuing the evaluation. I asked Sam more about the voices he heard. He said it was always the same voices telling him he is worthless and not good at anything. He described voices that are "always following me. There is nothing I can do about it." It became clear to me that Sam was paranoid and appeared to be having auditory hallucinations which started about halfway into the PAI.

During the interview portion of the meeting, I asked Sam directly about participating in mental health services. He denied any outpatient counseling history treatment yet, at the end of the interview, he said, "My counselor tells me to ignore the voices." I said, "What counselor?" He told me he was recently enrolled in a residential psychiatric treatment program. I pieced together that he was currently participating in an intensive outpatient program for dual diagnoses. He had both a substance abuse counselor and mental health counselor. Unsurprisingly, the PAI was completely invalid. As I began to fully realize that Sam's reality testing was not intact, I got that sinking feeling a therapist gets when your psychotherapy patient tells you they have intent and a plan for suicide. My anxiety began to quickly rise. I began thinking to myself, "I am thousands of miles away and have a psychotic sperm donor applicant. What do I need to do to protect him and help him? Protect myself?" I asked him if I could call his counselor or a family member. He would not allow me to call but did tell me his brother was picking him up from the appointment. I screened for suicide and homicide. He denied both. I had to let Sam leave without any intervention. I didn't know if he had an altered mental status from drugs or if he had a thought disorder. Clearly his reality testing was not intact.

After Sam left, I began to feel angry. How could the sperm bank not see that this man was not an appropriate candidate? They were putting me and their agency at risk of problems. And then my anxiety translated into fear, as it does, about what could happen. I was convinced I was going to be sued. Being a trailblazer in telehealth was no longer a great idea but a disaster. What was I thinking? I wasn't doing what my colleagues were doing. How was I going to explain this to a jury? And it was also such a waste of my time. It was going to take hours to complete the full report.

After some reflection and peer consultation, I settled down and realized this is why I am important and valuable. We are trained mental health professionals who can recognize and diagnose psychiatric problems. We know the difference between someone who is just a bit unusual and true mental illness. When I recounted this situation to the director of the sperm bank, she said, "So he's a little odd?". "No," I said, "This is a whole other ballgame." I then had to explain how a disconnection from reality was quite different than being "a little odd." The sperm bank followed my recommendation and did not accept Sam as a sperm donor. But what would have happened if a psychological evaluation wasn't a requirement for sperm donors? What would have happened if this sperm donor applicant went forward? A million disastrous outcomes come to mind. I wish Sam would have let me contact his counselor. I sometimes think of him and hope he is stable with good supports.

This case illustrates how best practice is to have a monitor for third-party evaluation, if conducted via telehealth. The donor coordinator was able to tell me that nobody was in the waiting room, validating that there were no real voices, and it was likely a psychotic process. She also checked up on the donor to see if he was becoming too agitated to continue the meeting. This case also demonstrates how much behavior we can actually observe via telehealth.

Case 3 (CE): The Nursery

A month into the pandemic, Leslie and Alex contacted me to begin couple's therapy. They had a 40-week stillborn baby in mid-March 2020 and were overwhelmed with grief. Leslie was on leave from her job as a dental assistant and Alex had been laid off from one job at a gym but was still working as a server, outside at a restaurant. I was hesitant to begin diving into such intense trauma and loss over video, yet there was no choice as the pandemic raged across the world.

In the first session, Leslie was in her bathrobe and her hair was in a messy bun on top of her head. I asked them if they wanted to share their story with me. Leslie agreed. Through tears she said that they had been expecting a girl and had named her Aspen. It was their first child. Leslie said she had always wanted to be a mother and had a miscarriage prior to her pregnancy with Aspen. Two days before Leslie's due date, she went to the hospital with contractions. She was sent home due to no dilation. The next day, also her husband's birthday, she said she didn't feel the baby moving and went to the hospital. Ultrasound revealed no heartbeat. Leslie and Alex returned home for one night to process this loss and Leslie gave birth the next day to Aspen. They said the hospital staff was kind to them, and Leslie showed me pictures taken at the hospital of them with their daughter. However, at the follow-up appointment at Leslie's obstetrician's office, her doctor entered the exam room and said "Where is your baby? Did you leave her at home?" Clearly, he did not remember what had happened which was deeply hurtful to Leslie and Alex. They were not able to do a memorial service or be with family for support due to COVID-19. Then, to add insult to injury, both Alex and Leslie got COVID-19.

As a psychologist and fertility counselor, all I could do was provide a safe place to hold their pain and observe their grief. Leslie slipped into a major depression and Alex became angry. They both began to binge drink and argue with each other. I encouraged them to not let their daughter's death break them, and to try to turn toward each other rather than against, while acknowledging grief is an individual journey. Seven months after the loss of Aspen, Leslie was pregnant again, and then miscarried. Their pain was exacerbated and neither of them could work. They began to divide family and friends into those who understood their grief and those who didn't. As their therapist, I started to feel helpless and was afraid I would end up in the category of those who didn't get it. I struggled to help them with the onslaught of difficulties. I wondered if my older, more experienced colleagues would do things differently.

As the couple approached their daughter's 1-year birthday and death, they began to drown deeper in sadness with anticipatory grief for that day. In our telecounseling session, they both appeared tearful at the start and began to talk about their fear of not ever being able to move forward. I knew at times that Leslie would sit in the nursery to reflect and cry. As I struggled to figure out what to do, I decided to trust my gut and try something on a whim. Because we were on video, I asked them to give me a tour of the nursery. We spent the whole therapy hour in the nursery. They showed me the crib, where the cat was now sleeping, the rocking chair with the handmade quilt, and all the clothes carefully organized and labeled by size. We went through every detail of the room.

This session created a monumental shift in the therapy. I believe they felt that I was able to witness their grief in a profoundly different way. By viewing Leslie's organization of the nursery and the meaning of all the knickknacks, I was able to join them in their experience in a new visually authentic way. The therapy seemed to get unstuck and while they were not without their ups and downs, Leslie and Alex began to move forward. We often talk about the cautions and limitations of telehealth but, perhaps, not as often about what it can do therapeutically that in-person office meetings cannot.

Conclusion

Overall, these three cases are examples of the advantages, risks and benefits that telehealth offers. As the world becomes more and more based in digital/video communication, it's critical that mental health professionals find effective ways to evolve their practice modalities. While the move to telehealth should not be taken without careful administrative, legal, and ethical decision-making, there are opportunities to expand our skill set to help more individuals and couples through their fertility journeys.

References

1. American Psychological Association. Ethical Principles of Psychologists and Code of Conduct. 2017. Available at: www.apa.org/ethics/code/ethics-code-2017.pdf [last accessed June 19, 2022].

2. American Psychological Association. The Standards for Educational and Psychological Testing. 2014. Available at: www.apa.org/science/programs/testing/standards [last accessed June 19, 2022].

3. Corey DM, Ben-Porath YS. Practical guidance on the use of the MMPI instruments in remote psychological testing. *Prof Psychol Res Pract* 2020;**51**:199–204.

4. Finger MS, Ones DS. Psychometric equivalence of the computer and booklet forms of the MMPI: a meta-analysis. *Psychol Assess* 1999;**11**:58–66.

5. Health Insurance Portability and Accountability Act (HIPAA). Pub., L,104–191. Health Insurance Portability and Accountability Act (HIPAA) Security Rule. 2013. Technical safeguards. 45 CFR § 164.312(e).

6. Joint Task Force for the Development of Telepsychology Guidelines for Psychologists. Guidelines for the practice of telepsychology. *Am Psychol* 2013;**68**:791–800.

7. Luxton DD, Pruitt LD, Osenbach JE. Best practices for remote psychological assessment via telehealth technologies. *Prof Psychol Res Practice* 2014;**45**:27–35.

8. Menton WH, Crighton AH, Tarescavage AM, Marek RJ, Hicks AD, Ben-Porath YS. Equivalence of laptop and tablet administrations of the Minnesota Multiphasic Personality Inventory-2 Restructured Form. *Assessment* 2019;**26**:661–669.

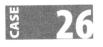

Nuts and Bolts of Fertility Counseling: Legal Issues and Practice Management

William Petok and Margaret Swain

Introduction

William (Bill) Petok: I have been a psychologist, primarily in private practice in Baltimore, Maryland since 1980. I'm also a Clinical Associate Professor of Obstetrics and Gynecology at the Sidney Kimmel Medical College of Thomas Jefferson University in Philadelphia, Pennsylvania. My graduate training at the University of Maryland, College Park emphasized a behavioral approach to problems. I did a subsequent postdoctoral year at the Family Therapy Institute of Washington, where I learned to approach people's problems from a systemic and strategic perspective. I was "invited" to work with fertility patients by my brother-in-law, Bill Schlaff, then in his REI fellowship at Johns Hopkins. The legal issues of reproductive medicine have always intrigued me, perhaps due to being married to an attorney. Over the years my wife, Barbara, and I have discussed the complex and difficult matters that patients and fertility counselors must consider as they proceed with the tasks of building a family. She never fails to say how difficult our work is compared to hers in pension and labor law. Of course, nothing could be further from the truth as all areas of law have their own complexities. And many areas of practice require knowledge of the law that governs your practice, but I think it's reasonable to assert that most don't require a knowledge of law as diverse as ours does. To that end, I've been fortunate to know and work with Peggy Swain on countless cases in which legal issues are discussed as they pertain to the specific case. As a result, I have gained a tremendous respect for the work our legal colleagues do.

Margaret (Peggy) Swain: I am an attorney in private practice in Baltimore, and am also a registered nurse. In a prior life, I worked as a clinical nurse for one of the first IVF programs here in town. After beginning my legal career, the physician with whom I had worked as a nurse, the incomparable Dr. Jairo Garcia, asked me if I would start an egg donor recruitment program. Of course, I said yes, even though I knew nearly nothing about the legal aspects of egg donation – at the time, the law was really just developing. As luck would have it, Andrea Braverman was hosting a program about egg donation, I signed up and the rest is history! Perhaps because my early history was through the lens of psychological concerns, support and education, I have always believed that the emotional aspects of assisted reproductive technology (ART) must be acknowledged and respected, as they inform all other components. Thanks to our colleagues in the mental health arena, we feel comfortable that our clients are well-prepared to manage the unique stressors and sometimes difficult situations that may arise during ART.

The legal paradigms surrounding parentage, consent, process and the like have become an integral part of third-party reproduction. As Bill says, there are very few areas of medicine and the mental health profession that are so closely intertwined with the law. It is only through an integrated team approach that we can accomplish our shared goals of secure, legally recognized, stable families and fair, ethical treatment of all involved in these arrangements.

The case presented below is a composite of several cases that we've worked on over the years. We've highlighted some of the more vexing issues and attempted to make them relevant for today's practicing fertility counselor. Some of the events are real but the people involved are fictitious.

Who Promised What?

Finding an egg donor can be a daunting task and in many cases the cost of using an agency is beyond the reach of some. Sometimes a donor is found from a relative or good friend. Sometimes the donor is "discovered" by happenstance. For example, two women meet at a baby shower and share stories of their own families, or lack thereof. The woman with children, feeling a connection with the childless woman, makes a generous gesture and offers to donate her eggs. They talk, get to know each other, and reach an agreement. The following case has similar elements. When an arrangement of this type takes place, there is no agency or program to guide the participants through the psychosocial and legal issues. Most REI programs will advise the women to seek legal counsel and provide the recipient with ASRM guidelines for the use of a donor and how she must be evaluated prior to any medical procedures being undertaken. That is exactly what happened here.

After meeting at a neighborhood get together, Janelle, 42, asked Sarah, 29, a married mother of three, to be her egg donor. She told Sarah how desperately she wanted to have a child and the great difficulties she and her husband had encountered. Now, with age and severely diminished ovarian reserve an issue, she knew that any child would be the result of an egg donation. Her doctor had confirmed this with her. The two women lived in the same community, and both immigrated to the United States (US) from the same Spanish-speaking country. After thinking it over Sarah decided to become the donor, in part because she felt for Janelle and the compensation would be helpful to her and her family. Janelle consulted with her physician who referred her to an attorney and told her that Sarah would have to be evaluated by a psychologist before he would proceed with a retrieval. Janelle had not fully appreciated the steps and cost necessary to achieve her dream, but she was already part way down that road.

When I received the initial referral, I asked about the language barrier. The referring clinic told me Sarah could have our meeting in English. But when I spoke with her on the telephone to schedule the meeting it became clear that while I might be able to interview her, I would be unable to administer a psychological test to her in English, a standard part of third-party consultations, because there were too many idiomatic expressions in the test protocol.

Sarah was referred to me for psychological evaluation and psychoeducational consultation. Prior to meeting with Sarah, I held a consultation session with Janelle. She told me that during her 14-year marriage she and her husband had tried in the last 5 years to conceive without success. She told me that Sarah was a "friend" for the past year whom she'd met through a third "friend." She told me her husband, Robert, had met Sarah and was "fine with it." She further told me that she had no desire for any ongoing relationship with Sarah. She said that her husband couldn't make it to our meeting because he had to work. I indicated that my normal procedure was to meet with both people in the relationship first but would catch up with him later.

The meeting with Janelle took place in my home office. During the consultation we discussed the usual broad range of issues. When I asked Janelle about her plans for disclosure about their use of a donor, she said that only her husband would know. I told her that certainly was a choice but wanted to offer her an alternative approach. I said that children understand the idea of "helper" at an early age and that was one way to begin

such a conversation with a donor-conceived child. I explained the advantages of providing a child with this information and the disadvantages of keeping secrets. I offered to provide her with a bibliography in Spanish if she wished. I finished by saying this was a very personal decision and that my goal was to give her the information so she could make an informed choice about how to approach disclosure. Often, when provided with reasons why disclosure is helpful to the child, a recipient will tell me something along the lines of "... I never thought about it like that." This was not the case here.

I neglected to ask her about a contract between the two women and what if any payment had been discussed. I knew the physician and the attorney involved and suspected they had discussed these issues with Janelle. My meeting with Sarah was scheduled for the next day. I knew her native language was not English, but the physician at the fertility center was fluent in Spanish, offered to provide a translator and I obtained a copy of the Minnesota Multiphasic Personality Inventory (MMPI) in Spanish.

During the evaluation I asked the usual questions about disclosure and privacy. Did the donor have an idea about what the recipient wished? What, if anything, would she explain to her family? How did she meet the recipient and how did she decide to become a donor? Her responses to some of the questions were disconcerting at a minimum. Sarah told me that upon hearing Janelle's story of infertility she'd asked if she could help her, telling me she "saw the anguish on her face. I told her I have a lot of kids."

Within 3 months Janelle had asked her to become a donor. There was no discussion of payment. When Sarah started her medical evaluation, she was informed that her expenses would be covered and that the donor fee would help cover those expenses. She told me her husband "did not get into this ..." but indicated that if she had to be paid "... to do a good deed, don't do it." She then told me that she thought Janelle was too focused on the child being her own and that Sarah thought Janelle was being selfish. She wished she felt more appreciation from Janelle for the help she was providing. "I told her she should choose someone who doesn't know her rather than me."

I finally asked her how she would feel if I told her it was not a good idea for her to be the donor. Would she be disappointed or relieved? She told me it would be OK if she could not do it. The lack of clarity about the compensation was a concern, as was the donor's feelings about the recipient. The fact that they lived two blocks apart in a community with many people from their country of origin suggested to me that they would see each other frequently, while shopping or out and about. That did not feel like a good situation.

Before the testing was started, Sarah asked when she would get her payment. I was unclear if there was a contract in place and deferred. I said that normally payment takes place in stages that begin after the medical and psychological evaluations are completed. Sarah was quite insistent that this was not correct. During the interview Sarah told me she had known Janelle for 2.5 months and another red flag was raised for me. While I hadn't seen the test results yet, I had an uneasy feeling about this arrangement.

My normal practice is to evaluate the donor before meeting with the spouse or significant other if there is one. My logic is that if the donor does not meet the necessary standards, the recipients will have not spent time and money trying to establish how that person might think or feel, if the arrangement was not going forward. In this case I never met either of the spouses.

As it turned out, I did not think Sarah was a good donor candidate for several reasons. Her MMPI profile had several spikes indicating a volatile personality. Then there was the misunderstanding about payment and Sarah's reaction to my explanation, which validated the MMPI finding. In addition, there was something unsettling about the difference in the accounts of how long the women had known each other. Finally, I knew the women lived near each other and would likely run into each other from time to time, potentially creating a difficult situation.

My letter to the fertility center, also delivered to Janelle's attorney, detailed why I recommended against Sarah going forward as a donor. Then the fireworks started!

I have two offices; one is in my home. My evaluation with Sarah was at the fertility center to accommodate the translator and to allow the physician to answer any questions on the spot. A week after she was informed that her donor was rejected, Janelle showed up at my home, while I was in my other office. My wife answered the door and indicated a phone number for Janelle to call if she wished to speak with me. I subsequently received a phone call from Janelle and a reporter threatening an exposé in the Spanish language press, both print and television. I immediately called both the attorneys, Janelle's whom I knew and the one representing Sarah, who also spoke her native language.

Issues Raised

This case raised issues of language competency, knowledge of the contract, understanding of secrecy versus privacy, how a disgruntled client could create havoc without a lawsuit, as well as general principles of sound business practice and cross discipline collaboration. These issues are also addressed in the companion *Clinical Guide* chapter volume.

Language Competency

I was trained on the MMPI and had used if for years but never in Spanish. Furthermore, my Spanish education ended in college and was so rudimentary it was embarrassing. But I knew the reproductive medicine practice and the lawyer who represented the intended parents, and had a great deal of respect for both. I knew the MMPI was available in Spanish so one problem was solved. But I thought I needed an interpreter so I could get the best picture of Sarah. Fortunately, the clinic had an interpreter who worked for the local circuit court and had the necessary experience to translate both in the interview and for any questions that might arise during testing. But would I have to pay for the service? That could eat into my fee significantly, not a pleasant thought.

Federal law requires medical practices to use interpreters. *Title VI of the Civil Rights Act of 1964* requires interpreters for all patients with limited English proficiency (LEP) based on national origin who receive federal financial assistance except for Medicare Part B. Just as in the case of wheelchair accessibility for disabled persons, not providing interpreters when needed is discrimination and is illegal. A case with similar components was presented by us in the first edition of this text [1]. But this was not a Medicare case, and I am technically not a medical professional. So, was I obligated to follow Title VI? As it turns out, psychologists are responsible for providing interpreter services [2]. Thankfully, the clinic absorbed the cost of the interpreter.

Most importantly, I had to trust that the interpreter was giving me accurate information and did not have some pre-existing relationship with the donor. A trained interpreter will likely give a better rendition of what is said than a family member or friend who perhaps has a vested interest in portraying the person in the best possible light. My goal was to provide the best possible evaluation/consultation without bias. I would have been lost without the services of the interpreter.

What Does the Contract Say?

I had not seen the contract between the two parties regarding the compensation. In fact, I rarely if ever see these contracts. Should I have seen this one? It might have helped me to understand what had been arranged in advance. But is that the job of the fertility counselor or the reproductive attorney? A waiver of conflict of interest is always recommended when a fertility counselor is providing services to both sides of an arrangement [1]. In this case such a waiver was a protection for the adverse outcome the recipient experienced. But would it have helped me to know about what agreements had taken place before I accepted the case? Based on the outcome it seems like it would have been a good idea but not necessary because I was protected, having a signed waiver of conflict of interest. Having a competent translator available allowed me to inquire if the prospective donor or recipient had any questions about the language of the consent/waiver.

Matters of Disclosure

An important consideration when evaluating a donor is the idea of privacy versus secrecy. It appeared to me that the desire on both parts was absolute secrecy. The case took place before direct-to-consumer genetic testing was widely available. As a result, I did not make a statement about the inability of anyone to offer anonymity. Today that would be a standard point of discussion recommended by the Ethics Committee of the American Society for Reproductive Medicine (ASRM) [3]. Specifically, ASRM recommends that donors be counseled about the risk of losing anonymity:

- Social media and future implications for identification.
- Understanding of the likelihood and implications of contact through direct-to-consumer deoxyribonucleic acid (DNA) websites and implications for the donors, their children, current or future partners, and their extended families [4].

Parenthetically, this sets the stage for discussing disclosure to a child and why that might be in the best interests of the child and the family.

While this may be complicated for some donors or recipients to understand, I have developed a script that seems to make the point. I will say, "If your donation/recipiency were to result in a pregnancy today, the child would be 13 years old in "year XXXX," at which time they will likely be studying biology in middle school and learning about DNA. Part of that study could involve taking a swab from you, your spouse, and the child for comparison. The results will identify to the child that one of his parents does not have a genetic connection. This will create a new set of issues for you as parents to address. Or your child, knowing they were donor-conceived, may use one of the genetic testing services to discover more about the donor." For this reason, it is difficult if not impossible to keep the donor anonymous.

Is Legal Action the Only Negative Consequence of an Evaluation "Gone Wrong?

As fertility counselors, we learn early on to do a variety of things to keep within ethical and legal boundaries. Practicing within your level of competence is critical, as is having the proper legal authority to offer the service you've been asked to provide. To do otherwise usually violates professional ethical standards and may violate state law. For example, in Maryland, to administer, score and interpret psychological tests such as the PAI or MMPI, the professional's degree must meet, among others, the following requirements: "Personality Assessment. Studies in this area shall include, but are not limited to, the construction, standardization, scoring, and interpretation of personality tests." (COMAR 10.58.11.03 et al.). A complaint to the Board will require demonstration that the license holder has completed the necessary education, supervision and examinations.

A complaint to the board of examiners for your profession is a stress-inducing event to say the least. Practicing to avoid such a complaint is critical. But will doing so prevent a disgruntled client from complaining? How will you be protected if you aggravate someone to the point they complain? Malpractice insurance is essential as part of risk management strategy that includes ethical practice. The policy I hold provides $25,000 reimbursement "per proceeding" before a licensing board and similarly an additional $7,500 for "other governmental regulatory body defense." Given the relatively low cost for malpractice insurance, compared with some other health care professionals, our recommendation is purchasing the maximum offered.

In this instance, I was clear about meeting the necessary legal requirements and holding a good policy to protect me financially should my board receive a complaint. But what about the threat from the reporter?

A close review of my malpractice insurance made it clear that I was covered for "assault and battery" if it happened on my work premises or if I was providing covered services off site. Did the threat to my reputation constitute an assault? Not according to my malpractice policy. Assault is the attempted touching of a person without his or her consent, including under those circumstances where the person feels fearful that a touching will occur. Even though the threat was going to "touch" my reputation, I was not protected by my insurance. And my business policy was focused on actual property I owned or leased for the purpose of carrying out my practice. It would be an underestimate to say I was concerned!

Reputation insurance is available, but most policies are too expensive for the average fertility counseling practice to afford. They tend to cover an actual loss in sales resulting from a brand-damaging incident. Clearly, a negative news report would have damaged my "brand!"

Why Is It a Good Idea to Have a Conversation with the Lawyers in the Arrangement?

The most important action I took was to consult with the two lawyers working on this case. The lawyer representing the donor was well-versed in the communities of origin for these two women. He also was able to talk with his client and ascertain that the interpreter had given me an accurate account. But most importantly he let me know that the verbal threat of an "exposé" was most likely nothing more than a threat and advised that I *not* respond to the reporter. I was grateful for the advice and my anxiety was quelled, somewhat.

Whether or not I should have inquired about the contractual offer prior to meeting with either party in retrospect seems like an obvious "yes." However, it is not my usual practice to do so. My assumption, perhaps incorrectly so, is that since I'm not a lawyer it's not my place to insert myself. At the same time, some knowledge of the contract would have been helpful when I was first presented with the question about the payment arrangement. My pre-existing relationship with one attorney was useful and speaks to the usefulness of developing those relationships in advance. This takes time but is well worth it for the ability to understand what has been arranged by the parties in advance.

It is not unusual for me to discuss common aspects of contracts with intended parents and gestational carriers during my consultations/evaluations. I use language that indicates that I am not giving legal advice. Instead, I am offering a look into what they may expect. For example, I will frequently say something like "most contracts contain language that discusses the use of social media during a pregnancy. Your lawyer and the other party's lawyer will help work that out. It might say something about what can be said about whom you are carrying for or whether or not you can put pictures of yourself on your feed while you are pregnant." Many individuals are unaware that this will be the case and are pleased that the issue was raised in advance so they can consider it before the contractual negotiations begin.

My knowledge of contractual language is the result of conversations with attorneys prior to and during the course of evaluations/consultations with their clients and has proved valuable in helping donors/gestational carriers have reasonable expectations about the process.

Summary

The fictitious case presented here raises a finite number of legal and risk management issues that a fertility counselor could face. Our goal was to offer a glimpse at some of them without being overwhelming. Clearly, a lot was learned from this case about the issues presented here, particularly regarding contracts that donors and recipients engage in, the use of interpreters, and competency when working with individuals from other communities than our own. Our best advice is to follow the guidelines provided by your profession on ethical practice, know the laws in your state governing your practice, be aware of any Federal regulations that could impact how you practice, and have a good legal consultant who knows reproductive law and maintain malpractice insurance. Good clinical supervision and/or consultation with another fertility counselor with more experience is always a good idea if you are stuck on something. And finally, don't be afraid to turn down a case if it feels over your head.

He that fights and runs away,
May turn and fight another day;
But he that is in battle slain,
Will never rise to fight again.

Tacitus [5]

References

1. Swain M, Petok W. Legal issues for fertility counselors. In: Covington SN, Ed. *Fertility Counseling: Clinical Guide and Case Studies.* Cambridge: Cambridge University Press, 2015, 296–310.

2. Searight HR, Searight BK. Working with foreign language interpreters: recommendations for psychological practice. *Prof Psychol Res Pract* 2009;**40**:444–451.

3. Daar J, Collins L, Davis J, et al. Interests, obligations, and rights in gamete and embryo donation: an Ethics Committee opinion. *Fertil Steril* 2019;**111**:664–670.

4. Practice Committee of the American Society for Reproductive Medicine and the Practice Committee for the Society for Assisted Reproductive Technology Guidance regarding gamete and embryo donation. *Fertil Steril* 2021;**115**:1395–1410.

5. Tacitus. No Title. *Quotesia*. Available at: https://quotesia.com/tacitus-quote/694265.%0A%0A Read; more at: https://quotesia.com/ tacitus-quote/694265/citation [last accessed June 19, 2022].

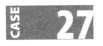

Ethical Platform of Assisted Reproduction

Jeanne O'Brien and Julianne Zweifel

Introduction

Jeanne O'Brien: I am a board-certified reproductive endocrinology and infertility specialist with a focused interest in reproductive genetics. The most challenging aspect of being an infertility specialist lies in the complexity of clinical decision-making and the ability to compassionately convey the disappointments that our innate biology brings us. As a part of a large assisted reproductive technology (ART) practice, I have been able to Chair the Ethics Committee and collaborate with many fertility specialists when faced with difficult clinical decisions. I also consider myself a life-long student. Motivated by the remarkable advances in genomics over the last decade and the relative absence of knowledgeable infertility specialists, I am pursuing a Masters in Genomics. My thoughts are shaped and influenced by the remarkable time we live in. One where science makes it possible to edit the genome despite the lack of a comprehensive ethical consensus regrading appropriate utilization. The present hope and hype of biomedical innovation in reproductive medicine and the recognition that innate biology lacks perfection are important themes in my life and in my writing.

Julianne Zweifel: I describe myself as a reproductive health psychologist, meaning that I am a clinical psychologist with training in human physiology and anatomy as well as subspecialty training in how physiology and psychology interact to influence reproductive health experiences. I've been practicing within the Department of Obstetrics and Gynecology at the University of Wisconsin School of Medicine and Public Health for nearly 20 years. My clinical work is with patients experiencing infertility, miscarriage, still birth, fetal health concerns, pregnancy termination and postpartum depression. It is emotionally hard work, but I love it.

It was within my role at the University of Wisconsin Ob/Gyn department that I became drawn to ethics. Coming out of graduate school, I would have described ethics as esoteric, old and dusty but, in my position as the department reproductive health psychologist, I was tasked with leading a monthly ethics discussion group that was attended by physicians, nurses, chaplains, attorneys and administrators, some of whom had formal ethics training. Through the requirement of researching and leading monthly ethics discussions, I developed a strong respect for the complexity, competing interests, nuance and importance of ethics as well as ways in which ethics are impacted by explicit and implicit bias. I've come to recognize that ethics and ethical debate is not for the timid and not for those who wish a quick and easy answer. I went on to become a member of the University of Wisconsin hospital ethics committee and more recently became a member of the American Society for Reproductive Medicine ethics committee.

We present two in-depth cases which exemplify both clinical complexity and the value of ethical frameworks in decision-making. It's our hope that the formal discussion of reproductive ethics and case presentations equip clinicians with the ability to perceive, analyze and address ethical complexities in assisted reproduction. It should be noted that these cases represent an amalgamation of clinical issues and ethical challenges occurring with developing reproductive technology, and not one specific event.

The first case allows consideration of hurdles that come with donor gametes, ART and genomics. Genomic information is intrinsically and permanently shared across individuals. Genomic ties cannot be erased, and they are no longer anonymous, especially when consumer genomic testing makes a guarantee of future anonymity impossible for both donors and recipients.

The second case explores how a treatment plan for infertility transformed over time into an odyssey for nonmedical sex-selection. It also provides an opportunity to consider new reproductive technologies such as polygenic risk predictors, which could soon be used for nonclinical reasons for embryo selection. The answers to the questions posed by these case studies will not be solely scientific.

Case Discussions

The Unsuspecting Sperm Donor is a BRCA2 Carrier

A healthy 32-year-old woman conceived with sperm from a de-identified donor. A routine prenatal ultrasound revealed the fetus had major structural brain abnormalities. The 22-week male had an underdeveloped brain for gestational age, agenesis of the corpus callosum and ambiguous genitalia. The patient elected to terminate the pregnancy after extensive multidisciplinary counseling. Following the termination, exome sequencing was performed to try and identify a genetic cause or pathogenic variant responsible for the fetal anomalies. *Exome sequencing* is a type of genetic test that involves sequencing and comparing the entire protein coding genes (exome) of the genetic parents and fetus simultaneously (exome trio). The sperm donor was not contacted to participate in this genetic testing, thus an exome comparison between the mother and fetus was performed (exome duo). The exome results indicated that the male fetus carried a pathogenic variant in a gene located on the X chromosome which is known to cause the clinical findings. The pathogenic variant was not detected in the maternal genes and most likely represented a de novo germline mutation (spontaneous). The sperm donor would not be a carrier of the X-linked pathogenic variant since he was a healthy adult.

While the de novo finding did not present ethical challenges, the exome sequencing of the fetus returned an additional, unexpected, result with significant repercussions. The fetus was also a carrier for BRCA2. The American College of Medical Genetics and Genomics (ACMG) classifies BRCA2 as a medically actionable disease gene variant and advises disclosure even in unconsented individuals when identified incidentally. ACMG considers the disclosure of findings for adult-onset conditions such as breast cancer is in the best interests of a child [1].

It remains unclear how best to handle actionable secondary findings in the prenatal context of donor-assisted conceptions. What are the responsibilities of the intended parent(s), medical professionals, and donor gamete banks in these cases? The exome duo revealed that only the fetus and not the genetic mother was found to have the pathogenic BRCA2 variant which is associated with hereditary breast and ovarian cancer. This means that the variant is most likely from the genetic contribution of the sperm donor. In this case, we have unintentionally identified the presence of a pathogenic cancer oncogene in an unconsented de-identified sperm donor. In most cases, clinicians will generally be notified very quickly when an ART pregnancy, especially one that is donor-conceived, is abnormal. This speaks to the pervasive and yet erroneous belief that ART guarantees a commercial product free of defects. The healthcare professional will need to quickly obtain directed genetic testing from the individuals who contributed to the pregnancy. This requires a multidisciplinary approach utilizing experts such as a social worker, genetic counselor, medical geneticist, specialized genomics laboratory, and medical director of the gamete bank. In the United States (US), the ART provider will rely on the medical director of the gamete bank to make appropriate notifications to a donor after an unintended finding.

More broadly, the increasing use of genomic testing prenatally and after birth to determine an etiology for a suspected genetic condition is generating new ethical issues, especially in donor-conceived pregnancies. Genetic testing in donor conceptions upends the directional and temporal flow of genetic bioinformation. A pathogenic finding often points away from the intended parents toward the donor as the potential source for the genetic variant. ART providers may not have timely access to gamete donors in order to obtain a specimen or stored DNA to complete genetic testing. Donor gamete providers need to recognize that future genomic investigations involving donors challenge traditional medical consent processes and may reveal personally relevant and important information for individuals who are not themselves patients.

The patient was unsure about what to do with her three remaining, transferable male embryos from this sperm donor. Each embryo has a 50% chance of being a carrier of the pathogenic BRCA2 variant. However, a male may be a silent carrier who remains unaffected by the BRCA2 gene. Genetic risks are difficult to fully predict; variable penetrance and expressivity means we remain unable to accurately predict the future, even of a cancer oncogene. What should she do? The patient can transfer an untested embryo and consider testing an ongoing pregnancy for BRCA2. It is technically possible but more difficult to conduct indirect testing with preimplantation genetic testing (PGT-M, Mendelian or single gene) of the remaining embryos for the BRCA2 variant. This is costly and not covered by insurance in most cases. She may decide to discard the remaining embryos and choose a new sperm donor. Of note, commercial sperm banks in the US do not routinely screen sperm donors for cancer oncogenes. Thus, a new sperm donor will also have a risk of carrying a cancer oncogene, although the likelihood will be low.

Ethicists would affirm the patient's right to know or not know the genetic status (BRCA2 positive or not) of her embryos. From an ethics perspective, it is interesting to examine and contrast the importance of passing on one's genetic material verses the effort to shield the offspring from serious health risks. Biogenetic parents who fail to produce unaffected embryos from IVF may elect to transfer a known BRCA2 positive embryo. A *Robertson reproductive autonomy argument* would support this parental choice, even if it were certain the offspring would be affected. Alternatively, a *virtue ethics perspective* would advise that a parent de-prioritize their desire for a genetic connection in favor of promoting a good health outcome for the child.

In our example however, where a sperm donor contributed to the generation of embryos, the contribution of the de-identified sperm donor may be devalued, and the donor sperm deemed a defective commercial product to be discarded. While few would argue that a parent should not be permitted to use a different sperm donor in a goal to have a healthy child, the "swapping" of donors can be viewed as de-humanizing the donor and as discussed in the accompanying *Clinical Guide* volume chapter, contributes to parents viewing children as "objects of our design." One could also consider the swapping of donors to be at odds with *virtue ethics*. Where do we draw the line between clinical health versus desired traits such as eye color, height or even intelligence? This question will challenge ART providers in the years to come.

In the case example, what are the responsibilities of the provider (and patient) to the sperm donor and the donor's family? During the informed consent process for genetic testing, the genetic mother had the option to decline the return of any secondary findings. The sperm donor was not part of the informed consent process. Does the sperm donor permanently relinquish all genetic autonomy? Is an informed consent valid for a finding that was not specifically discussed at the time of donation? Genetic testing of a fetus or a donor-conceived offspring done without prior consent from the gamete donor may have significant ramifications for the unconsented donor. Potential benefits include knowledge, the ability to utilize cancer screening and even the prevention of disease. The impact is magnified by the fact that successful gamete donors (especially sperm) will have many biogenic offspring. The finding in the gamete donor also sets off a cascade of potential counseling and testing among the donor's family members as well as other recipient families that have been created from the gamete donation. Implications also involve risk of insurance discrimination and family disruption.

This case also tests the boundaries of the traditional physician–patient relationship. The ART provider has no professional relationship with the sperm donor. It is reasonable to assume the presence of the BRCA2 variant is unknown in the sperm donor's family. The sperm

donor and family could benefit by preventing a severe health outcome. One court has held that a doctor must take "responsible steps . . . to assure that the information reaches those likely to be affected or it is made available for their benefit" [2]. Is it enough for the physician to notify the sperm bank?

The unexpected finding of the abnormal pregnancy at 22 weeks highlights a challenge for ART providers. In the US, infertility patients transition back to their obstetrician (OB) after the first 8 weeks of pregnancy. This transition of care almost always precedes a decision for further genomic testing during the pregnancy by a high-risk OB or geneticist. Thus, the counseling and consenting of the mother prior to genomic testing was not done by the reproductive endocrinologist (RE). The RE may well not even be aware that the pregnancy was terminated. As the bioinformation becomes available, the ART provider needs to play catch-up and also address patient concerns that something was done wrong or missed for this to happen.

Patients often do not recognize the role of luck in genomics. We all resist the idea that luck plays a role in our lives. The use of donor gametes creates an inflated sense of control. Recipients often fail to make a distinction between purchasing donor gametes screened to have a high likelihood of health and the random mistakes of genetics. It is helpful to discuss with patients that a 25-year-old can have a child with Down's syndrome (it is just not as likely compared to the risk in a 43-year-old). Even if we sequence all genetic parents prior to conception and only proceed when there are no known identified risks, children will still be born with birth defects and disabilities. Reproduction with or without donor gametes does not guarantee biologic perfection. While a goal of a healthy child is certainly understandable, as articulated in the corresponding *Clinical Guide* chapter, not everything in the world is open to what we may desire or devise.

When we look back from results to try and figure out why something happened, we are susceptible to assuming causation or cherry-picking data to confirm our preferred narrative. This is not chess where outcomes correlate tightly with decision quality. It is biology (genetics) randomly in action, and the uncertainty gives us room to deceive ourselves. Information is hidden from us in the genome despite the use of advanced technology to select for health. Some things are unknown to us still or even unknowable in severity prior to birth.

The psychology of loss factors in as we apply analytical frameworks to the recipient's decision-making in this case. In general, the use of donor gametes often means a recipient(s) has already grieved the loss of having a shared genetic child with a partner. How could the recommended medical treatment result in a new unimaginable problem? The way we field outcomes is path dependent. The recipient is coming from a path of need or failure (donor sperm), so an added dilemma of an affected pregnancy is even more difficult to comprehend. How we discuss and understand risks in medicine is often not consistent with how our patients understand risk. Physicians need to express some uncertainty regarding the health of all conceptions, including donor-assisted.

Our challenges are amplified against the backdrop of increasing sophistication and utilization of genomic testing. Genomic medicine is revolutionizing the practice of reproductive medicine. The prenatal exome creates a virtual image of the future child. A prenatal exome also has the potential to result in the discarding of additional embryos due to concerns that the embryos might be affected. Oftentimes, it is not possible to know with certitude how a predicted genomic risk will manifest after birth. The recipient's decision to terminate the severely affected pregnancy as well as discard the potentially affected remaining embryos without testing is ethically reasonable. It is worth considering the recipient's decision to receive secondary findings from the exome testing. She could have declined to receive information that related to adult-onset conditions. The decision is at odds with care-based ethics. Did the recipient act with moral equality and respect for the sperm donor? The commodification of gametes has profound implications. Parents would not be blamed for naturally conceiving a child with a rare recessive disease. However, clinics and sperm banks have been sued for providing gametes with previously unknown genetic defects.

What was the outcome of this case? The patient decided to discard the remaining transferable embryos due to the potential risk of carrying the BRCA2 gene. She started the IVF process all over with a new sperm donor. Using the ethical analysis strategy presented in the corresponding *Clinical Guide* chapter, the interests of the patient and the potential for an unborn child to be a BRCA2 carrier primarily influenced the decision and clearly align with Robertson's procreative liberty. The medical director of the sperm bank was notified of the secondary finding. The sperm bank assumes responsibility for all notifications owing to the established doctor–patient relationship as well as knowledge of the sperm donor's identity.

We have an obligation to continuously question the aim of scientific progress as well as to consider the judgment of a "good life." Is there a duty to have a healthy child or even manipulate genetics in the name of optimizing health and other offspring characteristics? How do we value diversity? Responses will vary by cultural, social, and religious perspectives.

Final Thoughts

1. Third-party reproduction requires all care providers to acknowledge the fundamental uncertainty in biology. ART does not guarantee a healthy outcome or any outcome for that matter.
2. What are the potential unintended consequences of selecting against certain genes or combinations of genes?
3. Will the ability of some parents to access genomic screening of embryos worsen existing health disparities? How can we address this problem?

What If Biology Fails to Deliver?

Reproductive technologies allow for the possibility of selecting, for nonmedical reasons, an embryo based solely on genetic sex. In 2015, through a worldwide survey of 66 countries, approximately 65% of respondents stated that aneuploidy screening (PGT-A) for sex chromosome selection was not allowed [3]. In the US, each practice determines its policy regarding nonmedical sex selection. A survey study conducted in 2017 reported that the majority of American Assisted Reproductive Technology (ART) clinics offer nonmedical sex selection [4]. Even when a practice has a clear policy, physicians and patients who initially utilize PGT-A for aneuploidy screening only, may slowly progress down a path of nonmedical sex selection. The reproductive ethicist, Judith Daar, aptly refers to the ART provider/practice policy whether to offer nonmedical sex selection as an example of a "threshold decision" [5]. It should be noted that routine PGT-A screening reports include genetic sex as part of the result and their wide application in ART means that clinicians frequently face patient requests for a particular genetic sex when it becomes time to select an embryo for transfer.

In this case, an ART provider in the US agreed on a "threshold decision" to not offer nonmedical sex selection. Thus, family balancing or the desire of having one child of a particular sex *alone* was not an indication to proceed with ART. Each patient must have a diagnosis of infertility first and have utilized appropriate less invasive treatments prior to proceeding with IVF with or without PGT-A. However, what occurred here evolved over the course of treatment, and demonstrates the complexity of decision-making for physicians and patients when the parental priority for success entails something more than just a healthy child.

The case begins with a 34-year-old female patient with a history of infertility due to polycystic ovarian syndrome (PCOS), who initially underwent ovulation induction therapy. After 6 months of unsuccessful treatment, IVF was recommended as the next option. PGT-A was not advised at that point. The couple were able to conceive naturally during a treatment break and subsequently have two healthy sons. Four years later, the couple returned to the fertility clinic to resume treatment after three spontaneous first trimester miscarriages. The patient is now 38 years old, and the physician recommends IVF with PGT-A due to the recurrent miscarriages. The couple clearly expressed a desire to transfer a female embryo, if available, but not a requirement. The physician considered this request consistent with the clinic's policy to allow patient autonomy when selecting among normal embryos for transfer. Hopefully, the physician and couple recognized that the ART process doesn't guarantee a female embryo for transfer.

The first IVF cycle resulted in five normal males and one normal female. The transfer of the female embryo was negative. The couple declined to use the male embryos and requested to proceed with another PGT-A cycle in one last attempt to obtain a female embryo. The treating physician asked the couple about the disposition of surplus embryos and the couple stated they intended to proceed with embryo donation. The physician agreed to the treatment request. Notably, this request to do an IVF cycle in order to obtain female embryos was not consistent with clinic policy. However, granting the couple's earlier request to transfer a female embryo from the first cycle, predictably created pressure on the physician to agree to a higher-level request to create embryos specifically for the purpose of transferring a female embryo. This is an example of the foot-in-the-door phenomenon, whereby agreeing to an initial request, the physician views themself as helpful and this, in turn, sets the physician up to feel compelled to continue their behavior pattern of being supportive or obliging. A repeat IVF cycle again generated a large number of normal embryos but only one female. The second transfer also failed. Despite expressing this would be the last cycle, the couple requested one last cycle to try and get the desired embryo. The last cycle generated no female

embryos. The patient experienced a minor surgical complication after the oocyte retrieval that required treatment.

The couple have now completed three IVF cycles and two failed transfers. They have 12 normal male embryos and have requested a fourth IVF cycle to make one last attempt. The treatment plan is now an odyssey to find an embryo of a specific genetic sex when more than enough embryos are available to have a third child.

The physician now acutely appreciates their role in facilitating this situation with no end in sight as well as the ethical dilemma of continuing to provide care. The physician sought the guidance of a reproductive Ethics committee. The discussion focused on the conflict between the patients' reproductive autonomy to continue the care plan and the physician's autonomy to decline to proceed. This case highlights the concept of balanced autonomy in decision-making proposed by King in the *Clinical Guide* companion chapter.

In this case, the ethics discussion centered on the couple's priority to have a child of a particular sex. As a staunch advocate of parental reproductive autonomy, Robertson would support the couple's request to cycle again. Contrasting views of virtue ethics and feminist ethics caution that this plan places the potential child at risk of harm and devaluation. Specifically, spending this amount of money to acquire a child of a desired sex positions future children as products of a predefined plan, lessening their inherent value as individuals and contributing to the commodification of children [6]. Further, parents spending this amount of money to ensure the preferred genetic sex may create considerable pressure for the child to conform to gender-based roles and behavior, thus potentially depriving the child the right to an open future.

The 2015 ASRM Committee opinion acknowledges the controversy of nonmedical sex selection and encourages practitioners to establish policies [3]. ESHRE also takes a middle ground but cautions about unnecessary extra procedures to fulfil nonmedical sex selection [7]. How should the physician who is now in conflict with the couple's desire to do one more cycle negotiate a conversation with patients who see their future through having a child of the desired sex? The physician must balance the patient's desire to control the outcome, while accepting the limitations of biology.

The recommendation of the Ethics committee in this case focused on a resolution for both the patients and the physician. The physician needed to establish a way to end the self-perpetuating treatment plan with a boundary.

153

The physician had not established a clear parameter to stop and the patients' assumed approval from that ambiguity. The physician would assist the couple in completing a final IVF cycle regardless of the outcome for embryo sex. The couple would need to proceed with embryo transfer as the next step.

We encourage ART providers to seek the assistance of an Ethics committee, whether it be within their practice setting or a local academic setting, when confronted with difficult clinical care decisions like this.

Final Thoughts

1. The initial plan did not include any discussion of failure. What if there are no normal embryos of the desired genetic sex for transfer? What if the subsequent transfer fails and you are left with only embryos of the wrong genetic sex? For all reproductive technologies, the counseling pretreatment should include both outcomes, success and failure. Providers and patients need to complete the thought experiment prospectively.
2. The physician failed to define clear boundaries prior to starting each treatment cycle.
3. How should the treating physician proceed now?
4. The couple have expressed a desire to proceed with embryo donation for the unused embryos. Should this influence the decision of the physician regarding another IVF cycle?

Ethical Challenges Ahead

We have an opportunity to apply principles from the nonmedical sex selection case to other types of patient preferences regarding embryo selection. Reproductive medicine providers will soon face requests to utilize polygenic risk predictors (PRS) to rank order embryos for transfer based on the likelihood of common diseases such as diabetes or coronary artery disease. The introduction of embryonic polygenic predictors will be a new threshold of choice for ART providers. Given an upper limit of approximately 65% for implantation of a selected embryo, PRS have the potential to push couples to do unnecessary additional IVF cycles for a predicted benefit which may actually not be accurate. Predicting risk is not perfect. There is also a fine line between parental reproductive freedom to maximize potential health and positional advantage or enhancement. The so-called slippery slope quickly leads from prevention (selecting against diabetes) to seeking an advantage (selecting for intelligence). However, Julian Savulescu suggests "the mere fact

that technology could be used non-therapeutically doesn't warrant a moratorium on its use" ([8], p. 477). In 2015, he was making the case that there was a moral imperative to continue preclinical gene editing research on human embryos. It is reasonable to conclude that Robertson would support wide parental latitude regarding ART methods that select for a potentially better embryo for transfer (PGT-A and PRS). Does the procreative benefit framework afford the same latitude for parental decisions regarding future germline gene editing?

How do we find a path forward regarding patient preferences for selecting embryos? Polkinghorne proposed that moving forward will involve the participation of three parties: the experts, the beneficiaries, and the general public [9]. As the experts, ART providers are best positioned to assess the potential benefits, risks, and unknowns, while the long-term risks remain to be seen. We must carefully weigh our objectivity regarding treatments and transformative technologies, as some may be so eager regarding the potential benefits (for their patients as well as themselves) that it will influence their judgment. Our patients and the resulting children comprise the community of special beneficiaries and may also include anyone who is likely to be impacted from treatment decisions. Lastly, the general public needs to be involved and educated about the potential risks and benefits of transformative reproductive technologies. In reaching a decision about the implementation of mitochondrial replacement therapy, the United Kingdom (UK) modelled a strategy for public engagement by which the Human Fertilization and Embryology Authority (HFEA) incorporated broad public consultation [10].

The key message is that the physician and patient will face many threshold decisions in the course of treatment. The case presented discusses nonmedical sex selection, but other important embryo selection decisions are emerging. If offered a test that would make it less likely a child will have diabetes, would patients want to utilize it? The ethical considerations of nonmedical sex selection, selecting against health risks and selecting for enhancements clearly differ but also have common important considerations.

How the provider frames the capabilities and limitations of a technology (i.e., PGT-A) in the original discussion is critical. Providers must convey that the desire to prefer one option over another, the plan to select the preferred option with the assistance of technology, and the belief that the desired outcome will occur is not always consistent with the nature of biological processes.

We as providers want our patients to be successful in achieving their family-building goals. However, it is critical to introduce the possibility that their hoped-for ideal may not be possible. It is a difficult acknowledgment of our own limitations to those who look to us for hope. Assisted reproductive technologies will not always result in a successful outcome. How do we determine the next step? How do we make a decision that is desirable and ethical? These are the questions which all reproductive clinicians must ask themselves.

References

1. Miller DT, Lee K, Gordon AS, et al. Recommendations for reporting of secondary findings in clinical exome and genome sequencing, 2021 update: a policy statement of the American College of Medical Genetics and Genomics (ACMG). *Genet Med* 2021;**23**(8):1–8.

2. Scheuner MT, Peredo J, Benkendorf J, et al. Reporting genomic secondary findings: ACMG members weigh in. *Genet Med* 2015;**17**(1):27–35.

3. Ethics Committee of the American Society for Reproductive Medicine. Use of reproductive technology for sex selection for nonmedical reasons. *Fertil Steril* 2015;**103**(6):1418–1422

4. Capelouto SM, Archer SR, Morris JR, et al. Sex selection for non-medical indications: a survey of current pre-implantation genetic screening practices among U.S. ART clinics. *J Assist Reprod Genet* 2018;**35**(3):409–416.

5. Daar J. The role of providers in assisted reproduction: potential conflicts, professional conscience, and personal choice. In: Francis L, Ed. *The Oxford Handbook of Reproductive Ethics*. Oxford: Oxford University Press, 2017, 242.

6. Hendl T. A feminist critique of justifications for sex selection. *J Bioeth Inq* 2017;**14**(3):427–438.

7. Dondorp W, De Wert G, Pennings G, et al. ESHRE Task Force on Ethics and Law 20: sex selection for non-medical reasons. *Hum Reprod* 2013;**28**(6):1448–1454.

8. Savulescu J, Pugh J, Douglas T, et al. The moral imperative to continue gene editing research on human embryos. *Protein Cell* 2015;**6**(7):476–479.

9. Polkinghorne JC. Ethical issues in biotechnology. *Trends Biotechnol* 2000;**18**(1):8–10.

10. Deech R. Reproductive autonomy and regulation – coexistence in action. Just reproduction: reimagining autonomy in reproductive medicine, special report. *Hastings Center Rep* 2017;**47**(6):S57–S63.

Index

Printed in the United States
by Baker & Taylor Publisher Services